Nanoparticulate Drug Delivery Systems

Nanoparticulate
Drug Delivery Systems

edited by

Deepak Thassu
UCB Pharma, Inc.
Rochester, New York, U.S.A.

Michel Deleers
UCB Pharma, Chemin du Foriest
Braine l'Alleud, Belgium

Yashwant Pathak
UCB Manufacturing, Inc.
Rochester, New York, U.S.A.

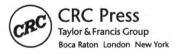

CRC Press
Taylor & Francis Group
Boca Raton London New York

CRC Press is an imprint of the
Taylor & Francis Group, an **informa** business

First published 2007 by Informa Healthcare, Inc.

Published 2019 by CRC Press
Taylor & Francis Group
6000 Broken Sound Parkway NW, Suite 300
Boca Raton, FL 33487-2742

© 2007 by Taylor & Francis Group, LLC
CRC Press is an imprint of Taylor & Francis Group, an Informa business

First issued in paperback 2019

No claim to original U.S. Government works

ISBN 13: 978-0-367-45311-4 (pbk)
ISBN 13: 978-0-8493-9073-9 (hbk)

Library of Congress Cataloging-in-Publication Data

Nanoparticulate drug delivery systems / edited by Deepak Thassu, Michel Deleers, Yashwant Pathak.
    p. ; cm. -- (Drugs and the pharmaceutical sciences ; v. 166)
  Includes bibliographical references and index.
  ISBN-13: 978-0-8493-9073-9 (alk. paper)
  ISBN-10: 0-8493-9073-7 (alk. paper)
  1. Drug delivery systems. 2. Nanoparticles. I. Thassu, Deepak. II. Deleers, Michel.
III. Pathak, Yashwant. IV. Series.
  [DNLM: 1. Drug Delivery Systems--methods. 2. Nanostructures. 3. Drug Carriers.
W1 DR893B v.166 2007 / WB 340 N184 2007]
  RS199.5.N36 2007
  615'.6--dc22   2006051461

I dedicate this book to my fellow scientists and my family: wife, Anu; daughter, Sakshi Zoya; son, Alex Om; and my dear parents, who taught me love, life, and compassion.

Deepak Thassu

To the loving memory of my father, who taught me honesty, humanism, and tolerance; to my wife, Dominique, for both her patience and complicity; and to my three children for their visions of life.

Michel Deleers

To the loving memories of my parents and Dr. Keshav Baliram Hedgewar, who gave a proper direction; my wife, Seema, who gave a positive meaning; and my son, Sarvadaman, who gave a golden lining to my life.

Yashwant Pathak

Foreword

The use of molecular or macromolecular entities and superstructures derived thereof for the delivery of drugs has a long history. Antibodies, for instance, were suggested early last century as a means to direct anticancer drugs to tumor cells in the body expressing the corresponding antigen. Their use in the form of monoclonals is now at the forefront of targeted therapy. Following advances in the discovery of cell receptors, receptor-binding macromolecules were added to the armamentarium of systems for the targeting of drugs. Parallel to these developments has been, since the early 1970s, the exploitation of liposomes as a delivery system for drugs and vaccines. These superstructures, formed spontaneously from amphipathic lipid molecules, together with a diverse collection of other promising superstructures derived from a huge variety of natural and synthetic monomeric or polymeric units, have evolved to sophisticated versions through the incorporation onto their surface of macromolecules that contribute to optimal pharmacokinetics of actives and their delivery to where they are needed. An ever increasing number of drug- and vaccine-delivery systems are being tested clinically, with many already marketed.

Recently, drug-delivery systems have been rediscovered as the biological dimension of nanotechnology. A leading article in a prestigious scientific journal tells us that "biologists are embracing nanotechnology—the engineering and manipulation of entities in the 1 to 100 nm range—and are exploiting its potential to develop new therapeutics and diagnostics." What else is new?, you might say! Nonetheless, the prefix *nano* (from the Greek word for *dwarf*) is a useful one because it helps define drug-delivery systems of a certain size range. Reflecting this trend of size definition, *Nanoparticulate Drug Delivery Systems* is a worthy attempt to bring together a wide range of drug-delivery systems for the delivery (targeted or otherwise), through a variety of routes of administration, of drugs, diagnostics, and vaccines in the treatment or prevention of disease, now encapsulated in the term "nanomedicine." Importantly, the book includes a wealth of the latest advances in the technology of nanoparticulates, including electrospinning, formation of microcrystals, production of liquid crystalline phases, and, last but not least, the technology of metallic nanoparticles. The editors, Deepak Thassu, Michel Deleers, and Yashwant Pathak, are to be complimented for both their judicial selection of nanosystems and choice of the international panel of contributors.

Gregory Gregoriadis
The School of Pharmacy
University of London
London, U.K.

Preface

For many decades, the interest in modifying drug-delivery systems has been a prominent thrust of pharmaceutical research. In recent years, due to tremendous expansion in the different scientific domains and skill sets, the scope has been widened to incorporate many faculties in the drug-delivery research covering physics, polymer sciences, electrical engineering, bioelectronics, genetics, biotechnology, and molecular pharmaceutics.

Pharmaceutical industry research culture is facing an uncertain future. Higher clinical development cost coupled with declining drug-discovery process and lower clinical success rates is decreasing the flow of new chemical entities in the research and development pipeline.

Due to the advent of analytical techniques and capabilities to measure the particle sizes in nanometer ranges, particulate drug-delivery systems research and development has been moving from the micro- to the nanosize scale. Significant research interests are geared towards utilizing the techniques where the particles can be reduced almost to nanometer ranges, thus reducing the dose and reactive nature of the molecule. This can deliver the drug at the targeted sites.

The book presented herewith is an attempt to describe the research efforts being done in this direction by the global scientific community. Nanoparticulate drug-delivery systems are a challenging area, and there are pulsating changes happening almost every day. This is an attempt to cover the recent trends and emerging technologies in the area of nanoparticulate drug-delivery systems.

The first chapter covers a complete overview of the nanoparticulate drug-delivery system, covering wide applications and evaluation of the nanoparticulate drug-delivery system in various fields. Chapter 2 encompasses formulations of nanosuspensions for parenteral delivery. The third chapter covers the polymer-based nanoparticulate drug-delivery systems. Chapters 4 to 6 focus on nanofibers, nanocrystals, and lipid-based nanoparticulate drug-delivery systems, respectively.

Chapters 7 to 10 discuss the engineering aspects and different techniques used for nanoparticulate drug-delivery systems, including nanoengineering, aerosol flow reactor, supercooled smectic nanoparticles, and metallic nanoparticles, respectively. Chapters 11 and 12 focus on biological requirements and the role of nanobiotechnology in the development of nanomedicines. Chapters 13 to 21 cover the applications of nanoparticulate drug-delivery systems, including lipid nanoparticles for dermal applications; gene carriers for restenosis; ocular, central nervous system, gastrointestinal applications; adjuvant for vaccine development; and transdermal systems.

It is our hope that this multiauthored book on nanoparticulate drug-delivery systems will assist and enrich readers in understanding the diverse types of nanoparticulate drug-delivery systems available or under development, as well as highlight their applications in the future development of nanomedicines. This book is equally relevant to those in academia and industry, as well as scientists working in pharmaceutical drug delivery worldwide. The text is planned so that each chapter represents an independent area of research and is easily followed without referring to other chapters.

We would like to express our sincere thanks to Tony Benfonte for the figures in Chapters 1 and 13 and to Linda Glather for reading the manuscript and suggesting corrections and punctuation. Special thanks to our editors, Stevan Zolo, Yvonne Honigsberg, and Sherri Niziolek, who helped us to get through the project successfully.

Last, but not least, we would like to express our sincere gratitude to all the authors who have taken time from their busy schedules to be part of this project and written wonderful chapters that added both the depth and value to this book.

Deepak Thassu
Michel Deleers
Yashwant Pathak

Contents

Contributors

María José Blanco-Prieto   Department of Pharmacy and Pharmaceutical Technology, University of Navarra, Pamplona, Spain

Heike Bunjes   Department of Pharmaceutical Technology, Institute of Pharmacy, Friedrich Schiller University Jena, Jena, Germany

Matthew D. Burke   Department of Pharmaceutical Development, GlaxoSmithKline, Research Triangle Park, North Carolina, U.S.A.

Sudhir S. Chakravarthi   Department of Pharmaceutical Sciences, University of Nebraska Medical Center, Omaha, Nebraska, U.S.A.

Joseph F. Chiang   Department of Chemistry and Biochemistry, State University of New York at Oneonta, Oneonta, New York, U.S.A., and Department of Chemistry, Tsinghua University, Beijing, China

Einat Cohen-Sela   Department of Pharmaceutics, School of Pharmacy, The Hebrew University of Jerusalem, Jerusalem, Israel

Sinjan De   Research and Development, Perrigo Company, Allegan, Michigan, U.S.A.

Michel Deleers   Global Pharmaceutical Technology and Analytical Development (GPTAD), UCB, Braine l'Alleud, Belgium

Hannele Eerikäinen   Pharmaceutical Product Development, Orion Corporation Orion Pharma, Espoo, Finland

Victoria Elazar   Department of Pharmaceutics, School of Pharmacy, The Hebrew University of Jerusalem, Jerusalem, Israel

Hila Epstein-Barash   Department of Pharmaceutics, School of Pharmacy, The Hebrew University of Jerusalem, Jerusalem, Israel

Socorro Espuelas   Department of Pharmacy and Pharmaceutical Technology, University of Navarra, Pamplona, Spain

Carlos Gamazo   Department of Microbiology, University of Navarra, Pamplona, Spain

Maria Rosa Gasco   Nanovector srl, Torino, Italy

Gershon Golomb   Department of Pharmaceutics, School of Pharmacy, The Hebrew University of Jerusalem, Jerusalem, Israel

Juan M. Irache   Department of Pharmacy and Pharmaceutical Technology, University of Navarra, Pamplona, Spain

K. K. Jain   Jain PharmaBiotech, Basel, Switzerland

Ashwath Jayagopal   Biomaterials, Drug Delivery, and Tissue Engineering Laboratory, Department of Biomedical Engineering, Vanderbilt University, Nashville, Tennessee, U.S.A.

Esko I. Kauppinen   NanoMaterials Group, Laboratory of Physics and Center for New Materials, Helsinki University of Technology, and VTT Biotechnology, Helsinki, Finland

Judith Kuntsche   Department of Pharmaceutical Technology, Institute of Pharmacy, Friedrich Schiller University Jena, Jena, Germany

Vinod Labhasetwar   Department of Pharmaceutical Sciences, University of Nebraska Medical Center, Omaha, Nebraska, U.S.A.

Anna Lähde   NanoMaterials Group, Laboratory of Physics and Center for New Materials, Helsinki University of Technology, Helsinki, Finland

Robert J. Lee   Division of Pharmaceutics, College of Pharmacy, NCI Comprehensive Cancer Center, NSF Nanoscale Science and Engineering Center for Affordable Nanoengineering of Polymeric Biomedical Devices, The Ohio State University, Columbus, Ohio, U.S.A.

Annick Ludwig   Department of Pharmaceutical Sciences, University of Antwerp, Antwerp, Belgium

Dmitry Luzhansky   Department of Corporate Technology, Donaldson Company, Inc., Minneapolis, Minnesota, U.S.A.

Rainer H. Müller   Department of Pharmaceutical Technology, Biotechnology, and Quality Management, Freie Universität Berlin, Berlin, Germany

Jan Möschwitzer   Department of Pharmaceutical Technology, Biotechnology, and Quality Management, Freie Universität Berlin, Berlin, Germany

Jean-Christophe Olivier   Pharmacologie des Médicaments Anti-Infectieux, Faculty of Medicine and Pharmacy, and INSERM, ERI 023, Poitiers, France

Giulio F. Paciotti   CytImmune Sciences, Inc., Rockville, Maryland, U.S.A.

Yashwant Pathak   UCB Manufacturing, Inc., Rochester, New York, U.S.A.

Manuela Pereira de Oliveira   Pharmacologie des Médicaments Anti-Infectieux, Faculty of Medicine and Pharmacy, and INSERM, ERI 023, Poitiers, France

Janne Raula   NanoMaterials Group, Laboratory of Physics and Center for New Materials, Helsinki University of Technology, Helsinki, Finland

Barrett E. Rabinow   Baxter Healthcare Corporation, Round Lake, Illinois, U.S.A.

Dennis H. Robinson   Department of Pharmaceutical Sciences, University of Nebraska Medical Center, Omaha, Nebraska, U.S.A.

V. Prasad Shastri   Biomaterials, Drug Delivery, and Tissue Engineering Laboratory, Department of Biomedical Engineering, Vanderbilt University, Nashville, Tennessee, U.S.A.

Jongwon Shim   Nanotechnology Research Team, Skin Research Institute, R&D Center, Amorpacific Corporation, Kyounggi, South Korea

Eliana B. Souto   Department of Pharmaceutical Technology, Biotechnology, and Quality Management, Freie Universität Berlin, Berlin, Germany

Lawrence Tamarkin   CytImmune Sciences, Inc., Rockville, Maryland, U.S.A.

Deepak Thassu   UCB Pharma, Inc., Rochester, New York, U.S.A.

Jaspreet K. Vasir   Department of Pharmaceutical Sciences, University of Nebraska Medical Center, Omaha, Nebraska, U.S.A.

Jun Wu   Division of Pharmaceutics, College of Pharmacy, The Ohio State University, Columbus, Ohio, U.S.A.

Xiaobin Zhao   Division of Pharmaceutics, College of Pharmacy, The Ohio State University, Columbus, Ohio, U.S.A.

1 Nanoparticulate Drug-Delivery Systems: An Overview

Deepak Thassu
UCB Pharma, Inc., Rochester, New York, U.S.A.

Yashwant Pathak
UCB Manufacturing, Inc., Rochester, New York, U.S.A.

Michel Deleers
Global Pharmaceutical Technology and Analytical Development (GPTAD),
UCB, Braine l'Alleud, Belgium

INTRODUCTION

Nanotechnology and nanoscience are widely seen as having a great potential to bring benefits to many areas of research and applications. It is attracting increasing investments from governments and private sector businesses in many parts of the world. Concurrently, the application of nanoscience is raising new challenges in the safety, regulatory, and ethical domains that will require extensive debates on all levels.

The prefix *nano* is derived from the Greek word *dwarf*. One nanometer (nm) is equal to one-billionth of a meter, that is, 10^{-9} m. The term "nanotechnology" was first used in 1974, when Norio Taniguchi, a scientist at the University of Tokyo, Japan, referred to materials in nanometers. The size range that holds so much interest is typically from 100 nm down to the atomic level approximately 0.2 nm, because in this range materials can have different and enhanced properties compared with the same material at a larger size. Figure 1 shows the nanometer in context (1). Nanotechnologies have been used to create tiny features on computer chips for the last 25 years. The natural world also contains many examples of nanoscale structures, from milk (a nanoscale colloid) to the sophisticated nanosized and nanostructured proteins that control a range of biological activities, such as flexing muscles, releasing energy, and repairing cells. Nanoparticles (NPs) occur naturally and have been in existence for thousands of years as products of combustion and cooking of food.

Nanomaterials differ significantly from other materials due to the following two major principal factors: the increased surface area and quantum effects. These factors can enhance properties such as reactivity, strength, electrical characteristics, and in vivo behavior. As the particle size decreases, a greater proportion of atoms are found at the surface compared to inside. For example, a particle size of 30 nm has 5% of its atoms on the surface, at 10 nm 20%, and at 3 nm 50% of the atoms are on surface (1). Thus, an NP has a much greater surface area per unit mass compared with larger particles, leading to greater reactivity. In tandem with surface area effects, quantum effects can begin to dominate the properties of matter as size is reduced to the nanoscale. These can affect the optical, electrical, and magnetic behavior of materials. Their in vivo behavior can be from increased absorption to high toxicity of nanomaterials.

METHODS OF MEASUREMENTS AND CHARACTERIZATION OF NANOMATERIALS

Nanometrology is the science of measurements at the nanoscale, and its application underlies all the nanoscience and nanotechnology. The ability to measure and

Thassu et al.

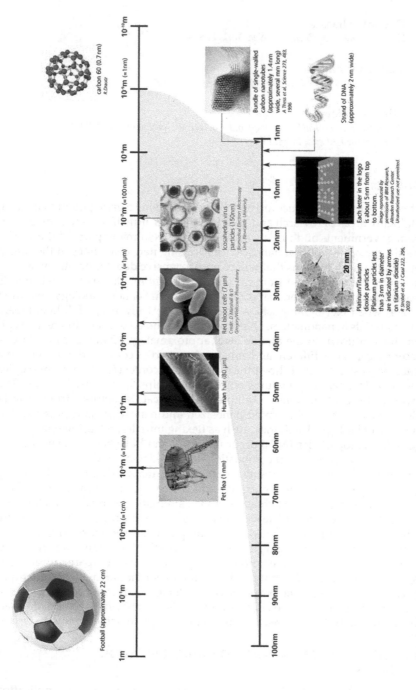

FIGURE 1 (*See color insert.*) Length scale showing the nanometer in context. The length scale of interest for nanoscience and nanotech-nologies is from 100 nm down to the atomic scale approximately 0.2 nm. *Source:* From Ref. 1.

characterize materials, as well as determine their shape, size, and physical properties at the nanoscale is vital for nanomaterials and devices. These need to be produced to a high degree of accuracy and reliability, to realize the applications of nanotechnologies. Nanometrology includes length and/or size (where dimensions are typically in nanometers) as well as measurement of force, mass, electrical, and other properties. Four commonly used techniques are: transmission electron microscopy (TEM), scanning electron microscopy (SEM), scanning probe techniques [scanning probe microscopy (SPM)], and optical tweezers (single-beam gradient trap).

Transmission Electron Microscopy
TEM is used to investigate the internal structure of micro- and nanostructures. It works by passing electrons through the samples and then using magnetic lenses to focus the image of the structure. TEM can reveal the finest details of the internal structure, in some cases the individual atoms. TEM with high-resolution transmission electron microscopy is the important tool for the study of NP.

Scanning Electron Microscopy
SEM uses the basic technology developed for TEM, but the beam of electrons is focused to a diameter spot of approximately 1 nm on the surface of the specimen and scanned repetitively across the surface. It reveals that the surface topography of the sample with the best spatial resolution currently achieved is on the order of 1 nm.

Scanning Probe Techniques (Scanning Probe Microscopy)
SPM uses the interaction between a sharp tip and a surface to obtain the image. The sharp tip is held very close to the surface to be examined and is scanned back and forth. As the tip is scanned across the sample, the displacement of the end of the cantilever is measured, using a laser beam. This can image insulating materials simply because the signal corresponds to the force between the tip and the sample, which reflects the topography being scanned. The scanning tunneling microscope brought a Noble prize for physics to Gerd Binnig and Heinrich in 1986. The atomic force microscope uses this SPM technique, which reflects the surface topography of the samples.

Optical Tweezers (Single-Beam Gradient Trap)
Optical tweezers use a single laser beam (focused by a high-quality microscope objective) to a spot on the specimen plane. The radiation pressure and gradient forces from the spot create an optical trap, which holds a particle at its center. Small interatomic forces and displacements can be measured by this technique. Samples that can be analyzed range from single atoms to micrometer-sized spheres to strands of DNA and living cells. Numerous traps can be used simultaneously with other optical techniques, such as scalpels, which can cut the particle being studied. Various analytical techniques utilized in nanometrology are enumerated in Table 1.

MANUFACTURE OF NANOMATERIALS
There are a wide variety of techniques that are capable of creating nanostructures with various degrees of quality, speed, and cost. These manufacturing approaches

TABLE 1   Analytical Techniques Used for Characterization of Nanoparticles

Name of the technique	Reference
Laser diffraction	(2)
Photon correlation spectroscopy	
Wide-angle X-ray scattering	
Differential scanning colorimetry	
Proton nuclear magnetic resonance spectroscopy	
Electron spin resonance	
Electron transmission microscopy	(3)
Sedimentation velocity analysis and EM	(4)
DLS and cryo-TEM	(5)
DLS and TEM	(6)
Flow cytometry and ELISA method	(7)
Fluorometry	(8)
Fluorescence and TEM	(9)

Abbreviations: DLS, dynamic light scattering; ELISA, enzyme-linked immunosorbent assay; EM, electron microscopy; NP, nanoparticle; TEM, transmission electron microscopy.

fall under two categories: bottom-up and top-down. Figure 2 illustrates the types of materials and products which can be manufactured using these two approaches (1).

Bottom-Up Manufacturing

Bottom-up manufacturing involves the building of nanostructures atom by atom or molecule by molecule. This can be done in three ways: chemical synthesis, self-assembly, and positional assembly.

Chemical synthesis is a method of producing raw materials, such as molecules or particles, which can then be used either directly in products in their bulk-disordered form or as the building blocks of more advanced ordered materials. Figure 3 represents the generic processes that are involved in the production of NPs (1):

1. Self-assembly is a production technique in which atoms or molecules arrange themselves into ordered nanoscale structures by physical or chemical interactions within the smaller units. The formation of salt crystals and snowflakes with their intricate structure are examples of the self-assembly process. Although self-assembly occurs in nature, in industry it is relatively new and not a well-established process (1).

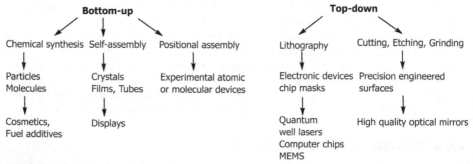

FIGURE 2   The use of bottom-up and top-down techniques in manufacturing nanoparticles. *Abbreviation*: MEMS, microelectromechanical system. *Source*: From Ref. 1.

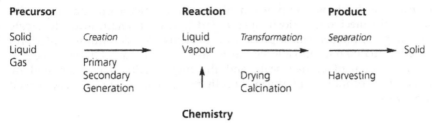

Chemistry

FIGURE 3 The generic processes that are involved in the production of nanoparticles. *Source*: From Ref. 1.

2. In positional assembly, atoms, molecules, or clusters are deliberately manipulated and positioned one by one. Techniques such as SPM for work on surfaces or optical tweezers in free space are used for this. Positional assembly is extremely laborious and rarely used as an industrial process.

Top-Down Manufacturing

Top-down manufacturing involves starting with a larger piece of material, and etching, milling, or machining a nanostructure from it by removing material. Top-down methods offer reliability and device complexity. These are higher in energy usage and produce more waste than the bottom-up methods.

Although the nanotechnologies have been used by industries for many decades (semiconductor and chemical industry), it is still very much at infancy stage. In recent years, the tools used to characterize materials (Table 1) have led to better understanding of the behavior and properties of matter on a very small scale. Increased knowledge of the relationship between the structure and properties of nanomaterials has enabled the production of materials and devices with higher performance and increased functionality. At the same time, there are uncertainties which need to be addressed about the direction that nanotechnology will take, and about the hazards to humans and the environment that are presented by certain aspects of this technology (10).

There are several good reports and reviews which cover the production and characterization of NPs and nanoparticulate drug-delivery systems (NPDDSs). Venkateswarlu and Manjunath (11) have discussed the preparation and characterization of clozapine NPs. They used hot homogenization and later ultrasonication method to formulate solid–lipid nanoparticles (SLNs) incorporating clozapine. Dingler and Gohla (12) have discussed the production of SLN and scaling up studies and Gasco (13) has patented a method for producing SLN. Mehnert and Mader (14) have written an excellent review about the SLN production and characterization. Many reviews are reported by Muller et al. (15) and others (2–5,16–18). Rigaldie et al. (19) have shown the high-hydrostatic-pressure technique to preserve and sterilize the spherulites, an NPDDS. Several papers and patents are reported by our group (20–26) and Rodriguez et al. described a high-pressure emulsification and homogenization process for NPDDS preparation (17).

Microfluidics is being explored for applications in NPDDS. It is based on instruments that are capable of transferring small volumes of liquids ranging from microliters to nanoliters. Microfluidic "lab-on-the-chip" technology requires an understanding of the forces that control fluid movement and reaction conditions and brings the potential benefits of miniaturization, integration, and automation.

Manufacturing such chips combines methods from microchip industry with expertise in fluid mechanics, biochemistry, and hardware engineering to create miniature integrated biochemical-processing systems. A microfluidics platform provides better quality data and allows shorter assay development times. Owing to the direct measurement at nanoscale and the high-quality data generated by microfluidics, this technology platform is finding a place in drug discovery as well as NPDDS (27–31).

DRUG-DELIVERY SYSTEMS

An ideal drug-delivery system possesses two elements: the ability to target and to control the drug release. Targeting will ensure high efficiency of the drug and reduce the side effects, especially when dealing with drugs that are presumed to kill cancer cells but can also kill healthy cells when delivered to them. The reduction or prevention of side effects can also be achieved by controlled release. NPDDS provide a better penetration of the particles inside the body as their size allows delivery via intravenous injection or other routes. The nanoscale size of these particulate systems also minimizes the irritant reactions at the injection site. Early attempts to direct treatment to a specific set of cells involved attaching radioactive substances to antibodies specific to markers displayed on the surface of cancer cells. Antibodies are the body's means of detecting and flagging the presence of foreign substances. Antibodies specific to certain proteins can be mass produced in laboratories, ironically using the cancer cells. These approaches have yielded some good results, and NPDDSs are demonstrating lot of potential in this area.

Lipid-Based Colloidal Nanodrug-Delivery Systems

Lipid nanocapsules are submicron particles made of an oily liquid core surrounded by a solid or semisolid shell. NPDDSs were primarily developed to combine the colloidal stability of solid particle suspensions in biological fluids and the solubilizing properties of liquids (32,33). SLNs were invented at the beginning of 1990s and are produced either by high-pressure homogenization or by microemulsion technique (34). SLNs consist of solid matrix and can be described as parenteral emulsions in which the liquid–lipid oil is replaced by a solid–lipid. Owing to their solid particle matrix, they can protect incorporated ingredients against chemical degradation (35) and allow modification of release of the active compounds (36). Homogenization followed by ultrasonication was used for the production of clozapine-loaded SLNs (11).

Colloidal drug carriers offer a number of potential advantages as delivery systems, such as better bioavailability for poorly soluble drugs. Other advantages of these SLNs include: use of physiological lipids, the avoidance of organic solvents in the preparation process, a wide potential application spectrum (oral, dermal, and intravenous), high-pressure homogenization as an established production method (which allows large-scale production), improved bioavailability, protection of sensitive drug molecules from the environment (water and light), and a controlled release characteristic (14). Common disadvantages of SLNs include: particle growth, unpredictable gelation tendency, unexpected dynamics of polymorphic transitions, and inherently low incorporation capabilities due to crystalline structure of the SLN (14). The key parameters in characterizing the SLN include: concentration, nanocapsule size and shape, thickness, and shell composition, defining the freeze-drying

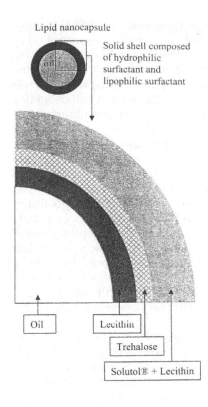

Lipid nanocapsule

Solid shell composed of hydrophilic surfactant and lipophilic surfactant

Oil

Lecithin

Trehalose

Solutol® + Lecithin

FIGURE 4 Proposed topology for lipid nanocapsules freeze-dried in the presence of trehalose. *Source*: From Ref. 37.

conditions such as cryoprotectant, pressure, and temperature cycle. Some of the factors for the formulation of the lipid NP are: the drug payload depends on the oil content, the evolution of the hydrophilic–lipophilic balance of solutol HS15 is the driving force of SLN formation (Fig. 4), and the SLN diameter depends on both the Foil/F solutol and the solutol HS15/Lipoid S 100 ratios (37). Besides nanoemulsions, nanosuspensions (38), mixed micelles and liposomes, melt-emulsified NP-based lipids, and solids at room temperature have been developed (15). The low incorporation capabilities were overcome by using liquid–lipid nanostructured carriers (39). Several excellent reviews and papers on the SLN are reported (14,38,40–44).

Recent Trends in Solid–Lipid Nanoparticle Research
Recently, a lipid-based solvent-free formulation process has been developed to prepare lipid nanocapsules in the nanometer range (32,45). This process takes advantage of the variation of the hydrophilic–lipophilic balance of an ethoxylated hydrophilic surfactant as a function of the temperature, leading to an inversion phase. In the first step, several temperature cycles applied around the inversion-phase temperature lead to droplet size decrease and homogenization. In a second step, fast cooling leads to the crystallization of the lecithin (introduced in the formulation both as lipophilic cosurfactant and constituting material of the rigid shell), which leads to the formation of a stable lipid nanocapsule suspension. This suspension can be freeze-dried and resuspended in an aqueous medium extemporaneously. The freeze-drying can alter the topology of the NPs; hence while doing so, the structure of the NPs needs to be preserved (37).

Jores et al. (2) have studied physicochemical investigations of SLN and oil-loaded SLN using nuclear magnetic resonance and electron spin resonance. They have investigated various techniques to evaluate and characterize them using photon correlation spectroscopy. Laser diffraction was used for particle size determination, and field flow fractionation with multiangle light scattering detection was used to separate the particles due to their Stokes radius. It helped in understanding the topography of the particles. Cryo-TEM was used to study the ultrastructure of the NPs.

SLNs have been shown to condense DNA into nanometric colloidal particles capable of transfecting mammalian cells in vitro (46). Compared with standard DNA carriers such as cationic lipids or cationic polymers, SLN offers several technological advantages such as a relative ease of production without organic solvents, the possibility of large-scale production with qualified production lines, good storage stabilities, possibility of steam sterilization, and lyophilization (47). In a study by Rudolph et al. (47), a diametric tyrosine aminotransferase (TAT) peptide derived from the arginine-rich motif of the HIV-1 TAT protein that functions as nuclear localization sequence and as a protein transduction domain could be used to substantially enhance gene transfer efficiency of SLN-based vectors, leading to gene expression levels even higher than observed for polyethylenimine (PEI) gene vectors. This might allow aerosol application of fragile gene delivery systems to lungs in the future studies.

The common ground of cationic liposome nanoemulsions (48) and SLNs for transfection is the need for cationic lipids to facilitate deoxyribonucleic acid (DNA) binding. In liposome formulations, these lipids are arranged as bilayers around an aqueous core. Interaction with DNA initiates structural rearrangements into different structures depending on the kind of lipid, lipid/DNA ratio, incubation media, and time (38). Tabatt et al. (49) have shown equipotency of SLNs and liposome formulated from the cationic lipids in in vitro DNA transfection efficiency.

A study by Kogure et al. (50) demonstrated the development of a multifunctional envelope-type nanodevice for a gene-delivery system. This contained membrane-permeable peptide R8 with less cytotoxicity. This system can incorporate various functional devices such as a specific ligand to a specific cell, intracellular sorting devices that permit endosomal escape, and nuclear localization. This lipid-based device can be a useful tool for gene delivery for gene therapy and biochemical research (Fig. 5: schematic steps for nanodevices). Lee et al. (51) reported an increased stability and controlled release of lovastatin by microencapsulating the drug-loaded lipid NPs. Several studies have shown the application of SLN formulation for the delivery of paclitaxel and its pro-drug for cancer treatment (52).

Hou et al. (53) have described the modified high shear homogenization and ultrasound techniques to produce SLNs. Model drug mifepristone was incorporated in SLNs, and the mean particle size was found to be 106 nm. The drug entrapment efficiency was more than 87% and showed relatively long stability, as the leakages were small. Olbrich et al. (54) described the potential delivery of hydrophilic antitrypanosomal drug diminazine diaceturate to the brain of infected mice formulating the lipid drug conjugate NP by combination of stearic and oleic acids. An excellent work on an in vivo evaluation of tobramycin SLNs and their duodenal administration is described by Cavalli et al. (55), and is further discussed in the following chapters in detail.

Williams et al. (56) have studied lipid-based NP formulation of SN38, a camptothecin analog used as antineoplastic drug. They showed improved drug loading

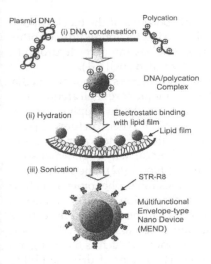

FIGURE 5 Three steps involved in constructing the multifunctional envelope-type nanodevice. *Source*: From Ref. 50.

and good lactone stability in the presence of human serum albumin (HSA). The NPDDS showed prolonged circulation in murine blood and better efficacy against a resistant model of human colon carcinoma in nude mice. It was also demonstrated that the blood half-life of SN38 was greatly prolonged by incorporation in NPs.

Nanoparticulate Polymeric Micelles as Drug Carriers

Polymeric micelles have attracted much attention in drug delivery, partly because of their ability to solubilize hydrophobic molecules, their small particle size, good thermodynamic solution stability, extended release of various drugs, and prevention of rapid clearance by the reticuloendothelial system (RES) (57). Critical micelle concentration (CMC), similar to low-molecular-weight surfactants, is the key characterization parameter for polymeric micelles. CMC is the concentration at which the amphiphilic polymers in aqueous solution begin to form micelles while coexisting in the equilibrium with the individual polymer chains or unimers. At CMC or slightly above the CMC, the micelles form loose aggregates and contain some water in the core (58). With further increases in amphiphilic polymer concentration, the unimer to micelle equilibrium shifts towards micelle formation. The micellar structure then becomes more compressed and stable, whereas residual solvent is excluded from the core, and the micelle size is reduced. The lower CMC values correlate to more stable micelles. This concept is especially important from the pharmacological point of view, as upon dilution with a large volume of the blood, micelles with high CMC values may dissociate into unimers and their content may precipitate out, whereas the micelles with low CMC are more likely to remain the same. Thus, to develop improved drug-delivery systems, amphiphilic molecules that are able to form more stable micelles with lower CMC values are appropriate candidates. A fascinating study reported by Djordjevic et al. (59) utilized scorpion-like amphiphilic macromolecules. They used indomethacin as a model drug for the study and reported this method as convenient for drug delivery while minimizing drug toxicity and maximizing the drug effectiveness.

Generally, the amphiphilic core/shell structure of polymeric micelles is formed from block copolymers, which are hydrophobic polymer chains linked to hydrophilic polymer chains (60). Association of the hydrophobic portions of the block copolymers creates the inner micelle core due to their cohesive interactions with each other in aqueous media (i.e., hydrophobic interactions), whereas the outer hydrophilic portions surround the inner hydrophobic core as a hydrated shell (61).

Polymeric micelles are self-assemblies of block copolymers in aqueous media. Many advantages have been demonstrated with their unique core shell architecture. Hydrophilic shells from the aqueous exterior segregate the hydrophobic cores. Hydrophobic drugs can be solubilized into the hydrophobic core structures of polymeric micelles at concentrations much higher than their intrinsic water solubility. Polymeric micelles are known to have high drug-loading capacity, high water solubility, and appropriate size for long circulation in the blood (62). The hydrophilic shell surrounding the micellar core can protect undesirable phenomena such as intermicellar aggregation, or precipitation, protein adsorption, and cell adhesion. The chemical composition of the polymeric micelles can be tailor-made to have desirable physicochemical properties for drug solubilization (63). The hydrophobic drug is incorporated into the hydrophobic core by interactions such as metal–ligand coordination bonding and electrostatic interaction. The extent of drug solubility depends on the compatibility between the drug and the micelle core (64). One of the limitations of drug-loaded polymeric micelles is low stability in aqueous solution, and the stability becomes even lower as the drug-loading content increases (65).

Various types of drugs can be loaded into the hydrophobic core of polymeric micelles by chemical conjugation or physical entrapolymeric micelles sent utilizing various interactions such as hydrophobic interactions, or ionic interactions, or hydrogen bonding. Furthermore, the hydrophobic core serves as a reservoir from which the drug is released slowly over an extended period of time. The hydrophobic inner core is solubilized by the hydrophilic shell, which prevents the inactivation of the core-encapsulated drug molecules by decreasing the contact with the inactivating species in the aqueous (blood) phase. As the outer hydrophilic part of the polymeric micelles interacts with biocomponents such as cells and proteins, it affects their pharmacokinetics and disposition, as well as their surface properties (66).

Polymeric Micelles and Solubilization of Drugs

Solubilization of drugs is a complex mechanism that involves different parameters, for example, hydrophobicity, molecular volume, crystallinity, flexibility, charge, and interfacial tension against water. The lack of water solubility hampers the use of many potent pharmaceuticals. Polymeric micelles are self-assembled nanocarriers with versatile properties that can be engineered to solubilize, target, and release hydrophobic drugs in a controlled release fashion. Unfortunately, their large-scale use is limited by the incorporation methods available. This poses a problem when sterile dosage forms are formulated. Polymeric micelles present a core shell architecture that results from the self-assembly of the amphiphilic block polymers in a selective solvent above a threshold concentration referred to as critical association concentration (67). Their structure is such that the core provides an isolated cargo space where hydrophobic drugs can partition. This is of great significance as many potent pharmaceuticals are highly hydrophobic by nature. The nanometric size of polymeric micelles varies from 10 to 100 nm and the flexible highly hydrated corona minimizes nonselective scavenging and rapid clearance by the monolayer phagocyte system. These drug carriers can extravasate and accumulate passively in regions presenting leaky vasculatures such as tumors, inflamed and infracted tissues (68).

Novel One-Step Drug-Loading Procedure for Nanocarriers

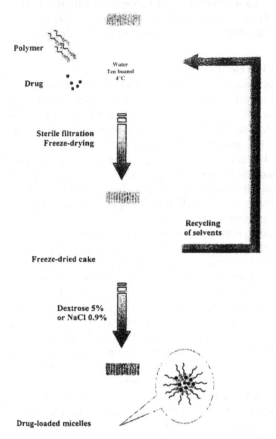

Polymer

Drug

Water
Ten buanol
4°C

Sterile filtration
Freeze-drying

Recycling
of solvents

Freeze-dried cake

Dextrose 5%
or NaCl 0.9%

Drug-loaded micelles

FIGURE 6 Scheme of the freeze-drying procedure for water-soluble amphiphilic nanocarriers. *Source*: From Ref. 44.

Recently, polymeric micelles have also been shown to distribute to defined cytoplasmic organelles (69) and increasing efforts are now directed at targeting the subcellular components (44). A simple method to have higher drug loading in the amphiphilic nanocarriers polymeric micelles was developed by Fournier et al. (44). Figure 6 shows the schematic production of polymeric micelles and its freeze-drying procedure.

Polymeric Micelles and Reticuloendothelial System
Polymeric micelles provide an attractive characteristic in that they can avoid uptake of the drugs by RES in vivo and hence these can circulate in the blood for a longer time. This advantage comes from the structure of a micelle, the hydrophilic portions of the amphiphilic block copolymer form the outer shell and are exposed to body fluid, and hence the micelles can be protected from phagocytic cells and plasma proteins in blood. Another important biological advantage of polymeric micelles is the EPR9-enhanced permeability and retention effect or passive targeting. As a result, polymeric micelles can slowly accumulate in malignant or inflamed tissues due to the elevated levels of vascular permeability factors in such cells (70). Polymeric micelles seem to be ideal carriers for poorly water-soluble drugs because of their

distinct advantages such as high solubility, long circulation of drug in blood, permeation of an anticancer drug by the EPR effect (71), and simple sterilization. They have two major disadvantages: physical instability upon dilution limits their pharmaceutical application and water-soluble drugs cannot be in the micelles.

Recent Trends in Polymeric Micelles Research

Francis et al. (72) have studied the polysaccharide-based polymeric micelles for the delivery of cyclosporine A. They demonstrated that coupling of hydrophobic groups to water-soluble polysaccharides significantly promotes the solubilizing power of either dextran or hydroxypropyl cellulose (HPC) toward cyclosporine A. The bioadhesive properties of HPC enhance the association of polymeric micelles toward caco-2 cell monolayers and facilitate internalization of the polymer and the transport of the drug. The polysaccharide-based polymeric micelles offer unique opportunities for the oral delivery of lipophilic drugs. Similar studies for cyclosporine have been reported using SLN (73), polycaprolactone NPDDS (74), poly-lactic acid polyethylene glycol NPs (75), and chitosan derivatives (76).

A new modality of drug targeting tumors is based on drug encapsulation in polymeric micelles followed by a localized triggering of the drug intracellular uptake induced by ultrasound, which is focused into the tumor volume (77). A rationale behind this approach is that drug encapsulation in polymeric micelles decreases a systemic concentration of free drug, diminishes intracellular drug uptake by normal cells, and provides passive drug targeting of tumors via enhanced penetration and retention effect as a result of abnormal permeability of tumor blood vessels (78). Drugs targeting tumors reduce unwanted drug interactions with healthy tissues (79). With micelle accumulation in the tumor interstitium, an effective intracellular drug uptake by the tumor cells should be ensured, making it possible for ultrasonic irradiation to be used (77). The in vitro and in vivo experiments have suggested that polymeric micelles can be degraded into unimers under the action of ultrasound, which may provide an additional advantage of in vivo sensitization of multidrug-resistant cells (80). It is suggested that this technique can be useful in treatment of ovarian carcinoma tumors of small size; hence early detection is necessary for tumor treatment.

POLYMER-BASED NANOPARTICULATE DRUG-DELIVERY SYSTEMS

Several polymers and nonlipid materials have been evaluated as carriers for drugs in the nanoparticulate forms. These materials have shown different properties and advantages when formulated as drug-delivery systems. A brief description of each of the polymeric systems follows.

Hydrogel-Based Nanoparticulate Drug-Delivery Systems

A progressively increasing interest has been paid to self-assembled hydrogel NPs from hydrophobized water-soluble polymers due to their potential biomedical and pharmaceutical applications (81). The NPs have shown various structural and rheological features in aqueous solutions depending on the structure of the parent water-soluble polymer, conjugated hydrophobic moiety or groups, and the degree of substitution. The formation of self-assembled NPs is theorized by a free-energy-minimized structure, sharing a common feature of assembly of polymeric micelles. However, there exists a difference in the interior structure between NPs and polymeric micelles formed from amphiphilic block copolymers. The interior of polymeric NPs consists of dispersed multiple hydrophobic island domains in a hydrophilic sea domain due to the random association of hydrophobic moieties conjugated to soluble macromolecules. Polymeric micelles provide one inner core of hydrophobic segments with a hydrophilic shell (82,83). The NPs formed from polymers containing moiety switching its hydrophilicity by external stimuli is expected to exhibit stimuli responsive surface property plus macroscopic hydrogel bulk property. These properties might lead to the accumulation of the NPs at a disease site and the change of drug-release behavior from slow-to-fast drug release. An interesting study using pullulan acetate/sulfonamide conjugates in self-assembled NPs responsive to pH change was reported by Na et al. (81).

Amphiphilic block copolymers are widely studied as potential NPDDSs as they are capable of forming aggregates in aqueous solutions (84,85). These aggregates are comprised of a hydrophilic shell and hydrophobic core. They are good vehicles for delivering hydrophobic drugs because the drugs are protected from possible degradation by enzymes. Changing the composition of hydrophobic and hydrophilic blocks on the polymer chains can vary the morphology of NPs produced from amphiphilic block copolymers. Various forms of morphologies such as sphere, vesicles, rods, lamellas, tubes, large compound micelles, and large compound vesicles have been reported. Some of these structures are good candidates for drug-delivery applications (86). Compared with normal shell micelles, vesicles with a hydrophilic core and hydrophobic layers are better for drug delivery. In the clinical studies, it has been shown that vesicles improve the treatment efficacy of anticancer drugs such as doxorubicin due to enhanced permeability and retention properties (87). The block copolymers comprised of commercial pluronic systems and biodegradable poly(lactic acid) are very good carriers for drug delivery and controlled release applications (88).

Zhang et al. (89) synthesized triblock copolymers of poly(caprolactone-co-lactide)–b-poly(caprolactone-co-lactide) (PCLLA–PEG–PCLLA) by ring-opening copolymerization of caprolactone and lactide in the presence of polyethylene glycol. They entrapped an anticancer drug, a camptothecin derivative by nanoprecipitation technique. The in vitro and in vivo evaluation of this NPDDS showed a potential for use with poorly soluble anticancer drugs. They demonstrated that the drug release from these systems can be controlled by controlling the particle size, as they found the larger the NPs size, the lower was the drug release. The body distribution of these NPs showed that the blood concentration can be maintained for a longer time, and the tissue body distribution was affected by the particle size (90). Several other groups have shown the application of the triblock copolymers for NPDDSs (91–93). Yoo and Park (94) have shown folate receptor-targeted PLGA–PEG micelles entrapping a high loading amount of doxorubicin, showing better uptake of the drug. The in vitro and in vivo studies have shown the accumulation of the drug in the tumor cells in a site-specific manner.

An excellent review on block copolymer micelles for drug delivery, design, characterization, and biological significance is written by Kataoka et al. (60). Another review on applications of poly(ethylene oxide) block copolymer–poly(amino acids) micelles is published by Lavasanifar et al. (95). Vriezema et al. (96–98) have reported some interesting methods to produce block copolymers.

NPs based on hydrogels are being developed for the delivery of macromolecules, and some of the candidates of hydrogel utilized for this purpose are enumerated in Table 2. Many polymeric carriers were reported useful in the

TABLE 2 Hydrogel Matrices

Based on natural materials	Synthetic polymers	Responsive polymers
Collagen	Poly(n-vinyl pyrrolidine)	Methacrylates
Gelatin	Poly(vinyl alcohol)	Poly(N-isopropylacrylamide)LCST
Starch	Poly(phosphazenes)	PEO–PPO–PEO Pluronics
Alginates	Poly[ethylene oxide-b-poly(propylene oxide)] copolymers	
	PEO–PPO–PAA graft copolymer	
Chitosans	PL(G)A/PEO/PI(GA) copolymers	PLGA–PEO–PLGA (LCST)
Dextrans	PVA-g-PLGA graft polymers	
	PEGT–PBT copolymers (polyactive)	
	MA–oligolactide–PEO–oligolactide–MA	

Source: From Ref. 104.

formulation of NPDDSs, especially in the treatment of cancer, for example, poly(2 ethyl-2-oxazoline) block-poly-caprolactone (99), polyalkyl cyanoacrylate polymers (100), PLGA NPs (101), polysaccharide decorated polyisobutyl cyanoacrylate NPs (102), and serum albumin NPs (103).

Dendrimer-Based Drug-Delivery Systems

Three-dimensional tree-like branched macromolecules possess some fascinating characteristics: a well-defined structure, a very narrow molecular weight distribution, a three-dimensional structure tuned by dendrimer generation and dendron structure, and flexibility for tailored functional groups with high density on the periphery (66). Studies of biomedical application of dendrimers are becoming more and more attractive especially in the field of nonviral gene vector and NPDDS (105,106).

Photodynamic therapy of cancer involves the systemic administration of photosensitizers to solid tumor tissues and local illumination with light of a specific wavelength, leading to photochemical destruction of cancer cells via generation of singlet oxygen or superoxide from molecular oxygen. Suitable carriers and delivery of photosensitizers should have a simple but effective strategy to realize high selectivity, high photodynamic efficacy, and have less side effects. It is a challenge to formulate the photosensitizers. Zhang et al. (107) reported the use of dendrimer polymeric micelles for the delivery of photosensitizers successfully.

Calcium Carbonate Nanoparticles

Ueno et al. (108) have reported the incorporation of hydrophilic drugs and bioactive proteins into solid calcium carbonate NPs. The size of the NPs was controlled by mixing speed and was around 105 to 128 nm. These $CaCO_3$ NPs were stable and sustained the release of the drug betamethasone phosphate.

Proticles: Protamine-Based Nanoparticulate Drug Carriers

Protamine is a nonantigenic and virtually nontoxic peptide from the sperm, the compound derived from salmon, the most widely used source, and has a molecular mass around 5000 g/mol. It can be used as a carrier system for delivery of DNA or oligonucleotides and it is being used as the cationic component. Several groups have described the applications of proticles as drug-carrier systems (109–112). In most studies, the peptide was employed together with relatively large double-stranded

DNA in a two-step procedure. In the first step, it is condensed with DNA into a compact particle and subsequently the complex was incorporated into protamine or suitable cationic liposomes. In some cases, transferring was also used. The term "proticles" was used to represent oligonucleotides/protamine NPs by Dinaure et al. (95).

Vogel et al. (109) showed inclusion of HSA in the proticles led to dramatic stability of the particles. They reported many advantages of this system such as: the proticle production by self-assembly is simple and rather rapid. The excipients used are nonantigenic and have very low toxicity and are well accepted in pharmaceutics. The particles are relatively stable in water and cell culture medium. They show an increased uptake by a variety of cells, as compared to naked oligonucleotides, and after cellular uptake, the oligodeoxyribonucleotide (ODN)/protamine NPs readily release the active agent. They reported two distinct disadvantages: first, they immediately show massive aggregation and precipitation when produced or transferred into solutions containing salts at physiological ionic strength or even at concentrations in the range of mmol/l, and secondly, those containing the more stable (phosphorothioates PTOs) instead of ODNs (diesters) do not release their nucleic acid after particle uptake by cells (109).

Chitosan-Based Nanoparticulate Drug-Delivery System
Chitosan, a polycationic polymer, comprising D-glucosamine and N-acetyl-D-glucosamine linked by b-(1,4)-glycosidic bonds, has been extensively researched for NPDDSs for delivering anticancer drugs, genes, and vaccines (113–116). In these applications, it is important to assess the effectiveness of uptake of the carrier and associated drug cargo into the target cells. Chitosan, being a natural polymer, is biocompatible. Chitosan NPs were also evaluated for ocular applications. The cationic polysaccharide chitosan showed excellent properties such as biodegradability, nontoxicity, biocompatibility, and mucoadhesiveness, which are desirable for the ocular delivery systems. An interesting study by Campos et al. (117) demonstrated that Chitosan NPs were able to interact and remain associated to the ocular mucosa for an extended period of time, thus promising carriers for enhancing and controlling the release of drugs to the ocular surface. A review published by Hejazi et al. (103) discusses various aspects of chitosan-delivery systems covering the availability, physicochemical, and biological properties of chitosan. The review covered various applications of chitosan-delivery systems for colon-specific delivery, as absorption enhancers, and for GI tract delivery systems including the NPDDS. Park et al. (119) have assessed the application of self-aggregates formed by modified glycol chitosan as a carrier for peptide drugs. They exhibited comparable biological activity to parenteral peptides. Fluorescein isothiocyanate (FITC)-labeled peptides were released from the self-aggregates in a sustained manner for approximately a day. A report using chitosan alginate combination nanospheres showed the utility of these nanospheres for drug-delivery systems formulation (120). Self-assembled NPs containing hydrophobically modified chitosan for gene delivery was reported by Yoo et al. (121). They demonstrated that modified glycol chitosan NPs composed of hydrophobized DNA enhanced the transfection efficiencies in vitro as well as in vivo. Kumar et al. (122) showed the application of chitosan-based NPs in treating allergic asthma.

Silicone Nanopore-Membrane-Based Drug-Delivery System
Top-down microfabrication techniques have been used to create nanopore membranes consisting of arrays of parallel rectangular channels, which range from 7 to 50 nm.

The original method was pioneered by Chu et al. (123) and consisting of two basic steps, surface micromachining of nanochannels into a thin film on the top of the silicon wafer and forming the nanopore membrane by etching away the bulk of the silicone wafer underneath the thin-film structure. The experimental and mathematical results have shown that the devices outfitted with silicone nanopore membranes can regulate the drug-delivery kinetics of a wide range of drugs. Moreover, the mechanism of release is attributable to a novel constrained diffusion mechanism provided by the precise geometry of the nanopore membrane itself, and no moving parts such as pistons are required. The drugs can likely be loaded into the device reservoir in a range of physical states, including solutions, crystalline, or micronized suspensions. Flexibility with respect to the physical form of encapsulated drugs provides options to substantially increase the loaded dose and duration of the therapy, as well as promoting approaches to increase stability of proteins, which are intrinsically unstable in an aqueous solution at body temperature (124–126).

Polyester Polysaccharide Nanoparticles
NPs can be prepared from preformed copolymers by methods such as emulsification-solvent evaporation, nanoprecipitation, or salting out, all of which require dissolution of polymers in organic solvents. Lemarchand et al. (127) reported a study using interfacial migration-solvent evaporation method leading to NP formation using a novel family of amphiphilic copolymers based on Dextran grafted with polycaprolactone side chains. They reported that these materials were found to be able to self-organize and precipitate in the presence of mixtures of water and ethyl acetate. Ethyl acetate in a water emulsion was stable and produced the best NPs.

Albumin and Gelatin Nanospheres
Since the first reports on the preparation of uniformly sized albumin microspheres in the early 1970s, these biodegradable, biocompatible particles have found various applications. Initially conceived as a diagnostic tool, albumin particles have been utilized as drug-carrier systems (128). More than 100 therapeutic and diagnostic agents were incorporated into albumin particles and have been investigated for intravenous, intramuscular, intra-arterial, and intra-articular administration. Albumin particles are well suited for drug targeting and drug delivery because of their lack of toxicity and antigenicity. Compared with other colloidal carrier systems such as liposomes, albumin nanospheres have better stability, shelf life, controllable drug-release properties, and higher loading properties for hydrophilic molecules due to drug-binding properties of native albumin. Albumin particles can be obtained by many methods. In a study by Muller et al. (128), they optimized the manufacturing techniques of albumin nanospheres with average diameter of 200 nm. They studied the effect of five different process variables on particle size, polydispersity, and yield, to optimize the preparation technique to reach sub-200-nm particles.

An interesting novel drug-delivery system for improved all-*trans* retinoic acid (atRA) therapy for external treatments of photo-damaged skin was developed. The research team prepared inorganic-coated atRA NPs using boundary-organized reaction droplets. The interfacial properties of organic architecture in atRA micelles were used to template the nucleation of inorganic materials. When administered, they found a boost in the production of hyaluronan among the intercellular spaces of the basal and spinous cell layers of the epidermis. Nano-atRA technology for atRA therapy could not only efficiently regulate keratinocyte cell proliferation and differentiation, but also markedly produce the additional benefit. Human skin severely injured by chronic ultraviolet irradiation may be completely repaired due to the accelerated turnover of skin tissue, which is induced by nano-atRA (129–131).

Antibody-modified gelatin NPs have been reported to be a carrier system for targeting the specific T-lymphocytes by Balthasar et al. (132). Gelatin NPs were formed by two-step desolvation process. They showed the utility of this system for targeting the lymphocytes.

Polymeric Nanocapsules as Drug Carriers

These were first prepared by solubilization of the outer shell material in an organic solvent (133). Interesting biopharmaceutical performances of drugs encapsulated in polymeric NPs have been reported for the oral (134), the parenteral (135,136), and the ocular routes (137). However, the industrial constraints of solvent handling, limited scale, and particular efforts needed to decrease residual solvent down to few parts per million induced high manufacturing costs.

A clear aqueous nanodispersion of porpofol, a lipophilic anesthetic agent, was developed by Chen et al. (138), which possessed physical and chemical stability. It had better red blood cell compatibility and improved microbial resistance compared with the marketed product diprivan that is an oil-based emulsion. They showed the new nanodispersion using a combination of poloxamer, PEG 400, polysorbate 80, propylene glycol, and citric acid known as TPI 213 F (138). An interesting study of the in vitro degradation of polymer poly-DL-lactic acid (PDLLA), poly-DL-lactic-co-glycolic acid (PLGA), and polyethylene-oxide-based NPs showed that it took two years to degrade the PDLLA-based NPs, whereas it took 10 weeks to degrade PLGA NPs (139).

Poly(methyl vinyl ether-co-maleic anhydride) (PVA/MA) is a biodegradable poly-anhydride widely used for developing polymeric micelles as NPDDSs which possess bioadhesive as well as mucoadhesive properties. Arbos et al. (140) reported the application of these in the formulation of NPDDSs and showed that the bioadhesive properties of these NPs appear to modulate gastrointestinal transit profiles. An interesting study was reported by Luu et al. (141) on developing polymeric micelles of nanostructured DNA delivery scaffold by electrospinning of PLGA (polylactide-co-glycolide) and PLA–PEG (poly(DL-lactide)-poly(ethylene glycol)). They showed that the release of plasmid DNA was sustained over 20 days, and the DNA released was structurally intact and capable of cell transfection and bioactivity. It was the first successful demonstration of plasmid DNA incorporation into a polymer scaffold using electrospinning. Other groups have also used the nanosized scaffold for drug delivery successfully for vascular endothelial growth factor (142), for osteotropic factors (143), and for plasmid DNA (144).

A hydrotropic polymer system using N,N-diethyl nicotinamide was reported to be useful for the NPDDS of the poorly water-soluble drug paclitaxel. The micelles ranged between 30 and 50 nm and could be easily redissolved in an aqueous system. They demonstrated higher loading capacity and physical stability compared with other polymeric micelles (66).

Son et al. (130) have shown the accumulation of doxorubicin-loaded glycol chitosan nanoaggregates in tumor cells by enhanced and permeation effects. Several other studies also reported the accumulation of drugs in tumor cells in vivo using NPDDSs (146,147). Aneed (148) has written an excellent overview of the current drug-delivery systems used for cancer gene therapy, covering both the viral and nonviral vectors for carrying the therapeutic genes.

Polystyrene Nanospheres

These monodisperse polystyrene microparticles, also called latex microspheres, are used in a wide range of immunodiagnostic assays, as size standards for calibration of equipolymeric micellesent, in cell biology applications, and so on. The physical adsorption of the polystyrene particles is used to bind ligands to the surface of the particles. Sakuma et al. (149) studied the mucoadhesion of polystyrene NPs having surface hydrophilic polymeric chains in the GI tract in rats. They reported that the muco-adhesion of poly(N-isopropylacrylamide) NPs strongly enhanced the absorption of salmon calcitonin. Another interesting study showing applications of polystyrene NPs was reported by Hayakawa et al. (150). To establish an effective tool for the prevention of HIV-1 transmission, lectin-immobilized polystyrene NPs were synthesized and examined for their HIV-1 capture activity. It showed that when concanavalin A was immobilized on the surface of polystyrene NPs (mean diameters of 400 nm) with poly(methacrylic acid) branches and incubated with HIV-1 suspension at room temperature for 60 minutes, the NPs achieved >3.3log and a 2.2log reduction of viral infectivity in HIV-1 suspension at a concentration of 2 and 0.5 mg/ml, respectively, demonstrating the potential of this technique for prevention of viral transmission (150). Similar studies were also reported by Akashi et al. (151). Ogawara et al. (152) wrote a review on hepatic disposition of polystyrene NPs and the implications for rational design of particulate drug carriers. The clearance of colloidal particles from the blood circulation occurs by phagocytosis and/or endothelial cells, mainly in the liver, spleen, and bone marrow. The relative distribution of the injected particles in these organs is known to depend on various factors such as the size and the surface properties of the particles, and the type of serum proteins adsorbed onto the surface of the particles. The basic principles behind their distribution characteristics into the RES, however, remain unclear (152). An interesting study reported by Ogawara et al. (153) showed that precoating with serum albumin has reduced the receptor-mediated hepatic disposition of polystyrene nanospheres. This technique can be used to prevent rapid clearance by the mononuclear phagocyte system in vivo.

SOME COMMERCIALLY AVAILABLE NANOPARTICLES
Melamine Nanospheres

The melamine (polymethylenemelamine) nanospheres and microspheres are made from cross-linked melamine and have some advantages depending on the application compared with polystyrene particles. They have a higher density (1.51 g/cm^3), are very stable, can be stored indefinitely, can be resuspended in water, do not swell or shrink in most organic solvents, and are heat resistant up to 300° C. These monodisperse (CV 1–2%) melamine microparticles are hydrophilic and can be suspended in water and their refractive index is 1.68. The surface of plain melamine microparticles is terminated with methylol groups, which could be readily functionalized in the desired manner (154).

Plain Polymethyl Methacrylate and Biodegradable
Polylactide Nanospheres

Plain polymethyl methacrylate particles are available as 10% suspension, when higher concentrations for production are necessary (154). Polylactide (PLA) is a biodegradable thermoplastic derived from lactic acid. It resembles clear polystyrene, provides good esthetics (gloss and clarity), but it is stiff and brittle and needs modifications for most practical applications (i.e., plasticizers increase its flexibility).

These particles are made from PLA with a density of 1.02 g/cm^3. They are supplied as 1% aqueous solution (10 mg/ml) and are stable at a neutral pH for at least three months. Degradation starts through basic or acidic pH or enzymatic hydrolysis.

Magnetic Plain Dextran Nanospheres

The super paramagnetic NPs on the basis of dextran with a size of 250 nm have a magnetite content of 90%. A permanent magnet can easily separate 50 and 100 nm particles from 130 and 250 nm particles. Such smaller sizes can only be separated by a "high gradient magnetic field" device.

Gold Nanospheres

Gold particles are of highest quality and can be used in the production of diagnostic tests as well as conjugation studies of proteins and antibodies. The particles have a very narrow size distribution (CV between 5% and 15% depending on size) and are available from 2 to 250 nm. The number of particles/ml is given in the product/ordering table. The solutions are stabilized with HAuCl$_4$. Gold and silver colloids or sols are available in a number of different sizes. There are 14 different gold colloid sizes and are offered in four packing sizes. The products are best stored at room temperature, although storage at 4°C is an option. However, temperatures too close to freezing will destabilize the sol, causing aggregation and product loss (154).

Silver Nanospheres

Silver nanospheres are of highest quality and can be used in the production of diagnostic tests as well as conjugation studies of proteins and antibodies. The particles have a very narrow size distribution (CV between 10% and 20% depending on size) and are available from 2 to 250 nm.

Silica Nanospheres

These mono-disperse silica particles with a density of 2.0g/cm^3 are simple to dispense and to separate. Although polystyrene particles ($d = 1.04$) are difficult to separate by centrifugation under a size of 500 nm, silica particles do set down easily and are easy to resuspend. The silica particles are stable in water and organic solvents, produced under a new dying method. Silica particles are easy to functionalize and available as fluorescent particles. They are useful for coupling of DNA, oligonucleotides, oligopeptides, proteins, lectins, and antibodies. The silica particles are also available with different functional groups as –NH$_2$, and –COOH, albumin, protein A, epoxy, NHS, NTA, and EDTA (154). Li et al. (155) have prepared and characterized porous hollow silica NPs for controlled release applications. They reported a novel method for preparing hollow silica nanospheres with a porous shell structure via the sol–gel route and using inorganic calcium carbonate NPs as a template with 100-nm diameter and a wall thickness 10 nm of the nanospheres. Several factors were found to affect the drug release rate from the nanospheres (155).

Alumina Nanospheres

Alumina nanospheres and microspheres have been used in various applications because of their size uniformity and high degree of spherical particles (as a result, high flowability and high packing density). Properties of alumina, such as high thermal conductivity, heat resistance, hardness, and so on, are useful in formulation. These particles are often used as fillers for thermal conductivity sheets. Alumina nanospheres are available with plain, amino, and carboxyl functional groups. The alumina microspheres and nanospheres can be prepared with many functional groups such as albumin, protein A, epoxy, NHS, NTA, EDTA, and many others. They are useful for coupling of DNA, oligonucleotides, oligopeptides, proteins, lectins, and antibodies.

Carbon Nanotubes

In the last 15 years, it has been an exciting time for the field of carbon nanomaterials. The discoveries of fullerenes and carbon nanotubes have attracted the attention of many researchers all over the world (156). Iijima (157) first discovered these in 1991. They are now commercially available and can be manufactured on large scales (158). There are several companies who manufacture the carbon nanotubes and gradually their prices are reducing. They have a great potential in the drug-delivery systems and many other applications (159).

DIVERSE AND EMERGING TRENDS IN NANOTECHNOLOGY APPLICATIONS

Nanotechnology is making a great impact in many areas and some of the major areas are as follows.

Biological Analysis and Discovery

The basic science behind identifying the presence of a particular gene or protein has been developing for some time. The introduction of nanofluidics offers an excellent opportunity to work with smaller amounts of material. It can be used to segregate proteins and nucleic acids (DNA and RNA) based on size and shape. Nanomembranes offer a great potential in this area (160). There are several groups working on the idea of passing a single DNA or RNA thread through a nanosized pore, forcing it to straighten out and pass through a base part of fundamental coding element of nucleic acid (161,162). Changing electrical gradients on either side of the structure containing the pore, or quantum tunneling current across the pore, could be used to identify the particular base that is passing through. The ability to sequence a whole genome, the sum total of genes in an organism in a matter of hours, has been proposed as a potential application of this approach. The impact of these techniques in formulation of drug-delivery systems and their therapeutic applications will be worth watching during the coming few years.

Nanoparticles Tagging

Another boon to analysis will likely come from the attaching of NPs to molecules of interest. NPs small enough to behave as quantum dots can be made to emit light at varying frequencies. These attached molecules can be spectroscopically measured and will allow many different molecules to be measured from the same single sample. Another similar approach relies on getting the molecules to bind nanowires that have stripes on them similar to bar codes. These detection technologies are getting closer to commercialization. These can also further be applicable in the development of drug-delivery systems (163).

Nanostructured Materials

Nanostructured materials coupled with liquid crystals and chemical receptors offer the possibility of cheap, portable biodetectors that might, for instance, be worn as a badge. Such a badge could change color in the presence of a variety of chemicals and would have applications in hazardous environments (163). These can also be explored as NPDDSs.

Single-Molecule Detection

There are methods to detect a single photon. If one can make a nanostructure such as a quantum dot which will emit a photon in the presence of a particular molecule, one can make a device that can detect a single molecule of a substance. Various groups are working in this direction. The key commercial aspects of the use of micro- and nanotechnology in biodetection relate to portability, cost, and sensitivity (164).

Protective Nanoparticles Against Pathogens

NPs are disruptive to bacteria and viruses simply by virtue of their physical nature. This has led to ideas of lacing fabrics in hospitals with such NPs or nanoparticulate creams that can be spread on the body or sprays that can be inhaled, protecting against various pathogens (163).

Nanotubes and Cellular Manipulation

Nanotubes and cellular manipulation hold a great promise of being useful in bio- logical applications and as NPDDSs. There are tubes small enough to suck out a nucleus from a cell and place it into another. This is the technique behind cloning but nanotubes are finer still and offer the potential of making probes and delivery mechanisms that can be even more precise (165,166).

Nanoengineered Prosthetics

There are several devices which can be plugged into parts of central nervous sys- tems (CNSs), designed for processing visual or auditory information. Nanotechnology is changing all that: there is a potential for replacing a few of our organs for seeing, hearing, and touch, although connecting to CNS and avoiding classical problems of rejection will be a challenge. Synergies between our application areas, materials with greatly improved strength and designer surface properties offer potential for use in all manner of implants, from artificial hearts to hip implants. All these will have excellent potential in NPDDSs in the near future (163).

Thiomer Nanoparticles

Thiolated polymers designated as thiomers are thiol side-chain-bearing polymers. Owing to the introduction of these functional groups, thiomers exhibit comparatively stronger mucoadhesive, cohesive, enzyme inhibitory, and permeation-enhancing properties. They have excellent potential in the formulation of the NPDDSs. Several attempts are going on developing NPDDSs for insulin and calcitonin using thiomer NPs. A nasal delivery system for human growth hormone, a pulmonary delivery system for vasoactive intestinal peptide, a noninvasive delivery system for the KLH antigen, and nasal delivery systems for amyloid-binding peptides are being gener- ated and researched using thiomer polymeric NPs (154,167–169).

Nanostructured Monoliths

Functional nanostructured monoliths are being developed and optimized for the analysis of protein and peptides by nano-HPLC–MS/MS. Ring-opening metathesis polymerization (ROMP) is employed to develop nanostructured separation media. ROMP is a living polymerization technique capable of controlling polymerization at a molecular level. These show a better performance of protein and peptide analysis using nanocoupling techniques. Demand for nanoseparation phases is increasing heavily as nanocoupling techniques, particularly nano-HPLC-MS, are becoming more important.

Antibody-Coated Nanospheres

The 0.7 to 0.9 μm goat antimouse IgG-coated polystyrene particles are prepared by using passive adsorption; the coated particles are stable for several years under proper storage conditions. Antibody-coated polystyrene particles have antibody contents 14 μg/mg solid, 0.2 μg/cm^2, 1.5×10^4, IgG/particle, and binding capacity to IgG-FITC 4 μg/mg. These can be used for targeted delivery of drugs (170).

Nanocrystallites

An interesting application of nanotechnology was reported by Yin et al. (171) where they used pluronic in spray-drying to produce the nanocrystallites of the drug needing improved bioavailability or improved solubility. They utilized Pluronic F127 and developed several combinations of drug with pluronic, and spray-dried these combinations using the organic solvent.

Nanohybrids

A novel method of delivering nonionic poorly water-soluble drugs such as camptothecin was developed and reported by Tyner et al. (172). Camptothecin was first incorporated into micelles derived from negatively charged surfactants. The negatively charged micelles were then encapsulated in NPs of magnesium–aluminum hydroxides by an ion-exchange process. The resulting structures were termed nanohybrids. They released camptothecin rapidly with complete release within 10 minutes at both 4.8 and 7.2 pH. The encapsulation process allowed almost three times the drug loading and has excellent potential for drug-delivery applications. This complex was shown to provide similar cytotoxic characteristics to naked drug but the nanohybrids can be administered in a dose-controlled fashion due to good dispersion of the complexes in water. The ability to attach targeting biologically active molecules to the outside surface of the nanohybrids as well as the potential controlled release properties of the complexes indicate that these hybrids can be used for specific delivery of poorly soluble nonionic drugs (172).

Another interesting study from the same group was reported for the application of the nanohybrids as a nonviral vector for gene delivery. The nanohybrids were synthesized by the intercalation of a full gene and promoter encoding green fluorescent protein between layers of an inorganic host. The nanohybrids were delivered to 9L Glioma cells, JEG3 Choriocarcinoma placental cells, and cardiac myocytes. All cells were able to internalize and tolerate the nanohybrids and expressed the gene with some cell lines having up to 90% transfection efficiency (173). The nanohybrids mimic key features of viral delivery systems. Unlike other reported inorganic vectors, the host encapsulates the DNA molecule between the inorganic layers, protecting it from premature recognition or degradation. In addition, the presence of hydroxyl group on the host surface provides the means to link biologically active molecules to the exterior surface of the nanohybrids, suggesting the possibility of targeting the drug-delivery systems. Other advantages of nanohybrid systems include less foreign DNA and the ability to deliver multiple genes to cells. In addition, use of the nanohybrids is expected to increase control of the expression level of target genes by regulating the amount of DNA introduced into the cells. Such dose control is difficult to achieve in viral vectors. Preparation of viral constructs can be time-consuming and tedious. As the nanohybrids are applicable to a wide range of genes, they may be prepared through a simple one-step process, thus greatly shortening the amount of time needed to produce a functional vector (173).

Nanocontainer Technology
Nanotechnology promises new avenues to medical diagnosis, treatment, and drug delivery. In this respect, there are some special injectable nanovehicles that are programmable towards specific targets and are able to evade the immune defense and are versatile enough to be suited as carriers of complex functionality. Biotin-functionalized (poly-(2-methyloxazoline)-b-poly(dimethyl siloxane)-b-poly(2-methyl oxazoline) triblock copolymers were self-assembled to form nanocontainers, and biotinylated targeting ligands were attached by using Streptavidin as a coupling agent. Specifically, fluorescence-labeled nanocontainers were targeted against the scavenger receptor A1 from macrophages, an important cell in human disease. In human and transgenic cell lines and in mixed cultures, receptor binding of these generic carriers was followed by vascular uptake. Low nonspecific binding supported the stealth properties of the carrier while the cytotoxicity was absent. These versatile carriers appear to be promising for diagnostic and therapeutic drug-delivery purposes (174).

Electrospun Nanofibers as Drug-Delivery Systems
Electrostatic spinning is a versatile technique applied to various micro- and nanofabrication areas using numerous polymers. The technique involves jetting a liquid stream of a drug/polymer solution to a potential between 5 and 30 kV; fibers at submicrometer diameters can be formed when electrical forces overcome the surface tension of the drug/polymer solution at the air interface (termed a Taylor cone) such that a jet forms (175). As the jet accelerating through the electric field, two possible outcomes have been hypothesized: (*i*) radial forces become increasingly important leaning to splaying of the solution stream or (*ii*) a continuous single filament is generated based on bending instability (176). As the solvent evaporates, fiber can be collected on the screen to give a nonwoven fabric or collected on a spinning mandrill. The fiber diameter is a function of solution surface tension, dielectric constant of polymer solution, feeding rate, and electrostatic field. The nature of the polymer can also direct the use of the electrospun fibers, with water-soluble polymers giving rise to immediate release dosage forms and water insoluble giving sustained release systems. A report by Verreck et al. (177) has used these nanofibers for the release of itraconazole. The fiber diameter ranged from 500 nm to a few micrometers. They showed that complete release of the poorly soluble drug can be achieved and the rate of drug release can be tailored, showing applications of these nanofibers for wound healing, buccal, and topical applications (178).

FUTURE DIRECTIONS

The majority of commercial NP applications in medicine are geared towards drug delivery. In biosciences, NPs are replacing organic dyes in applications that require high photostability as well as high multiplexing capabilities. There are some new developments in directing and controlling the functions of nanoprobes, for example, driving magnetic NPs to the tumor and then making them either release the drug load or just heating them in order to destroy the surrounding tissue. The major trend in further development of nanomaterials is to make them multifunctional and controllable by external signals or by local environment, thus essentially turning them into nanodevices (164).

REFERENCES

1. The Royal Society. Nanoscience and nanotechnologies: opportunities and uncertainties. London: Royal Society, 2004:4.
2. Jores K, Mehnert W, Mader K. Physicochemical investigations on solid–lipid nanoparticles and on oil loaded solid–lipid nanoparticles: a nuclear magnetic resonance and electron spin resonance study. Pharm Res 2003; 20:1274.
3. Maestrell F, Mura P, Alonso MJ. Formulation and characterization of triclosan sub-micron emulsions and nanocapsules. J Microencapsul 2004; 21:857.
4. Lochmann D, Vogel V, Weyermann J, et al. Physicochemical characterization of protamine-phosphorothioate nanoparticles. J Microencapsul 2004; 21:625.
5. Geze A, Putaux JL, Choisnard L, Jehan P, Wouessidjewe D. Long term shelf stability of amphiphilic B-cyclodextrin nanospheres suspensions monitored by dynamic light scattering and cryo-transmission electron microscopy. J Microencapsul 2004; 21:607.
6. Wang X, Dai J, Chen Z, et al. Bioavailability and pharmacokinetics of cyclosporine A-loaded pH sensitive nanoparticles for oral administration. J Control Release 2004; 97:421.
7. Yoo HS, Park TG. Biodegradable nanoparticles containing protein–fatty acid complexes for oral delivery of salmon calcitonin. J Pharm Sci 2004; 93:488.
8. Mo Y, Lim LY. Mechanistic study of the uptake of wheat germ agglutinin-conjugated PLGA nanoparticles by A549 cells. J Pharm Sci 2004; 93:20.
9. Alphandary HP, Aboubaker M, Jaillard D, Couvreur P, Vauthier C. Visualization of insulin loaded nanocapsules: in vitro and in vivo studies after oral administration to rats. Pharm Res 2003; 20:1071.
10. Hoet P, Hohlfeld IB, Salata OV. Nanoparticles—known and unknown health risks. J Nanobiotechnol 2004; 2:12.
11. Venkateswarlu V, Manjunath K. Preparation, characterization and in vitro release kinetics of clozapine solid–lipid nanoparticles. J Control Release 2004; 95:627.
12. Dingler A, Gohla S. Production of solid–lipid nanoparticles (SLN): scaling up feasibilities. J Microencapsul 2002; 19:11.
13. Gasco MR. Method for producing solid–lipid microspheres having narrow size distribution. US Patent 5,250,236, 1993.
14. Mehnert W, Mader K. Solid–lipid nanocapsules production, characterization and applications. Adv Drug Deliv Rev 2001; 47:165.
15. Muller RH, Mader K, Gohla S. Solid–lipid nanoparticles (SLN) for controlled drug delivery–a review of the state of the art. Eur J Pharm Biopharm 2000; 50:161.
16. Beck RCR, Pohlman AR, Guterres SS. Nanoparticles-coated microparticles: preparation and characterization. J Microencapsul 2004; 21:499.
17. Rodriguez SG, Allemann E, Fessi H, Doelker E. Physicochemical parameters associated with nanoparticles formation in the salting out, emulsification-diffusion and nanoprecipitation methods. Pharm Res 2004; 21:1428.
18. Liao X, Wiedmann TS. Measurement of process-dependent material properties of pharmaceutical solids by nanoindentation. J Pharm Sci 2004; 94:79.

19. Rigaldie Y, Largeteau A, Lemagnen G, et al. Effects of high hydrostatic pressure on several sensitive therapeutic molecules and a soft nano-dispersed drug delivery system. Pharm Res 2003; 20:2036.
20. Fruhling J, Penasse W, Brassine C, et al. Intracellular penetration of liposomes containing a water insoluble antimitotic drug in L1210 cells. Eur J Cancer 1980; 16:1409.
21. Laurent G, Laduron C, Ruysschaert JM, Deleers M. Inhibition of cationic liposomes of ³H-thymidine incorporation into DNA of L1210 cells. Res Commun Chem Pathol Pharmacol 1981; 31:515.
22. Hecq J, Deleers M, Fanara D, Vranckx H, Amighi K. Preparation and characterization of nanocrystals for solubility and dissolution rate enhancement of Nifedipine. Int J Pharm 2005; 299:167–177.
23. Hecq J, Deleers M, Fanara D, et al. Preparation and in vitro/in vivo evaluation of nano-sized crystals for dissolution rate enhancement of UCB-35440-3, a highly-dosed poorly water soluble weak base. Eur J Pharm Biopharm 2006; 64:360–368.
24. Vranckx H, Demoustier M, Deleers M. Pharmaceutical composition comprising nano-capsules. US Patent 05500224, March 19, 1996.
25. Fanara D, Grognet P, Berwaer M, Deleers M. Use of pharmaceutical compositions capable of being gelled in Periodontology. US Patent 6471970, WO 09956726, EP 01073414, October 29, 2002.
26. Fanara D, Berwaer M, Deleers M. Pharmaceutical compositions capable of being gelled. US Patent 6464987, WO09956725, EP01073415, October 15, 2002.
27. LaVan DA, McGuire T, Langer R. Small scale systems for in vivo drug delivery. Nat Biotechnol 2003; 21:1184.
28. Saltzman WM, Olbricht WL. Building drug delivery into tissue engineering. Nat Rev 2002; 11:177.
29. Ziaie B, Baldi A, Lei M, Gu Y, Siegel RA. Hard and soft micromachining for biomems: review of techniques and examples of applications in microfluidics and drug delivery. Adv Drug Deliv Rev 2004; 56:145.
30. Su YC, Lin L. A water powered microdrug delivery system. J Electrochem Syst 2004; 13:75.
31. McAllister DV, Allen MG, Prausnitz MR. Microfabricated microneedles for gene and drug delivery. Annu Rev Biomed Eng 2000; 2:289.
32. Heurtault B, Saulnier P, Benoit JP, Proust JE, Pech B, Richard J. Lipid nanocapsules, preparation, method and use as a medicine. Patent No. W001/64328, 2000.
33. Heurtault B, Saulnier P, Pech B, Benoit JP, Proust JE. Interfacial stability of lipid nanocap-sules. Colloids Surf B Biointerfaces 2003; 30:225.
34. Muller RH, Dingler T, Schneppe T, Gohla S. In: Wise D, ed. Handbook of Pharmaceutical Controlled Release Technology. New York: Marcel Dekker, 2000:359.
35. Jenning V, Korting MS, Gohla S. Vitamin A loaded solid lipid nanoparticles for topical use: drug release properties. J Control Release 2000; 66:115.
36. Muhlen AZ, Schwarz C, Mehnert W. Solid–lipid nanoparticles (SLNs) for controlled drug deliver–drug release and release mechanism. Eur J Pharm Biopharm 1998; 45:149.
37. Dulieu C, Bazile D. Influence of lipid nanocapsules composition on their aptness to freeze drying. Pharm Res 2005; 22:285.
38. Muller RH, Jacobs C, Kayser O. Nanosuspensions as particulate drug formulations in therapy rational for development and what we can expect for the future. Adv Drug Deliv Rev 2001; 47:3.
39. Jores K, Mehnert W, Drechesler M, Bunjes H, Johann C, Madder K. Investigations on the structure of solid–lipid nanoparticles (SLN) and oil loaded solid lipid nanoparticles by photon correlation spectroscopy, field flow fractionation and transmission electron microscopy. J Control Release 2004; 95:217.
40. Muller RH, Radtke SA, Wissing SA. Solid–lipid nanoparticles (SLN) and nanostructured lipid carriers (NLC) in cosmetic and dermatological preparations. Adv Drug Deliv Rev 2002; 54:131.
41. Muller RH, Radtke M, Wissing SA. Nanostructured lipid matrices for improved micro-encapsulation of drugs. Int J Pharm 2002; 242:121.
42. Chesnoy S, Huang L. Structure and function of lipid DNA complexes for gene delivery. Annu Rev Biophys Struct 2000; 29:27.

43. Merdan T, Kopecek J, Kissel T. Prospects for cationic polymers in gene and oligonucleotides therapy against cancer. Adv Drug Deliv Rev 2001; 47:165.
44. Fournier E, Dufresne MH, Smith DC, Ranger M, Leroux JC. A novel step drug loading procedure for water soluble amphiphilic nanocarriers. Pharm Res 2004; 21:962.
45. Heurtault B, Saulnier P, Pech B, Proust JE, Benoit JP. A novel phase inversion based process for the preparation of lipid nanocarriers. Pharm Res 2002; 19:875.
46. Tabatt K, Sameti M, Olbrich C, Muller RH, Lehr CM. Effect of cationic lipid and matrix lipid composition on solid–lipid nanoparticles mediated gene transfer. Eur J Pharm Biopharm 2004; 57:155.
47. Rudolph C, Schillinger U, Ortiz A, Tabatt K, Plank C, Muller RH, Rosenecker J. Application of novel solid–lipid (SLN) gene vector formulations based on a dimeric HIV-1 TAT peptide in vitro and in vivo. Pharm Res 2004; 21:1662.
48. Liu F, Yang J, Huang L, Liu D. New cationic lipid formulation for gene transfer. Pharm Res 1996; 13:1856.
49. Tabatt K, Kneuer C, Sameti M, et al. Transfection with different colloidal systems: comparison of solid–lipid nanoparticles and liposomes. J Control Release 2004; 97:321.
50. Kogure K, Moriguchi R, Sasaki K, Ueno M, Futaki S, Harashima H. Development of a nonviral multifunctional envelop-type nanodevice by a novel lipid film hydration method. J Control Release 2004; 98:317.
51. Lee KE, Cho SH, Lee HB, Jeong SY, Yuk SH. Microencapsulation of lipid nanoparticles containing lipophilic drug. J Microencapsul 2003; 20:489.
52. Stevens PJ, Sekido M, Lee RJ. A folate receptor targeted lipid nanoparticles formulation for a lipophilic paclitaxel prodrug. Pharm Res 2004; 21:2153.
53. Hou DZ, Xie CS, Huang KJ, Zhu CH. The production and characteristics of solid–lipid nanoparticles (SLNs). Biomaterials 2003; 24:1781.
54. Olbrich C, Gessner A, Schroder W, Kayser O, Muller RH. Lipid–drug conjugate nanoparticles of the hydrophilic drug diminazene-cytotoxicity testing and mouse serum absorption. J Control Release 2004; 96:425.
55. Cavalli R, Bargoni A, Podio V, Muntoni E, Zara GP, Gasco MR. Duodenal administration of solid–lipid nanoparticles loaded with different percentages of tobramycin. J Pharm Sci 2003; 92:1085.
56. Williams J, Lansdown R, Sweitzer R, Romanowski M, LaBell R, Ramaswami R, Unger E. Nanoparticle drug delivery system for intravenous delivery of topoisomerase inhibitors. J Control Release 2003; 91:167.
57. Kabanov AV, Batrakova EV, Alakhov VY. Pluronic block copolymers as novel polymer therapeutics for drug and gene delivery. J Control Release 2002; 82:189.
58. Torchilin VP. Structure and design of polymeric surfactant-based drug delivery systems. J Control Release 2001; 23:137.
59. Djordjevic J, Barch M, Uhrich E. Polymeric micelles based on amphiphilic scorpion like macromolecules: novel carriers for water insoluble drugs. Pharm Res 2005; 22:24.
60. Kataoka K, Harada A, Nagasaki Y. Block copolymer micelles for drug delivery: design, characterization and biological significance. Adv Drug Del Rev 2002; 54:113.
61. Kakizawa Y, Katakoa K. Block copolymer micelles for delivery of genes and related compounds. Adv Drug Del Rev 2002; 54:203.
62. Rosler A, Vandermeulen GM, Klok HA. Advanced drug delivery devices via self assembly of amphiphilic block copolymers. Adv Drug Del Rev 2001; 53:95.
63. Huh KM, Lee SC, Cho YW, Lee J, Jeong JH, Park K. Hydrotropic polymer micelle system for delivery of paclitaxel. J Control Release 2005; 101:59.
64. Kwon GS, Katakoa K. Block copolymers micelles as long circulating drug vehicles. Adv Drug Del Rev 1995; 16:295.
65. Burt HM, Zhang X, Toleikis P, Embree L, Hunter WL. Development of copolymers of poly(D,L lactide) and methoxypolyethylene glycol as micellar carriers for paclitaxel. Colloids Surf B Biointerfaces 1999; 16:161.
66. Fisher M, Vogtle F. Dendrimers: from design to application—a progress report. Angew Chem Int Ed Engl 1999; 38:885.
67. Dufresne MH, Fournier F, Jones MC, Ranger M, Leroux JC. Block copolymers micelles–engineering versatile carriers for drugs and biomacromolecules. In: Gurny R, ed.

Challenges in Drug Delivery for the New Millennium. Saint Priest: Bulletin Technique Gattefosse'96, 2003:103.

68. Kwon G, Suwa S, Yokoyama T, Okano T, Sakurai Y, Katakoa K. Enhanced tumor accumulation and prolonged circulation times of micelles forming poly(ethylene oxide-aspartate) block copolymer–adriamycin conjugates. J Control Release 1994; 29:17.

69. Savic R, Luo L, Eisenberg A, Maysinger D. Micellar nano-containers distribute to defined cytoplasmic organelles. Science 2003; 300:615.

70. Maeda H, Wu J, Sawa T, Matsumura Y, Hori K. Tumor vascular permeability and EPR effect in macromolecular therapeutics: a review. J Control Release 2000; 65:271.

71. Brigger I, Dubernet C, Couvreur P. Nanoparticles in cancer therapy and diagnosis. Adv Drug Deliv Rev 2002; 54:631.

72. Francis MF, Cristea M, Yang Y, Winnik FM. Engineering polysaccharide-based polymeric micelles to enhance permeability of cyclosporine A across caco-2 cells. Pharm Res 2005; 22:209.

73. Ugazio E, Cavalli R, Gasco MR. Incorporation of cyclosporine A in solid–lipid nanoparticles (SLN). Int J Pharm 2002; 241:341.

74. Varela MC, Guzman M, Molpeceres J, Aberturas MDR, Puyol DR, Puyol MR. Cyclosporine loaded polycaprolactone nanoparticles: immunosuppression and nephrotoxicity in rats. Eur J Pharm Sci 2001; 12:471.

75. Gref R, Quellec P, Sanchez A, Calvo P, Dellacherie E, Alonso MJ. Development and characterization of Cy-A loaded polylactic–polyethylene glycol PEG micro and nanoparticles: comparison with conventional PLA particulate carriers. Eur J Pharm Biopharm 2001; 51:111.

76. Campos AMD, Sanchez A, Alonso MJ. Chitosan nanoparticles: a new vehicle for the improvement of the delivery of drugs to the ocular surfaces, application to cyclosporine A. Int J Pharm 2001; 224:159.

77. Gao ZG, Fain HD, Rapoport N. Controlled and targeted tumor chemotherapy by micellar-encapsulated drug and ultrasound. J Control Release 2005; 102:203.

78. Wu J, Akaike T, Hayashida K, Okamoto T, Okuyama A, Maeda H. Enhanced vascular permeability in solid tumor involving peroxynitrite and matrix metalloproteinases. Jpn J Cancer Res 2001; 92:439.

79. Torchelin VP, Lukyanov AN, Gao A, Papahadjopoulos B. Immunomicelles: targeted pharmaceutical carriers for poorly soluble drugs. Proc Natl Acad Sci USA 2003; 100:6039.

80. Kabanov AV, Batrakova EV, Alakhov VY. An essential relationship between ATP depletion and chemosensitizing activity of Pluronic block copolymers. J Control Release 2003; 91:75.

81. Na K, Lee KH, Bae YH. pH sensitivity and pH dependent interior structural change of self assembled hydrogel nanoparticles of pullulan acetate/oligo-sulfonamide conjugate. J Control Release 2004; 97:513.

82. Cammas S, Suzuki K, Sone C, Sakurai Y, Kataoka K, Okano T. Thermo responsive polymer nanoparticles with a core shell micelle structure as site specific drug carriers. J Control Release 1997; 48:157.

83. Chung JE, Yokoyama M, Yamato M, Aoyagi T, Sakurai Y, Okano T. Thermo responsive drug delivery from polymeric micelles constructed using block copolymers of poly (N-isopropylacrylamide) and poly(butylmethacrylate). J Control Release 1999; 62:115.

84. Panyam J, Labhasetwar V. Biodegradable nanoparticles for drug and gene delivery to cells and tissues. Adv Drug Deliv Rev 2003; 55:329.

85. Vauthier C, Dubernet C, Fatal E, Alphandary HP, Couvreur P. Poly(alkylcyanoacrylates) as biodegradable materials for biomedical applications. Adv Drug Deliv Rev 2003; 55:519.

86. Discher DE, Eisenberg A. Polymeric vesicles. Science 2002; 297:967.

87. Harrington KJ, Lewanski CR, Stewart JSW. Liposomes as vehicles for targeted therapy of cancer. Part 2. Clinical development. Clin Oncol 2000; 12:16.

88. Xiong XY, Tam KC, Gan LH. Release kinetics of hydrophobic and hydrophilic model drugs from Pluronic F127/poly(lactic acid) nanoparticles. J Control Release 2005; 103:73.

89. Zhang L, Hu Y, Jiang X, Yang C, Lu W, Yang YH. Camptothecin derivative-loaded poly(caprolactone-co-lactide)-b-PEG-b-poly(caprolactone-c)-lactide nanoparticles and their bio-distribution in mice. J Control Release 2004; 96:135.

90. Moghimi SM, Hunter AC, Murray JC. Long circulating and target specific nanoparticles: theory to practice. Pharmacol Rev 2001; 53:283.
91. Shenderova A, Burke TG, Schwendeman SP. Stabilization of 10-hydroxy camptothecin in poly(lactide-co-glycolide) microsphere delivery vehicles. Pharm Res 1997; 14:1406.
92. Hu Y, Jiang X, Ding Y, et al. Preparation and drug release behaviors of nimodipine-loaded poly(caprolactone)-poly-(ethylene oxide) polylactide amphiphilic copolymer nanoparticles. Biomaterials 2003; 24:2395.
93. Riley T, Stolnik S, Heald CR, et al. Physicochemical evaluation of nanoparticles assembled from poly(lactic acid) poly(ethylene glycol) (PLA–PEG) block copolymers as drug delivery vehicles. Langmuir 2001; 17:3168.
94. Yoo HS, Park TG. Folate receptor targeted biodegradable polymeric doxorubicin micelles. J Control Release 2004; 96:273.
95. Lavasanifar A, Samuel J, Kwon GS. Poly(ethylene oxide) block poly(L-amino acid) micelles for drug delivery. Adv Drug Deliv Rev 2002; 54:169.
96. Vriezema DM, Hoogboom J, Velonia K, et al. Vesicles and polymerized vesicles from thiophene containing rod coil block copolymers. Nolte Angew Chem Int Ed 2003; 42:772.
97. Vriezema DM, Kros A, Gelder RD, Cornelissen JJLM, Rowan AE, Roeland JM. Electroformed giant vesicles from thiophene containing rod coil diblock copolymers. Macromolecules 2004; 37:4736.
98. Vriezema DM, Araganoes MC, Elemans HAAW, Cornelissen JJLM, Rowan AE, Roeland JM. Self assembled nanoreactors. Chem Rev 2005; 105:1455.
99. Lee SC, Kim C, Kwon IC, Chung H, Jeong SY. Polymeric micelles of poly(2-ethyl-2-oxazoline)-block–poly(caprolactone) copolymer as a carrier for paclitaxel. J Control Release 2003; 89:437.
100. Vauthier C, Dubernet C, Chauvierre C, Brigger I, Couvreur P. Drug delivery to resistant tumors: the potential of poly(alkyl cyanoacrylate) nanoparticles. J Control Release 2003; 93:151.
101. Mu L, Feng SS. A novel controlled release formulation for the anticancer drug paclitaxel (Taxol): PLGA nanoparticles containing vitamin E TPGS. J Control Release 2003; 86:33.
102. Chauvierre C, Labarre D, Couvreur P, Vauthier C. Novel polysaccharide decorated poly(isobutyl cyanoacrylate) nanoparticles. Pharm Res 2003; 20:1786.
103. Wartlick H, Schmitt SS, Strebhardt K, Kreuter J, Langer K. Tumor cell delivery of antisense oligonucleotides by human serum albumin nanoparticles. J Control Release 2004; 96:483.
104. Crommelin DJA, Strom G, Jiskot W, Stenekes R, Mastrobattista E, Hennink WE. Nanotechnological approaches for the delivery of macromolecules. J Control Release 2003; 87:81.
105. Ihre HR, Gagne L, Frechet JMJ, Szoka FC. Polyester dendritic systems for drug delivery applications: in vitro and in vivo evaluations. Bioconjug Chem 2002; 13:453.
106. Liu MJ, Kono K, Frechet R. Water soluble dendritic unimolecular micelles, their potential as drug delivery agents. J Control Release 2000; 65:121.
107. Zhang GD, Harada A, Nishiyama N, et al. Polyion complex micelles entrapping cationic dendrimer porphyrin: effective photosensitizer for photodynamic therapy of cancer. J Control Release 2003; 93:141.
108. Ueno Y, Futagawa H, Takagi Y, Ueno A, Mizushima Y. Drug incorporating calcium carbonate nanoparticles for a new delivery system. J Control Release 2005; 103:93.
109. Vogel V, Lochmann D, Weyermann J, et al. Oligonucleotide-protamine-albumin nanoparticles: preparation, physical properties and intracellular distribution. J Control Release 2005; 103:99.
110. Dinaure N, Lochmann D, Demirhan I, et al. Intracellular tracking of protamine/antisense oligonucleotides nanoparticles and their inhibitory effect on HIV-1 transactivation. J Control Release 2004; 96:497.
111. Lochmann D, Vogel V, Weyermann J, et al. Physicochemical characterization of protamine phosphorothioate nanoparticles. J Microencapsul 2004; 21:643.
112. Ando T, Yamasaki M, Suzuki K. Protamines: Isolation, Characterization, Structure and Function. Berlin: Springer, 1973.
113. Huang M, Khor E, Lim LY. Uptake and cytotoxicity of Chitosan molecules and nanoparticles: effects of molecular weight and degree on deacetylation. Pharm Res 2004; 21:344.

114. Janes KA, Fresneau MP, Marazuela A, Fabra A, Alonso MJ. Chitosan nanoparticles as delivery systems for doxorubicin. J Control Release 2001; 73:255.
115. Ma ZS, Lim LY. Uptake of Chitosan and associated insulin in the caco-2 call monolayers: a comparison between Chitosan molecules and Chitosan nanoparticles. Pharm Res 2002; 19:1488.
116. Illum L, Gill IJ, Hinchcliffe M, Fisher AN, Davis SS. Chitosan as a novel nasal delivery system for vaccines. Adv Drug Deliv Rev 2001; 51:81.
117. Campos AM, Diebold Y, Carvalho EL, Sanchez A, Alonso MJ. Chitosan nanoparticles as new ocular drug delivery systems: in vitro stability, in vivo fate and cellular toxicity. Pharm Res 2004; 21:803.
118. Hejazi R, Amiji M. Chitosan based gastrointestinal delivery systems. J Control Release 2003; 89:151.
119. Park JH, Kwon S, Nam JO, et al. Self assembled nanoparticles based on glycol Chitosan bearing 5 B-cholanic acid for RGD peptide delivery. J Control Release 2005; 95:579.
120. De S, Robinson D. Polymer relationships during preparation of Chitosan-alginate and poly-L-lysine-alginate nanospheres. J Control Release 2003; 89:101.
121. Yoo HS, Lee JE, Chung H, Kwon IC, Jeong SY. Self assembled nanoparticles containing hydrophobically modified glycol Chitosan for gene delivery. J Control Release 2005; 103:235.
122. Kumar M, Kong X, Behera AK, Hellermann GR, Lockey RF, Mohapatra SS. Chitosan IFN-c-pDNA nanoparticles (CIN) therapy for allergic asthma. Gene Vaccines Ther 2001; 1:3.
123. Chu WH, Chin R, Huen T, Ferrari M. Silicone membrane nano-filters from sacrificial oxide removal. J Micro Electrochem Syst 1999; 8:34.
124. Martin F, Walczak R, Boiarski A, et al. Tailoring width of microfabricated nanochannels to solute size can be used to control diffusion kinetics. J Control Release 2005; 102:123.
125. Desai TA. Microfabrication technology for pancreatic cell encapsulation. Expert Opin Biol Therap 2002; 2:633.
126. Desai TA, Hansford D, Ferrari M. Characterization of micromachined silicone membranes for immunoisolation and bioseparation applications. J Membr Sci 1999; 159:221.
127. Lemarchand C, Couvreur P, Besnard M, Costantini D, Gref R. Novel polyester–polysaccharide nanoparticles. Pharm Res 2003; 20:1284.
128. Muller BG, Leuenberger H, Kissel T. Albumin nanospheres as carriers for passive drug targeting: an optimized manufacturing technique. Pharm Res 1996; 13:32.
129. Yamaguchi Y, Nagasawa T, Nakamura N, et al. Successful treatment of photodamaged skin of nano scale atRA particles using novel transdermal delivery. J Control Release 2005; 104:29.
130. Lim SJ, Kim CK. Formulation parameters determining the physicochemical characteristics of solid–lipid nanoparticles loaded with all *trans*-retinoic acid. Int J Pharm 2002; 243:135.
131. Lim SJ, Lee MK, Kim CK. Altered chemical and biological activities of all *trans* incorporated in solid–lipid nanoparticles powders. J Control Release 2004; 100:53.
132. Balthasar S, Michaelis K, Dinauer N, Briesen VH, Kreuter J, Langer K. Preparation and characterization of antibody modified gelatin nanoparticles as carrier system for uptake in lymphocytes. Biomaterials 2005; 26:2723.
133. Couvreur P, Barratt G, Fattal E, Legrand P, Vauthier C. Nanocapsule technology: a review. Crit Rev Ther Drug Carrier Syst 2002; 19:99.
134. Dalencon F, Amjaud Y, Lafforgue C, Derouin F, Fessi H. Atovaquone and rifabutine loaded nanocapsules: formulation studies. Int J Pharm 1998; 153:127.
135. Hubert B, Atkinson J, Guerret M, Hoffman M, Devissaguet JP, Maincent P. The preparation and acute antihypertensive effects of a nanoparticular form of darodipine, a dihydropyridine calcium entry blocker. Pharm Res 1991; 8:734.
136. Barrat G, Puisieux F, Yu WP, Foucher C, Fessi H, Devissaguet JP. Anti meta-static activity of MDP-L-alanyl cholesterol incorporated into various types of nanocapsules. Int J Immuno-Pharmacol 1994; 16:457.
137. Calvo P, Alonso MJ, VilaJato JL, Robinson JR. Improved ocular bioavailability of Indomethacin by novel ocular drug carriers. J Pharm Pharmacol 1996; 48:1147.

138. Chen H, Zhang Z, Almarsson O, Marier JF, Berkovitz D, Gardner CR. A novel lipid free nanodispersion formulation of propofol and its characterization. Pharm Res 2005; 22:356.

139. Zweers MLT, Engbers GHM, Grijpma DW, Feijen J. Vitro degradation of nanoparticles prepared from polymers based on DL-lactide glycolide and poly(ethylene oxide). J Control Release 2004; 100:347.

140. Arbos P, Campenero MA, Arangoa MA, Renedo MJ, Irache JM. Influence of the surface characteristics of PVM/MA nanoparticles on their bioadhesive properties. J Control Release 2003; 89:19.

141. Luu YK, Kim K, Hsiao BS, Chu B, Hadjiargurou M. Development of a nanostructured DNA delivery scaffold via electro-spinning of PLGA and PLA–PEG block copolymers. J Control Release 2003; 89:341.

142. Murphy WL, Peters MC, Kohn DH, Mooney DJ. Sustained release of vascular endothelial growth factor from mineralized poly(lactide-co-glycolide) scaffolds for tissue engineering. Biomaterials 2000; 24:2521.

143. Whang K, Goldstick TK, Healy KE. A biodegradable polymer scaffold for delivery of osteotropic factors. Biomaterials 2000; 24:2545.

144. Perez C, Sanchez A, Putnam D, Ting D, Langer R, Alonso MJ. Poly(lactic acid)–poly(ethylene glycol) nanoparticles as new carriers for the delivery of plasmid DNA. J Control Release 2001; 75:952.

145. Son YJ, Jang JS, Cho YW, et al. Biodistribution and antitumor efficacy of doxorubicin loaded glycol Chitosan nano-aggregates by EPR effect. J Control Release 2003; 91:135.

146. Nigavekar SS, Sung LY, Llanes M, et al. ^{3}H dendrimer nanoparticles organ/tumor distribution. Pharm Res 2004; 21:476.

147. Balogh LP, Nigavekar SS, Cook AC, Minc L, Khan MK. Development of dendrimer gold radioactive nano-composites to treat cancer microvasculature. Pharma Chem 2003; 2:94.

148. Aneed AE. An overview of current delivery systems in cancer gene therapy. J Control Release 2004; 94:1.

149. Sakuma S, Sudo R, Suzuki N, Kikuchi H, Akashi M, Hayashi M. Mucoadhesion of polystyrene nanoparticles having surface hydrophilic polymeric chains in the gastrointestinal tract. Int J Pharm 1999; 177:161.

150. Hayakawa T, Kawamura M, Okamoto M, Baba M, et al. Concanavalin A-immobilized polystyrene nanospheres capture HIV-1 virions and gp120: potential approach towards prevention of viral transmission. J Med Virol 1998; 56:327.

151. Akashi M, Niikawa T, Serizawa T, Hayakawa T, Baba M. Capture of HIV-1 gp120 and virions by lectin immobilized polystyrene. Bioconjug Chem 1998; 9:50.

152. Ogawara KI, Higaki K, Kimura T. Major determinants in hepatic disposition of polystyrene nanospheres: implication for rational design of particulate drug carriers. Crit Rev Ther Drug Carrier Syst 2002; 19:45.

153. Ogawara KI, Furumoto K, Nagayama S, et al. Precoating with serum albumin reduces receptor-mediated hepatic disposition of polystyrene nanospheres: implications for rational design of nanoparticles. J Control Release 2004; 100:451.

154. Bernkop-Schnurch A, Kast CE, Guggi D. Permeation enhancing polymers in oral delivery of hydrophilic macromolecules: thiomer/GSH systems. J Control Release 2003; 93:95.

155. Li ZZ, Wen LX, Shao L, Chen JF. Fabrication of porous hollow silica nanoparticles and their applications in drug release control. J Control Release 2004; 98:245.

156. Zhou O, Shimoda H, Gao B, Oh S, Fleming L, Yue G. Materials science of carbon nanotubes: fabrication, integration and properties of macroscopic structures of carbon nanotubes. Acc Chem Res 2002; 35:1045.

157. Iijima S. Helical microtubules of graphitic carbon. Nature 1991; 354:56.

158. Maurin G, Stepanek I, Bernier P, Colomer JF, Nagy JB, Henn F. Segmented and opened multiwalled carbon nanotubes. Carbon 2001; 39:1273.

159. Nanotechnology Now. Nanotubes survey, April 2003.

160. Nam JM, Thaxton CC, Mirkin CA. Nanoparticles based bio bar codes for the ultrasensitive detection of proteins. Science 2003; 301:1884.

161. Mahtab R, Rogers JP, Murphy CJ. Protein sized quantum dot luminescence can distinguish between "straight," "bent" and "kinked" oligonucleotides. J Am Chem Soc 1995; 117:9099.

162. Cao YC, Jin R, Nam JM, Thaxton CS, Mirkin CA. Raman dye labeled nanoparticles probes for proteins. J Am Chem Soc 2003; 125:14676.
163. CMP Scientifica. Nanotech: The tiny revolution. copyrighted, 2001.
164. Salata OV. Applications of nanoparticles in biology and medicine. J Nanobiotechnol 2004; 2:3.
165. Pankhurst QA, Connolly J, Jones SK, Dobson J. Applications of magnetic nanoparticles in biomedicine. J Phys D Appl Phys 2003; 36:R167.
166. Reich DH, Tanase M, Hultgren A, Bauer LA, Chen CS, Meyer GJ. Biological applications of multifunctional magnetic nanowires. J Appl Phys 2003; 93:7275.
167. Kast CE, Guggi D, Langoth N, Bernkop-Schnurch A. Development and in vivo evaluation of an oral delivery system for low molecular weight heparin based on thiolated polycarbophil. Pharm Res 2003; 20:931.
168. Bernkop-Schnurch A, Hoffer MH, Krum K. Thiomers for oral delivery of hydrophilic macromolecular drugs. Expert Opin Drug Deliv 2004; 1:87.
169. Leitner VM, Guggi D, Krauland AH, Bernkop-Schnurch A. Nasal delivery of human growth hormone: in vitro and in vivo evaluation of a thiomer/GSH microparticulate delivery system. J Control Release 2004; 100:87.
170. Commercially available nanoparticles and nanospheres for medical applications. www.microspheres-nanospheres.com.
171. Yin SX, Franchini M, Chen J, et al. Bioavailability enhancement of a COX-2 inhibitor BMS-347070, from a nanocrystalline dispersion prepared by spray drying. J Pharm Sci 2005; 94:1598.
172. Tyner KM, Schiffman SR, Giannelis EP. Nanohybrids as delivery vehicles for camptothecin. J Control Release 2004; 95:501.
173. Tyner KM, Roberson MS, Berghorn KA, et al. Intercalation, delivery and expression of the gene encoding green fluorescence protein utilizing nanohybrids. J Control Release 2004; 100:399.
174. Broz P, Benito SM, Saw CL, et al. Cell targeting by a generic receptor targeted polymer nanocontainer platform. J Control Release 2005; 102:475.
175. Reneker DH, Chun I. Nanometer diameter of polymer, produced by electrospinning. Nanotechnology 1996; 7:216.
176. Kath DS, Robinson KW, Attawia MA, Ko FW, Laurencin CT. Bioresorbable nanofiber based systems for wound healing: optimization of fabrication parameters. Transactions of the 28th Annual Meeting for the Society of Biomaterials, 2002:143.
177. Verreck G, Chun I, Peeters J, Rosenblatt J, Brewster ME. Preparation and characterization of nanofibers containing amorphous drug dispersions generated by electrostatic spinning. Pharm Res 2003; 20:810.
159. Verreck G, Chun I, Rosenblatt J, et al. Incorporation of drugs in an amorphous state into electrospun nanofibers composed of a water insoluble non-biodegradable polymer. J Control Release 2003; 92:349.

2 Nanosuspensions for Parenteral Delivery

Barrett E. Rabinow
Baxter Healthcare Corporation, Round Lake, Illinois, U.S.A.

HISTORICAL INTRODUCTION

Need

The need for nanosuspensions as a dosage form was recognized as a means to administer therapeutic quantities of water-insoluble dosage forms (1). The continuing need for such a tool was reinforced with the uptake of high-throughput receptor-based screening assays employed by the pharmaceutical industry during the 1990s. This technique searches for drugs that exhibit strong binding to hydrophobic target receptor pockets and therefore produces drug leads that tend to be poorly water soluble (2). It was not only the kind of molecule that changed, but also the vast numbers of such drug leads that emerged from discovery efforts, that compelled a solution to the resulting formulation conundrum. Typically, these in vitro assays were conducted in dimethyl sulfoxide, to obviate problems of water insolubility during the preliminary discovery phase. With progression to animal studies, however, nontoxic vehicles were sought that would permit assessment of the toxicity of the drug candidate itself, without interfering effects due to the vehicle (3,4). Nanosuspensions commended themselves as suitable candidates because: (*i*) solvents were not needed, (*ii*) small particulate size permitted intravenous delivery, and (*iii*) the solid crystal phase permitted high loading, which permitted the animal studies to be conducted at many multiples of the intended dose in man.

Predecessor Technology

Equally important as the demand of applications was the ready availability of building blocks for implementation of the new technology. Homogenizers had been in use since the late nineteenth century for homogenization of milk, and more recently in the latter half of the twentieth century for commercial production of intravenous lipid emulsions. Therefore, such issues of cleanability, sterilizability, noncontamination of fluid processing streams with hydraulics, and so on, had been long resolved. It remained for more efficient valve designs to be developed, transmitting more of the energy to the particle (5). Similarly, milling equipment for particulates, as, for example, the paint industry, was available and amenable to the changes necessary for pharmaceutical use. This was accomplished by developing cross-linked polystyrene grinding media that was smaller and relatively noncontaminating, resulting in smaller drug particles (6). Precipitation and crystallization techniques were much older, but significant chemical engineering understanding and optimization occurred during the last century (7). Supercritical fluid processing (8) was commercially developed relatively recently. Substantial understanding of the role of surfactants, both for formulation stabilization (9) and for impacting pharmacokinetics (10), became clarified. Here, lessons were learned from earlier developed drug-delivery platforms, liposomes and emulsions, regarding prolonging circulation times of particulate dosage forms.

Combination of Component Technologies

The component technologies described above were often combined to improve performance and overcome individual deficiencies, in the development of nanosuspensions. Thus, nanosuspensions were lyophilized for greater stability (11), formulated with soluble molecular analogs (12), applied to liquid drugs to form emulsions (13), and combined in matrix pellet formulations (14) and multivesicular lipid systems (15). To reduce particle size to the nanometer range, supercritical fluid techniques were combined with an ultrasonic vibrating surface to enhance mixing and atomize the jet into nanodroplets (16), or sprayed into quenching surfactant solutions (17). Taxol nanosuspensions were prepared by emulsion templating, that is dissolving drug into a volatile solvent, homogenizing in an aqueous solution containing suitable stabilizers, and evaporating solvent to recover nanosuspensions (18). Finally, rapid precipitation and homogenization were synergistically combined to obtain stable nanosuspensions (19). Homogenization cracks crystals along their defect planes, induced by rapid precipitation, to reduce their size further. Additionally, the mechanical shock of homogenization often induces conversion of the unstable, initially formed polymorph resulting from precipitation, to the more thermodynamically stable polymorph.

FORMULATION APPROACHES AND MANUFACTURING METHODS
Strategy

The preparation of stable nanosuspensions must recognize the thermodynamic forces at work. For a given mass of drug substance, as particle size is reduced, surface area is increased. In an aqueous medium, this significantly increases the surface free energy of the drug system. Strong, and therefore stable bonds within the drug crystal lattice, on the one hand, and intermolecular hydrogen bonds of water molecules, on the other hand, are disrupted. Instead, they are replaced by a large interfacial area of hydrophilic water molecules in proximity with a hydrophobic drug surface. Such a system will tend to reduce the energetically unfavorable area by particle growth and by aggregation. Ostwald ripening represents one mechanism by which this may occur. By the Ostwald–Freundlich equation, smaller particles have a higher surface energy than larger particles (20). This leads to greater dissolution of smaller particles with consequent increasing size of larger particles. As a result, the distribution of the suspension shifts to increasing particle size. To address this as well as irreversible agglomeration, formulation strategy is designed to stabilize particle size over time.

Utilization of surfactant excipients is an essential part of formulation strategy. The particular surfactants are selected to be compatible with both phases, and so interpose themselves between the hydrophobic drug surface on one side and the aqueous media on the other. The effectiveness of their interaction is measured by the reduction in surface free energy. An ionically charged surfactant will provide electrostatic repulsion of neighboring particles, which will tend to inhibit aggregation. However, if the particles overcome this long-range r^{-2} repulsion (where r is the interparticulate distance), as by addition of a salt to increase dielectric shielding, they may still approach each other too closely. They may thus be subject to the short-acting (r^{-6}), but much stronger, attractive London dispersion forces resulting from instantaneous dipole polarization interactions (21). Under this circumstance, the particles will aggregate. To forestall this likely possibility, a second type of surfactant, designed to prevent too close contact by nonelectrostatic means, is also used in combination with an ionic surfactant. This may be a neutral, block copolymer type of molecule having hydrophobic and hydrophilic domains, for example, poloxamers. As particles bearing such surfactants approach each other, the movement of their polymeric chains becomes constrained, entailing a loss of entropy. This steric repulsion therefore is used synergistically with ionic repulsion to minimize aggregation over time.

Precipitation

Precipitation is accomplished by dissolving the drug in a suitable solvent and then mixing with a nonsolvent, effecting supersaturation with resultant precipitation. This is a two-part process: initially, solid-phase nuclei must form from molecules in solution, and subsequently crystals will grow. Conditions such as choice of solvent, temperature, order, and speed of addition are chosen to achieve different goals. To prepare drug crystals as small as possible, rapid creation of many nuclei is optimized while minimizing subsequent growth. To accomplish this, the drug solution may be added rapidly to the nonsolvent, effecting nearly immediate supersaturation and growth of many nuclei (22). Because of the preponderance of nonsolvent relative to drug solution, growth is limited. This order of addition is opposite to what is typically accomplished in pharmaceutical technology, where the goal is to achieve large, pure crystals by slower growth.

Despite attempts at optimization, it is found that precipitation alone is unable to generate suitable particles. The particle size is usually too large for injectable applications, and the distribution tends to be nonuniform. Furthermore, because of the speed of formation, such suspensions are typically not thermodynamically stable and tend to evolve over time. The metastable distribution may tend to grow in size if crystalline, or evolve to a crystalline form if formed initially in the amorphous state. If crystalline, rapidly formed precipitates also tend to have many lattice defects, and needle-like morphology.

Homogenization

Piston gap homogenization had been used for comminution of liquid-phase systems, such as emulsions and liposomes. Haynes (1) first described the use of the technique for size reduction of solid crystalline drugs in the presence of surfactant. The technique currently involves passage of a drug suspension under high pressure (5000–50,000 psi) through a variably adjusted, narrow gap. As the velocity of the fluid must increase through the stricture, the pressure drops in accordance with Bernoulli's principle. The pressure drop causes water vapor bubbles to form in the gap, but these subsequently collapse as the fluid enters a higher-pressure area. The rapid pressure collapse causes cavitations, which provides the energy to crack the particles. The greatest size reduction occurs in the first few passes of the suspension through the gap, with diminishing benefit thereafter. This may result from initial cracking of the crystals along defect planes, which become exhausted as the crystals become smaller. It is observed that increasing pressure usually decreases the ultimate particulate size. Size reduction of the suspension, as by jet milling, and prewetting of the slurry with surfactant are helpful ancillary techniques that can be used (23). The mean size of the particles attainable with this approach is typically 300 nm to 2 μm. Such suspensions may be terminally sterilized by autoclaving if the drug withstands heat. If the drug is heat-sensitive, aseptic production starting from sterile raw materials is possible.

Combined Precipitation/Homogenization

Precipitation may be combined with homogenization to overcome disadvantages associated with either technique alone. Heat-sensitive drugs may be dissolved in solvent, which is then aseptically filtered. Microprecipitation downstream of the filter will provide sterile crystals which may then be passed through a homogenizer. It is found that combining both techniques produces particles that are significantly smaller than can be attained by either technique alone. Furthermore, with precipitation alone, it often happens that the initially obtained precipitate proves to be unstable, undergoing further change. This may involve an amorphous to crystalline conversion or simply crystal growth over time. It is found, however, that subsequent homogenization arrests this growth by providing the energy necessary to overcome the activation barrier between the initially formed precipitate and the thermodynamically stable material.

IN VITRO AND IN VIVO PREDICTION OF STABILITY
AND PHARMACOKINETICS
Formulation Selection

Rational decision-making for formulation development of a poorly water-soluble compound proceeds sequentially by determining the most appropriate method for the compound. If the simpler approaches of pH adjustment, salt preparation, use of cosolvents, or use of lipids prove ineffective, then nanosuspensions may be considered. This approach is reserved for the most difficult compounds which have high crystal energy (high melting temperature) (24), in addition to high log P, as well as a requirement for high loading. For these compounds, successful formulation with nanosuspensions can be expected, provided the appropriate surfactant package is utilized, and sterilization issues can be addressed.

Molecular Determinants of Particle Size

Prior to embarking upon a specific nanosuspension program, the strategy for successful formulation can be determined by evaluation of the molecular structure with regard to Figure 1. The log of the water solubility (measured or calculated,

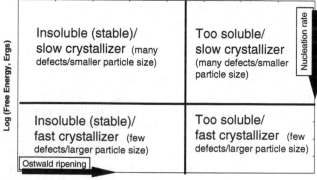

FIGURE 1   Planning formulation strategy of nanosuspensions based on molecular flexibility and solubility. Suitable candidates are insoluble and stable to growth via Ostwald ripening. Additionally, the nucleation rate is a measure of the defect number of the crystals, which determines friability and ability to form smaller particles.

with regard only to the structure, without need for melting point) is plotted along the horizontal axis. Too high a water solubility will lead to Ostwald ripening (increase of the particle size of the population). Along the vertical axis is plotted entropy, a measure of the degrees of freedom of the molecule, as an indicator of the disorder likely to be in the crystal. Crystal defects are an important consideration both where nanosuspensions are manufactured by growth, for example, crystallization, as well as by attrition, by milling, or homogenization. In the case of crystallization processes, it is the smaller, more rigid molecules, with less entropy to lose, that fit more readily, and therefore rapidly, into the growing crystal lattice (21). This could lead to a too rapid crystallization rate, resulting in particles that are excessively large. For attrition processes, on the other hand, it is known that impact force cracks crystals along their defect planes (25–28); smaller particles will result where there are many defects. The molecular gas-phase entropy, as calculated by vibrational mode analysis of the structure, is indicative of the defect rate and is plotted along the vertical axis. For molecules that are predicted to be too soluble (greater than several hundred ppm solubility), other formulation approaches may be more appropriate. If nanosuspensions must be used, then lyophilization should be considered for stability. Particular surfactant packages and more attention to processing conditions should be anticipated for molecules that crystallize quickly, to ensure successful formulation (29).

In Vitro Dissolution

It is also advantageous to be able to predict the in vivo pharmacokinetic behavior of the suspension. This can be done experimentally after the formulation has been made by injecting a bolus of the nanosuspension into a solution and plotting the resulting light transmittance. Physical persistence of particles will decrease transmittance, indicating slow solubility rate. Besides the extreme examples of compounds that do not dissolve at all, and those that dissolve virtually instantaneously, are those whose dissolution rate is dependent upon particle size or infusion rate. A plasma-simulating solvent may better approximate the in vivo case. It is found that the dissolution rate can also be calculated a priori by knowing only the surfactants used in the formulation and the structure of the molecule, by utilizing the Stokes–Einstein and Ostwald–Freundlich equations (29,30). Thus, before undertaking development, the in vivo pharmacokinetics can be estimated to determine the suitability of the approach.

Pharmacokinetic Profiles

Possible pharmacokinetic profiles of injectable drugs are shown in Figure 2. Based upon in vitro dissolution, a fast or slow-dissolving nanosuspension may be indicated. A fast dissolving formulation will yield a pharmacokinetic profile essentially identical to an a priori solution formulation (prepared with, e.g., high solvent level or extreme pH) of the drug (31,32). As a result, the tissue distribution will also be equivalent, as in the case for flurbiprofen (33). In contrast, the nanoparticles of a slow-dissolving formulation may be phagocytized first by the fixed macrophages of the liver and spleen (34). As they are subsequently dissolved within the cell, the drug will be slowly released. The resulting IV depot effect will yield a relatively low C_{max}, an apparent dip in the plasma curve within approximately 30 minutes of injection, followed by a distinct rise in the plasma concentration, peaking at around six hours for the rat, followed by a prolonged tail-off lasting over one hundred hours (Fig. 2A).

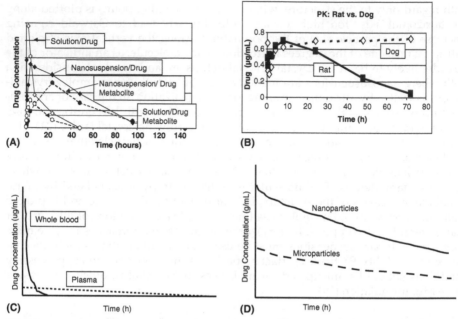

FIGURE 2 Schematic in vivo pharmacokinetic (PK) profiles of nanosuspensions. (**A**) Comparison of pharmacokinetic profiles for slow-dissolving nanosuspension versus solution formulations for both parent compound and metabolite. (**B**) Comparison of PK profile of slow-dissolving nanosuspension for rat versus dog. (**C**) Comparison of PK profile of slow-dissolving nanosuspension in plasma versus whole blood. (**D**) Comparison of plasma PK profiles of nanoparticles versus microparticles, administered subcutaneously.

The half-life is noticeably longer in the dog (Fig. 2B). Where metabolites are also tracked, it is observed that their growth is delayed, and their elimination is prolonged (Fig. 2A). In comparison with microparticulate suspensions administered subcutaneously, nanosuspensions may demonstrate a higher C_{max} and AUC (Fig. 2D). This occurs because dissolution of injected particles in a depot site often constitutes the rate-determining step for migration into the blood compartment. As particle size is reduced, surface area is increased, which increases dissolution rate. Often, appreciably higher drug concentrations appear in a whole blood assay as compared with plasma (Fig. 2C), assuming that the density of the nanosuspension is sufficiently greater than that of plasma. This may suggest red cell binding, but could also be indicative of uptake by circulating macrophages.

SAFETY OF INJECTABLE NANOSUSPENSIONS

The specification of safe levels of nanoparticulate suspensions that may be administered intravenously may be defined rationally in view of a wide database that has by now been accumulated. To place this into perspective, 40 years ago concerns were expressed about particulate matter in intravenous solutions, where extreme examples with dire consequences were exaggerated for that relatively new dosage form (35). Safety of injected particulates will be considered from two perspectives: (*i*) potential vascular occlusion as a function of the size, number, and composition of the particles and (*ii*) monocyte phagocytic system response.

In Vivo Distribution as a Function of Particle Size

Pharmacokinetics of organ distribution is dependent on particle size and rate of infusion. Nonmetabolizable particles larger than 7 μm are trapped in the pulmonary vasculature for extensive periods of time. In the lung, alveolar macrophages provide a mechanism for passing particles less than 12 μm (36) through the capillary walls permitting excretion into the sputum out of the lung. The extensive collateral circulation of the pulmonary vasculature appears to mitigate the potential blockage of capillaries by particles, with anticipated reduction of blood flow, if the particle load is kept sufficiently low (37).

However, there is evidence of capillary occlusion in the lungs of recipients of transfusion of unfiltered blood, which can contain particles of 20 to 500 μm in size. This effect was eliminated with the use of Dacron® wool depth filters of 40 to 80 μm. This suggests both an approach to deal with high particulate burdens of therapeutic nanosuspension dosage forms, as well as acceptability of particles <40 μm from such products (37).

If not dissolved initially, particles smaller than 7 μm escape from their initial lung sequestration rather quickly (38), within minutes, and undergo phagocytosis by the fixed macrophage cells of the liver and spleen (39,40). This is a normal behavior of these cells when presented with microbes and foreign material of size less than about 8 μm. In several rat studies, no evidence of an inflammatory reaction was found. Histologically, a low incidence of focal myocardial degeneration was found with 10 and 40 μm particles. Apparently safe levels of 8×10^6 particles/kg of size 0.4 to 10 μm or 4×10^5 particles/kg of particles of size 40 μm could be administered.

By way of comparison, Optison™ (Amersham Health) is an approved albumin microsphere suspension for echocardiographic imaging. Although the residence time in the body is very short because of the ultrasound-induced disruption of the particles, there is a load of smaller particles resulting from disintegration of the primary particles that must be cleared by the monocyte phagocytic system (MPS). The particle size mean diameter is 2.0 to 4.5 μm, with 93% less than 10 μm, but with a range extending upward to 32 μm. The concentration is 5×10^8 to 8×10^8 microspheres/mL, with a maximal recommended dose of 8.7 mL per contrast study (41). The maximum number of particles that can be injected for this approved product is therefore 7×10^9, or $9.9 \times 10^7 \text{ kg}^{-1}$.

Additionally, macroaggregated albumin injection is an approved product, routinely used in diagnostic imaging. The aggregated particles are formed by denaturing human albumin in a heating and aggregation process. Each vial contains four to eight million particles. By light microscopy, more than 90% of the particles are between 10 and 70 μm, whereas the typical average size is 20 to 40 μm; none is greater than 150 μm. The suggested range of particle numbers for a single injection is 200,000 to 700,000 with the recommended number being approximately 350,000 (42). By way of comparison, the USP <788> microscopic test for particulate matter in small-volume parenteral intravenous solutions permits 300 particles >25 μm. Therefore, conformance of IV drug nanosuspensions to the limits contained within the USP <788> standard will ensure significant safety factors relative to the current practice of pulmonary perfusion of radiographic particulate injections.

The above analysis addresses the high size end of the particle size distribution of a nanosuspension drug formulation. The mean value is far smaller, below 1 μm. Table 1 summarizes maximal IV levels of tolerated doses, reported in the literature.

TABLE 1 Maximal Levels of Injected Particles with Outcomes

Particle size (µm)	Protocol (particle dose/kg)	Outcome
1.3	Bolus, 6×10^9	PK study (43)
0.5–1.17	Bolus, 1.6×10^{12}	PK study (45)
0.4,4,10	Rats, bolus, 8×10^6	Well tolerated (39)
3.4	Dogs, bolus, 1×10^{10}	Well tolerated (48)
3.7	Dogs, repet. bolus, 2.4×10^8	Well tolerated (40)
3.4	Dogs, 2 min bolus, 8.9×10^7	Well tolerated (36)
2.0–4.5	Humans, bolus, 9.9×10^7	Optison, approved product (41)
0.4	Rats, bolus, 2.5×10^{12}	Well tolerated (Jerome Gass, Baxter Healthcare, personal communication)
0.4	Dogs, infusion, 1.3×10^{12}	Well tolerated (Jerome Gass, Baxter Healthcare, personal communication)

Response of the Monocyte Phagocytic System

The majority of the animal studies performed in the literature involved inert, non-metabolizable polystyrene, cross-linked styrene divinyl-benzene, or latex microspheres. A metabolizable drug nanoparticulate will be processed through the phagolysosomes of the macrophages much faster than will inert particles (51). This poses much less burden on the macrophages and enables them to cycle faster. If the reticuloendothelial system becomes overloaded by phagocytic activity, then reticuloendothelial blockage could occur (52), but only if the phagocytic overload is continued and heavy (53,54), because these cells can digest all biodegradable substances (55). Clinically, administration of liposomal doxorubicin (a cytotoxic agent and macrophage targeter) did not result in more frequent opportunistic infections in patients with AIDS-related Kaposi's sarcoma compared to patients treated with combinations of doxorubicin, bleomycin, and vincristine (56). This probably results from the compensatory increase in macrophage numbers and activity when subjected to high phagocytic loads (57).

APPLICATIONS OF PARENTERAL FORMULATIONS
Regional Anesthetics

Pursuing a local or regional anesthetic agent for post-op or chronic pain, Boedeker et al. (58) investigated the anesthetic effect of a lecithin-coated tetracaine-HI nanosuspension. It was produced by sonication, having 80% of the particle size distribution between 100 and 500 nm (by Coulter counter) and no particles >5 µm. About 0.3 cm³ of sample was infiltrated subcutaneously in rats' tails, and local anesthesia was detected with a hemostat. Animals served as their own controls by testing both proximally and distally to the injection site. Rats injected with 10% lecithin-coated tetracaine nanocrystals showed a tail block distal to the injection site lasting 43.4 ± 1.2 hours ($n = 9$), whereas those injected with 1% tetracaine solution had a mean tail block time of 8.5 ± 1.8 hours ($n = 5$). Both these groups regained a positive response to tail clamping distal to the injection site, thus ruling out nerve injury as the mechanism of local anesthesia. Those rats receiving 10% tetracaine solution either died within 10 minutes or developed wet gangrene of the tail. Negative controls of lecithin membranes without drug and 5% dextrose showed no anesthetic effect. No evidence of gross local tissue damage or systemic toxicity was observed with the nanosuspensions. Comparison of inflammation scores, based on neutrophilic accumulation, revealed no statistically significant difference in the level of tissue inflammation for the 10% nanosuspension versus 1% solution. All agents reached the noninjected control level of inflammation by 14 days (59). The nanosuspension thus provided sustained release without peaks in delivery of what would otherwise be a toxic concentration of the drug.

Because of the potential for neurotoxicity from the nanosuspension depot if placed proximal to nerves, a neurotoxicity study was conducted. Exposure of the rat sciatic nerve, followed by extra fascicular administration of the test and control articles to the fascia surrounding the nerve, and reclosure of the wound was performed. At 72 hours, the sciatic nerves were excised, fixed, stained, and scored microscopically for edema. There was no statistical difference between the 10% tetracaine nanosuspension, the 1% tetracaine solution which is used clinically, or 5% dextrose. All of the agents, however, caused statistically significant, although minimal, neural edema when compared to noninjected nerve (60).

Intradermal toxicity of a lecithin-coated suspension of dezocine, prepared similarly to that for tetracaine above, was evaluated in a rat model. It was compared with that for Dalgan®, a commercial solution formulation of the analgesic, consisting of 1.5% dezocine in a 30/70 propylene glycol/water mixture (61). Twenty rats were studied in each of the four groups, receiving 0.05 mL ID injections onto the shaved midback. Skin reactions were evaluated for 72 hours using the following criteria: discoloration 0 to 2; blanching 0 to 2; ulceration 0 to 2; eschar formation 0 to 2, with 0 being no effect and 2 the most severe. A cytotoxic index was calculated by multiplying the total score above by the area of injury. The index for 250 µg microcrystal dezocine at 6.0 ± 0.7 was significantly ($p < 0.01$) less than that for 250 µg Dalgan injection, which had an index of 24.2 ± 1.4. Negative control groups of lecithin membranes and 10% dextrose had still lower cytotoxicity indexes at 1.8 ± 0.3 and 0.6 ± 0.2, respectively. Despite having less cytotoxicity, the microcrystal dezocine formulation resulted in a significantly ($p < 0.01$) extended plateau of analgesia of 334 ± 16.9 minutes versus 48 ± 7.5 minutes for Dalgan. Thus, the intensity and duration of analgesia were prolonged while rendering the drug more tissue-compatible.

Intravenous
Malignant Hyperthermia

Phospholipid-coated nanosuspensions of dantrolene and sodium dantrolene were studied for treatment of malignant hyperthermia (62). The currently available dosage form, Dantrium® Intravenous, is a lyophilized formulation which must be reconstituted slowly to produce a 0.33 mg/mL solution, thus requiring a large administration volume of about 600 mL, at an alkaline pH of 9.5, as well as including mannitol (63). The administration-related issues are particularly onerous in the setting of an intraoperative emergency maneuver. To increase loading of this poorly water-soluble drug in a readily reconstituted format, either dantrolene or its sodium salt was coated with egg phospholipid prepared by homogenization using a microfluidizer. Following lyophilization, rapid reconstitutability within one minute to produce 10% to 15% suspensions was enabled for both the dantrolene nanosuspension (NS-D) and the sodium dantrolene nanosuspension (NS-NaD). Particle sizes of 300 to 800 nm for NS-NaD and 500 to 800 nm for NS-D were measured.

Dissolution of both nanosuspensions was rapid. A formal comparison for NS-NaD yielded pharmacokinetics equivalent to that for the solution formulation of the drug. A strain-gauge transducer of forelimb adduction measured the dose–response curves. These were also comparable, and are summarized as the effective dose necessary to produce 50% and 95% of the plateau response, as well as the magnitude of the plateau response. Similar values were also found in normal swine. Although the NS-D formulation gave a slightly higher ED_{50} twitch depression than Dantrium in malignant hyperthermia-susceptible swine (1.0 ± 0.2 vs. 0.6 ± 0.1 mg/kg), the more important ED_{95} was statistically equivalent (3.5 ± 0.4 vs. 2.7 ± 0.5). ED_{95} is more significant because the drug is dosed to near-plateau effect. The nanosuspensions successfully treated or prevented malignant hyperthermia in swine models.

With NS-NaD, 2.5 mg/kg IV bolus in swine was observed to cause pulmonary artery (PAP) hypertension as well as systemic hypotension. This was similar to the response seen with the injection of undissolved dantrolene powder. The systemic hypotension was eliminated with addition of a 6 μm filter, and the PAP increase was significantly reduced but not eliminated. NS-D, on the other hand, produced only minimal PAP increase when injected at the same rate with a 2 μm filter. It was suspected that postinfusion aggregation of particles was responsible for these effects, 19% of the NS-NaD being observed in aggregates of greater than 3 μm diameter, following 200× dilution. In contrast, no aggregation was seen for NS-D following dilution.

Earlier, it had been demonstrated that agglomeration of injected particles could sometimes be seen after fast (1 mL/5 sec) but not after slow (1 mL/min) injection of nanoparticles, essentially leading to plug flow (64,65). Additional explanation was provided by Ward and Yalkowski (66) who found that plug flow occurred where the injection rate matched the blood flow rate. If one injected either slower or faster than this rate, faster dissipation of the bolus would occur. The safer strategy is slower infusion (66). In dogs, rapid IV bolus up to 10 mg/kg of unfiltered NS-D could be administered with no PAP change, suggesting that swine may be a more sensitive model than the dog.

Antifungal
Preclinical Studies with Drug-Susceptible Fungal Strain
When formulated as a nanosuspension, the antifungal agent itraconazole could be IV dosed to the rat with no mortality at nearly 10 times the LD_{50} of the commercially available hydroxypropyl-β-cyclodextrin-solubilized drug, Sporanox® (Janssen Pharmaceutical Products, L.P.). This may occur because of reduced C_{max}, and therefore reduced C_{max}-induced toxicity, inasmuch as the slowly dissolving itraconazole particles are initially sequestered by the MPS. Subsequently, the drug is released over prolonged therapeutic, yet apparently, subtoxic levels. This safety profile permitted a much greater dose to be administered to rats and dogs. In *Candida albicans*-challenged immuno-suppressed rat models, the greater dose resulted in higher drug levels at the site of infection in the kidney which significantly reduced colony counts in that organ. In fact, colony counts of zero were found with sufficiently high doses of the nanosuspension. Treatment with Sporanox® resulted in a decrease in the colony-forming units, but they did not decline to zero. These results are consistent with the work of Andes (67), who found that for drugs of the azole class, the AUC/MIC ratio is the critical pharmacokinetic/pharmacodynamic parameter associated with treatment efficacy. Here, AUC is the area under the drug plasma curve and MIC is the minimum inhibitory concentration. Efficacy of azoles is independent of peak concentration.

Preclinical Studies with Drug-Resistant Fungal Strain
Animal results suggest that higher dosing, achievable with nanosuspensions, may cause a reconsideration of the in vitro–in vivo correlation of antifungal susceptibility

testing. Current guidelines for interpretive breakpoints of MIC for mucosal *Candida* infections are: susceptible ≤0.125 µg/mL; susceptible, dependent upon dose (S-DD): 0.25 to 0.5 µg/mL; and resistant ≥1.0 µg/mL (68). That is to say, the fungal infection should be clinically treatable if the results of the susceptibility testing indicate an MIC ≤ 0.125 µg/mL; and itraconazole should not be clinically effective if the MIC ≥ 1.0 µg/mL. Between 0.25 and 0.5 µg/mL, the organism may be considered susceptible, dependent upon dose (S-DD). It is clear, however, that these guidelines were formulated with assumptions made about the dose of itraconazole that can be administered, dependent upon current approved drug labeling. If greater dosing becomes clinically achievable through nanosuspensions, then the interpretive breakpoints of MIC, corresponding to what is considered treatable, may be revised upward.

Preliminary animal results suggest that efficacy toward fungal strains, conventionally considered resistant to itraconazole, can be demonstrated for itraconazole nanosuspensions. Thus, a prednisolone immuno-compromised rat model was challenged with a *Candida* strain considered resistant to itraconazole by the above guidelines (MIC = 16 µg/mL). Survival of the majority of the nanosuspension-treated animals was observed by the end of the 10-day experiment, whereas all of the Sporanox®-treated animals had died (69).

Clinical Study

The pharmacokinetics of itraconazole nanosuspension has been studied clinically in allergenic hematopoietic stem cell transplant recipients over a 14-day intravenous course of treatment (70). On days five and six prior to the transplant, 200 mg of nanosuspension was given IV every 12 hours followed by 200 mg every 24 hours for the next 12 days. Steady state was not reached, and the therapeutic level of 500 µg/L was maintained in five of the six cases for at least nine days after treatment cessation. The pharmacokinetic parameters found are compared in Table 2 with those of the commercial Sporanox® solution, as listed in the Physicians' Desk Reference (71) and other literature.

It is seen that in comparison with the solution formulation Sporanox®, the nanocrystal suspension occupied a larger volume of distribution and was cleared more slowly to give a longer half-life and larger area under the plasma concentration curve for the first 24 hours, AUC_{24}. This pharmacokinetic behavior is consistent with sequestration in the MPS depot, causing reduced clearance and increased volume of distribution. Subsequent release results in greatly prolonged delivery for the nanosuspension, as shown by half-life and more efficient utilization of the drug, as manifested by higher AUC.

The clinical results confirmed the animal data and suggest that the daily dosing established for Sporanox® may be reduced to a frequency commensurate with the prolonged half-life of the nanosuspension. The maintenance of therapeutic

TABLE 2 Comparison of Clinical Pharmacokinetics Between Itraconazole Nanosuspension and Sporanox®

	Itraconazole nanosuspension	Sporanox
V_{ss} (L)	1677 ± 827	796 ± 185
Cl (L/hr)	3.35 ± 1.8	22.9 ± 5.7
$t_{1/2}$ (hr)	346 ± 225 terminal	35.4 ± 29.4 mean and 30 terminal (72)
AUC_{24} (µg hr/L)	51558 ± 10635	30605 ± 8961

levels for nine days following termination of treatment is especially interesting, and suggests utility when patients migrate from intravenous to oral dosing, following hospital discharge, for example. Having a reliable internal depot of drug would be useful during the transition process to ensure continuity of delivered dose. Further clinical studies would be needed to confirm this point.

Anticancer: Paclitaxel
Characterization and Manufacture
Abraxane™ for Injectable Suspension is an approved, commercialized nanosuspension formulation. As shown by transmission electron microscopy, it consists of a core of paclitaxel, surrounded by an albumin shell with an overall mean size of 130 nm, spanning a range of about 100 to 200 nm (73). It is manufactured by adding a methylene chloride solution of paclitaxel to an aqueous solution of human serum albumin, using low-speed homogenization. The albumin migrates to the aqueous–solvent interface of the emulsion that is created. Application of high-pressure homogenization reduces the particle size and cross-links the albumin coating via the disulfide bonds, thus stabilizing the particle. The methylene chloride is then volatilized, leaving an aqueous suspension of nanoparticles. The particles consist of an amorphous paclitaxel core coated by a 25-nm thick shell of albumin with bound paclitaxel. The particle size is sufficiently small so as to be sterile-filtered (18). Importantly, Abraxane is formulated without Cremophor EL, which has been associated with a host of problems including sensitivity reactions, the need to infuse over prolonged periods of time, leaching of plasticizer from infusion sets, and so on.

Pharmacokinetics
Clinical pharmacokinetic studies for Abraxane have defined parameters relative to Taxol® summarized in Table 3 (74,75). The shorter 30-minute duration of infusion of Abraxane understandably results in higher plasma C_{max} than that for Taxol® administered with a three-hour infusion. The near-equivalence of half-lives, although not observed earlier for mice, reflects a similar terminal elimination rate of drug from the tissue compartment. Ibrahim et al. have attributed the reduced AUC of the nanosuspension to possibly several factors. The first is faster partitioning of the nanosuspension paclitaxel out of the vascular compartment, in comparison with Taxol®. It is known that Cremophor micelles reduce the free paclitaxel plasma fraction available for cellular partitioning, thus reducing tissue distribution from the central blood compartment. Not being formulated with Cremophor, Abraxane might be expected to exit the circulation faster. The second reason involves increased endothelial transcytosis via albumin-mediated gp60 receptor uptake of the particles (76).

Clinical Trial
Abraxane and Taxol® were studied head to head in a Phase III trial involving 460 breast cancer patients. Taxol® was administered using the standard protocol of

TABLE 3 Comparison of Clinical Pharmacokinetics Between Abraxane Paclitaxel Nanosuspension and Taxol®

Drug/dose	C_{max} (ng/mL)	$AUC_{(0-\infty)}$ (ng hr/mL)	$t_{\frac{1}{2}}$ (hr)	Cl (L/hr/m^2)
Abraxane (135 mg/m^2/ 30 min)	6100	6427	15	21
Taxol (135 mg/m^2/3 hr)	2170	7952	13	18

175 mg/m^2 by 3-hour infusion, including premedication with steroid and antihistamines to inhibit Cremophor-related hypersensitivity. In contrast, Abraxane was given at 260 mg/m^2 over a shorter duration 30 minutes, without premedication or G-CSF support. Despite the more aggressive protocol for Abraxane, the toxicity was no worse: there were no hypersensitivity reactions; neutropenia decreased; whereas neuropathy increased somewhat. This is significant given the correlation established between the duration of plasma paclitaxel concentrations exceeding 0.1 µmol/L with decline of absolute white blood cell count (74,75,77). In this trial, Abraxane also produced a higher tumor response rate versus paclitaxel (33% vs. 19%) and a longer time to tumor progression (21.9 wk vs. 16.1 wk) (78).

The improved efficacy of the nanosuspension may be surprising in view of the purported benefit of Cremophor EL in inhibiting the P-glycoprotein efflux pump, thereby enhancing drug level in tumor cells (79). The alleged benefit of this is probably overrated, inasmuch as Cremophor is retained in the central blood compartment, and therefore does not enter the tumor tissue (80). There are ancillary benefits to not formulating with Cremophor. As corticosteroids do not have to be taken as premedication, there is the possibility for combining paclitaxel with IL-2 or interferon for treatment of metastatic melanoma, renal cell carcinoma, and so on. The current Cremophor-containing formulation cannot be used because steroids, used for premedication, lyse lymphokine activated killer (LAK) cells, thus mitigating the benefits of the cytokines (18).

Intrathecal Delivery

Regional delivery of water-insoluble drugs offers the possibility of increasing local therapeutic concentrations while decreasing systemic side effects. In early work, epidural injection of a 10% butamben suspension intended for chronic cancer pain was well tolerated in dogs and humans (44,81). As a treatment modality for intractable brain tumors, the technique of direct injection into the ventricles of the brain is known as convective enhanced delivery. In addition to simply placing the drug within the central nervous system, this pressure gradient microinfusion of drug overcomes diffusion barriers associated with high intratumoral interstitial pressures and disordered tumor vasculature. As a result, drug is more rapidly distributed throughout the target volume (46). As an example of this application, intrathecal delivery of nanosuspension busulfan to a mouse model of neoplastic meningitis led to a significant increase in survival (47,49). The pharmacokinetics was determined in patients afflicted with neoplastic meningitis, who received the drug both by an Ommaya reservoir for intraventricular delivery and via lumbar puncture. The drug was well tolerated and resulted in delayed progression of disease (50).

CONCLUSIONS

Growth in the applications of nanosuspension technology has occurred in response to the voluminous number of water-insoluble drug candidates that have emerged from discovery programs. The inherent high loading of this dosage form distinguishes it from liposomes, emulsions, cyclodextrins, and polymeric nanoparticles, permitting dosing in animal toxicity studies at the required multiples of anticipated human exposure. Parenteral applications for subcutaneous, intramuscular, intradermal, intravenous, epidural, and intrathecal delivery have been studied in animals, with enhanced efficacy. At the same time, the safety profile has been observed to be improved in many cases when compared to conventional solution forms of the drugs. This occurs due to deletion of noxious excipients, change in the pharmacokinetic profile, or regional delivery, thus minimizing systemic toxicity. These therapeutic and safety benefits have been demonstrated for several drugs for different disease indications in clinical trials. On the basis of the successful clinical applications, it is anticipated that growth of this formulation tool will accelerate.

REFERENCES

1. Haynes DH. Phospholipid-coated microcrystals: injectable formulations of water-insoluble drugs. US Patent No. 5,091,188, 1992.
2. Lipinski CA, Lombardo F, Dominy BW, Feeney PJ. Experimental and computational approaches to estimate solubility and permeability in drug discovery and development settings. Adv Drug Deliv Rev 1997; 23:3.
3. Weiner M, Bernstein IL. Adverse Reactions to Drug Formulation Agents. New York: Marcel Dekker, 1989.
4. Gad SC. Vehicles and excipients. In: Gad SC, ed. Drug Safety Evaluation. New York: Wiley, 2002 (chapter 13.8).
5. Pandolfe WD. Development of the new Gaulin Micro-Gap™ homogenizing valve. J Dairy Sci 1982; 65:2035.
6. Merisko-Liversidge E, Liversidge GG, Cooper E. Nanosizing: a formulation approach for poorly-water-soluble compounds. Eur J Pharm Sci 2003; 18:113.
7. Myerson AS, Ginde R. Crystals, crystal growth, and nucleation. In: Myerson AS, ed. Handbook of Industrial Crystallization. Boston: Butterworth-Heinemann, 1992.
8. Knutson BL, Debenedetti PG, Tom JW. Preparation of microparticulates using supercritical fluids. In: Cohen S, Bernstein H, eds. Microparticulate Systems for the Delivery of Proteins and Vaccines. New York: Marcel Dekker, 1996:89–126.
9. Holmberg K, Jonsson B, Kronberg B, Lindman B, eds. Surfactants and Polymers in Aqueous Solution. 2nd ed. Sussex: Wiley, 2003.
10. Stolnik S, Illum L, Davis SS. Long circulating microparticulate drug carriers. Adv Drug Del Rev 1995; 16:195.
11. Peters K, Leitzke S, Diederichs JE. Preparation of a clofazimine nanosuspension for intravenous use and evaluation of its therapeutic efficacy in murine *Mycobacterium avium* infection. J Antimicrob Chemother 2000; 45:77.
12. Illig KJ, Wolf GL, Bacon ER, et al. A nonsurfactant wetting agent for the preparation of very small nanoparticle suspensions of an iodinated contrast agent. Pharm Tech 1999; 92–104.
13. Haynes D. Microdroplets of water-insoluble drugs and injectable formulations of containing same. US Patent No. 4,725,442, 1988.
14. Vergote GJ, Vervate C, Van Driessche I, et al. An oral controlled release matrix pellet formulation containing nanocrystalline ketoprofen. Int J Pharm 2001; 219:81.
15. Solis R, Belaredj S, Rogue V, et al. Encapsulation of nanosuspensions into Depofoam® particles. Abstract # 5141. In: 28th International Symposium on Controlled Release of Bioactive Materials, San Diego, CA, June 23–27, 2001.
16. Chattopadhyay P, Gupta RB. Production of antibiotic nanoparticles using supercritical CO_2 as antisolvent with enhanced mass transfer. Ind Eng Chem Res 2001; 40:3530.
17. Pace GW, Vachon MG, Mishra AK, et al. Process to generate submicron particles of water-insoluble compounds. US Patent No. 6,177,103, 2001.
18. Desai NP, Tao C, Yang A, et al. Protein stabilized pharmacologically active agents, methods for the preparation thereof and methods for the use thereof. US Patent No. 6,749,868, 2004.
19. Kipp JE, Wong JCT, Doty MJ, Rebbeck CL. Microprecipitation method for preparing submicron suspensions. US Patent No. 6,607,784 B2, 2003.
20. Kipp JE. Pharmaceutical nanotechnology review: the role of solid nanoparticle technology in the parenteral delivery of poorly water-soluble drugs. Int J Pharm 2004; 284:109 (chapters 16 and 17).

21. Moore WJ. Physical Chemistry. 3rd ed. Englewood Cliffs, NJ: Prentice-Hall, 1962.
22. Estrin J. Precipitation processes. In: Myerson AS, ed. Handbook of Industrial Crystallization. Boston: Butterworths/Heinemann, 1993:131–149.
23. Muller RH, Benita S, Bohm B, eds. Emulsions and Nanosuspensions for the Formulation of Poorly Soluble Drugs. Stuttgart: Medpharm Scientific Publishers, 1997.
24. Yalkowsky SH. Techniques of Solubilization of Drugs. New York: Marcel Dekker, 1981:1–14.
25. Huttenrauch R. Fundamentals of pharmaceutics. Acta Pharm Technol 1988; 34:1.
26. Grant D, York P. Entropy of processing: a new quantity for comparing the solid state disorder of pharmaceutical materials. Int J Pharm 1986; 30:161.
27. Duddu SP, Grant D. The use of thermal analysis in the assessment of crystal disruption. Thermochim Acta 1995; 248:131.
28. Griffith AA. Phil Trans Roy Soc London, Ser A 1921; 221:163.
29. Kipp J. Baxter Healthcare Corp., unpublished data, 2004.
30. Lee RW, Shaw JM, McShane J, Wood RW. Particle size reduction. In: Liu R, ed. Water-Insoluble Drug Formulation. Denver: Interpharm 2000:455–492.
31. Viernstein H, Stumpf C. Similar central actions of intravenous methohexitone suspension and solution in the rabbit. J Pharm Pharmacol 1992; 44:66.
32. Clement MA, Pugh W, Parikh I. Tissue distribution and plasma clearance of a novel microcrystal-encapsulated flurbiprofen formulation. Pharmacologist 1992; 34:204.
33. Pace SN, Pace GW, Parikh I, Mishra AK. Novel injectable formulations of insoluble drugs. Pharm Tech 1999 March; 116.
34. Moghimi SM, Hunter AC, Murray JC. Long-circulating and target-specific nanoparticles: theory to practice. Pharmacol Rev 2001; 53:283.
35. Garvan JM, Gunner BW. The harmful effects of particles in intravenous fluids. Med J Aust 1964; 2:1.
36. Kanke M, Simmons GH, Weiss DI, et al. Clearance of ^{41}Ce labelled microspheres from blood and distribution in specific organs following intravenous and intraarterial administration in beagle dogs. J Pharm Sci 1973; 6:508.
37. Barber TA. Patient issues related to particulate matter. In: Barber TA, ed. Pharmaceutical Particulate Matter, Analysis and Control. Buffalo Grove, IL: Interpharm Press, 1993 (chapter XII).
38. Singer JM. J Res Soc 1969; 6:561.
39. Gesler RM, Garvin PJ, Klamer B, et al. The biological effects of polystyrene latex particles administered intravenously to rats—a collaborative study. Bull Parent Drug Assoc 1973; 27:101.
40. Schroeder HG. Distribution of radiolabeled subvisible microspheres after intravenous administration to beagle dogs. J Pharm Sci 1978; 67:508.
41. Optison Product Description, Amersham Health.
42. DraxImage MAA Kit for the preparation of Technetium Tc 99m Albumin Aggregated Injection. Product insert, February 2002.
43. Wilkins DJ, Meyers PA. Br J Exp Pathol 1966; 47:568.
44. Shulman M. Treatment of cancer pain with epidural butyl-amino benzoate suspension. Reg Anesth 1987; 12:1.
45. Schoenberg MD, Gilman PA, Mumaw VR, Moore RD. The phagocytosis of uniform polystyrene latex particles (PLP) by the reticuloendothelial system (RES) in the rabbit. Brit J Exptl Path 1961; 42:486.
46. Hall WA, Rustamzadeh E, Asher AL. Convection-enhanced delivery in clinical trials. Neurosurg Focus 2003; 14:1.
47. Grossman SA, Krabak MJ. Leptomeningeal carcinomatosis. Cancer Treatment Rev 1999; 25:103.
48. Slack JD. Acute hemodynamic effects and blood pool kinetics of polystyrene microspheres following intravenous administration. J Pharm Sci 1981; 70:660.
49. Archer GE et al. Intrathecal busulfan treatment of human neoplastic meningitis in athymic nude rats. J Neuro-Oncol 1999; 44:233.
50. Quinn JA, Glantz M, Petros W, et al. Phase I trial of intrathecal Spartaject busulfan for patients with neoplastic meningitis. Abstract No. 318. In: Eighth ASCO Annual Meeting, Orlando, FL, May 18–21, 2002.

51. Kreuter J. Nanoparticles. In: Kreuter J, ed. Colloidal Drug Delivery Systems. New York: Marcel Dekker, 1994 : 219–342, ch. 5.
52. Daemen T, Hofstede G, Ten Kate MT, et al. Liposomal doxorubicin-induced toxicity: depletion and impairment of phagocytic activity of liver macrophages. Int J Cancer 1995; 61:716.
53. VanEtten EWM. Administration of liposomal agents and blood clearance capacity of the mononuclear phagocyte system. Antimicrob Agents Chemother 1998; 42:1677.
54. Bakker-Woudenberg IAJM. Administration of liposomal agents and the phagocytic function of the mononuclear phagocytic system. Int J Pharm 1998; 162:5.
55. Pesko LJ. Physiological consequences of injected particulates. In: Knapp JZ, Barber TA, Lieberman A, eds. Liquid- and Surface-Borne Particle Measurement Handbook. New York: Marcel Dekker, 1996.
56. Bogner JR. Liposomal doxorubicin in the treatment of advanced AIDS-related Kaposi sarcoma. J Acquir Immune Defic Syndr 1994; 7:463.
57. Daemen T, Regts J, Meesters M, et al. Toxicity of doxorubicin entrapped within long-circulating liposomes. J Control Release 1997; 44:1.
58. Boedeker BH, Lojeski EW, Kline MD, et al. Ultra-long duration local anesthesia produced by injection of lecithin-coated tetracaine microcrystals. J Clin Pharmacol 1994; 34:699.
59. Kline MD, Boedeker BH, Mattix ME, et al. Intradermal toxicity of lecithin-coated microcrystalline tetracaine. Anesthesiology 1992; 77:A800.
60. Boedeker BH, Kline MD, Mattix ME, et al. Peripheral neurotoxicity of lecithin-coated tetracaine microcrystals. Anesthesiology 1993; 79:A825.
61. DeMeo R, Haynes D, Bikhazi G. Comparing efficacy and intradermal toxicity of lecithin-coated microcrystal dezocine. Anesthesiology 1993; 79:A865.
62. Karan SM, Lojeski EW, Haynes DH, et al. Intravenous lecithin-coated microcrystals of dantrolene are effective in the treatment of malignant hyperthermia: an investigation in rats, dogs, and swine. Anesth Analg 1996; 82:796.
63. Lojeski EW, Karan SM, Boedeker BH, et al. Lecithin-coated dantrolene sodium microcrystals vs. dantrolene sodium: dose–response to muscular twitch in swine. Anesthesiology 1993; 79:A438.
64. Kreuter J, Tauber U, Illi V. Distribution and elimination of poly(methyl-2-C^{14}-methacrylate) nanoparticle radioactivity after injection in rats and mice. J Pharm Sci 1979; 68:1443.
65. Borchard G, Kreuter J. The role of serum complement on the organ distribution of intravenously administered poly(methyl methacrylate) nanoparticles: effects of pre-coating with plasma and with serum complement. Pharm Res 1996; 13:1055.
66. Ward G, Yalkowsky S. Studies in phlebitis. J Parenter Sci Technol 1993; 47:161.
67. Andes D. In vivo pharmacodynamics of antifungal drugs in treatment of candidiasis. Antimicrob Agents Chemother 2003; 47:1179.
68. Rex JH, Pfaller MA, Galgiani JN, et al. Development of interpretive breakpoints for antifungal susceptibility testing: conceptual framework and analysis of in vitro–in vivo correlation data for fluconazole, itraconazole, and *Candida infections*. Clin Infect Dis 1997; 24:235.
69. Rabinow BE, White RD, Glosson J, et al. Enhanced efficacy of NANOEDGE itraconazole nanosuspension in an immunosuppressed rat model infected with an itraconazole-resistant *C. albicans* strain. Abstract #R6184. In: Amer. Assn. of Pharm. Sci. Ann. Meeting, Salt Lake City, Utah, October 26–30, 2003.
70. Donnelly JP, Mouton JW, Blijlevens NMA, et al. Pharmacokinetics of a 14 day course of itraconazole nanocrystals given intravenously to allogeneic haematopoietic stem cell transplant (HCST) recipients. Abstract #A-32. In: 41st Interscience Conference on Antimicrobial Agents and Chemotherapy, Chicago, IL, December 16–19, 2001.
71. SPORANOX® (Itraconazole) Injection. Approved labeling. In: PDR 58 ed Physicians' Desk Reference®. Montvale, NJ: Thomson PDR, 2004:1772.
72. Willems L, van der Geest R, de Beule K. Itraconazole oral solution and intravenous formulations: a review of pharmacokinetics and pharmacodynamics. J Clin Pharm Therap 2001; 26:159.
73. Blum JL, Beveridge R, Robert N, et al. ABI-007 Nanoparticle paclitaxel: demonstration of anti-tumor activity in taxane-refractory metastatic breast cancer. Abstract 64. Proc Am Soc Clin Oncol 2003.

74. Ibrahim NK, Desai N, Legha S, et al. Phase I and pharmacokinetic study of ABI-007, a cremophor-free, protein-stabilized, nanoparticle formulation of paclitaxel. Clin Cancer Res 2002; 8:1038.
75. Taxol® (paclitaxel) Injection. Direction insert. Princeton, NJ: Bristol-Myers Squibb Oncology 2003.
76. Desai N, Trieu V, Yao R, et al. Increased endothelial transcytosis of nanoparticle albumin-bound paclitaxel (ABI-007) by endothelial gp60 receptors: a pathway inhibited by Taxol. Poster AO 066. In: 27th San Antonio Breast Cancer Symposium, San Antonio, TX, December 2004.
77. Huizing MT, Keung ACF, Rosing H, et al. Pharmacokinetics of paclitaxel and metabolites in a randomized comparative study in platinum-pretreated ovarian cancer patients. J Clin Oncol 1993; 11:2127.
78. Lee D. Current trials of a nanoparticle albumin-bound taxane formulation in metastatic breast cancer. Clin Breast Cancer 2004 Feb; 391.
79. Woodcock DM, Jefferson S, Linsenmeyer ME, et al. Reversal of the multidrug resistance phenotype with cremophor EL, a common vehicle for water-insoluble vitamins and drugs. Cancer Res 1990; 50:4199.
80. Sparreboom A, Verweij J, Van der Burg MEL, et al. Disposition of Cremophor EL in humans limits the potential for modulation of the multidrug resistance phenotype in vivo. Clin Cancer Res 1998; 4:1937.
81. Shulman M. Effect of epidural and subarachnoid injections of a 10% butamben suspension. Reg Anesth 1990; 15:142.

3 Nanoparticles Prepared Using Natural and Synthetic Polymers

Sudhir S. Chakravarthi and Dennis H. Robinson
Department of Pharmaceutical Sciences, University of Nebraska Medical Center, Omaha, Nebraska, U.S.A.

Sinjan De
Research and Development, Perrigo Company, Allegan, Michigan, U.S.A.

INTRODUCTION

Ideally, biologically active agents should be encapsulated within nanoparticles using polymers with well-defined physical and chemical properties. These polymers protect the active ingredient and, after local or systemic administration, potentially target and then release the drug in a controlled, predictable manner. The use of polymeric nanoparticle for drug delivery is a strategy that aims to optimize therapeutic effects while minimizing adverse effects. The purpose of this chapter is to highlight the major factors related to the use of nanoparticles fabricated from synthetic or natural polymeric materials that have been used in drug delivery and imaging. A comprehensive review of this area of research is beyond the scope of this chapter and hence the readers are referred to other reviews in the areas for additional information (1–3).

POLYMERIC CARRIERS USED TO PREPARE NANOPARTICLES

Polymers used in controlled drug delivery, including nanoparticles, may be classified as either (*i*) natural and synthetic, or (*ii*) biodegradable and nonbiodegradable. Examples of naturally occurring biodegradable and biocompatible polymers used to prepare nanoparticles include: cellulose, gelatin, pullulan, chitosan, alginate, and gliadin. The characteristics and performance, particularly in vivo, of nanoparticles prepared using natural polymers may be less predictable as these polymers may vary widely in chemical composition and hence, physical properties. In addition, natural polymers are often mildly immunogenic. Conversely, it is possible to synthesize polymers with precise chemical composition, resulting in highly predictable physical properties such as solubility, permeability, and rates of biodegradation. As a result, synthetic polymers are also more easily designed for specific applications, such as controlled rates of dissolution, permeability, degradation, and erosion, as well as for targeting. Examples of synthetic biodegradable polymers used to prepare nanoparticles include: polylactide (PLA), poly-(lactide-co-glycolide) (PLGA), polyanhydrides, poly-ε-caprolactone, and polyphosphazene. Biodegradability and biocompatibility are important properties of polymeric materials that are to be injected or implanted into the body. Nonbiodegradable polymeric nanoparticles may be used for controlled drug delivery and also in the complimentary field of diagnostic imaging. Examples of nonbiodegradable, synthetic polymers used in drug delivery include polymethyl methacrylate while polystyrene particles have been used as diagnostic agents.

Natural Biodegradable Polymers Used to Prepare Nanoparticles
Alginates
Alginates are linear, unbranched polysaccharides composed of random chains of guluronic and mannuronic acids (4). In aqueous media, the sodium ions from salts of these anionic, heteropolymers exchange with divalent cations, such as calcium, to form water-insoluble gels (5). Because of the favorable conditions during manufacture, alginates are ideal carriers for oligonucleotides (6), peptides (7), proteins (7), water-soluble drugs, or drugs that degrade in organic solvents. Alginates are non-immunogenic and available in a wide range of molecular weights as characterized by their inherent viscosity. Alginate nanoparticles are prepared by extruding an aqueous sodium alginate solution through a narrow-bore needle into an aqueous solution of a cationic agent, such as calcium ions, chitosan, or poly-L-lysine. These cations cross-link the guluronic and mannuronic acids to form an egg-box structure that forms the core of the gel matrix. In vivo, therapeutic agents are released when the matrix redissolves due to the reversible exchange of divalent cations with monovalent ions, especially sodium present in physiological fluid. A disadvantage of the use of alginates is that this reversible ion exchange may result in the rapid release of the therapeutic agent. However, an example of the use of alginate nanoparticles to sustain antibacterial drug levels above the minimum inhibitory concentration in the liver, lungs, and spleen after pulmonary administration was demonstrated using isoniazid, rifampicin, and pyrazinamide (8). One method to prolong release from alginate particles is to coat them with a cationic polymer, for example, poly-L-lysine or chitosan. In this application, the mass ratio of alginate to cationic polymer is critical in terms of release characteristics and particle size (9).

Chitosan
Chitosan is a natural polymer obtained by deacetylation of chitin, a component of crab shells. It is a cationic polysaccharide composed of linear $\beta(1,4)$-linked D-glucosamine. The various methods used to prepare chitosan-based nanoparticles and their applications have been extensively reviewed (10). Chitosan can entrap drugs by numerous mechanisms including chemical cross-linking, ionic cross-linking, and ionic complexation (11).

Gelatin
Gelatin is a natural, biodegradable protein obtained by acid- or base-catalyzed hydrolysis of collagen. It is a heterogenous mixture of single- or multi-stranded polypeptides composed predominantly of glycine, proline, and hydroxyproline residues and is degraded in vivo to amino acids. Gelatin nanoparticles are prepared by a two-step, desolvation process (12). Briefly, this coacervation procedure involves the addition of either another more water-soluble polymer or, a water-miscible nonsolvent for gelatin, to an aqueous gelatin solution above its gel temperature of about 40°C. The concentrated gelatin liquid particles are isolated and hardened by chemical cross-linking with glutaraldehyde. Alternately, these particles can be prepared using a simple o/w emulsion or w/o/w microemulsion method. Gelatin nanoparticles have been used to deliver paclitaxel, methotrexate, doxorubicin, DNA, double-stranded oligonucleotides, and genes. PEGylation of the particles significantly enhances their circulation time in the blood stream (13) and increases their uptake into cells by endocytosis. Antibody-modified gelatin nanoparticles have been used for targeted uptake by lymphocytes (14).

Pullulan
Similar to dextran and cellulose, the glucans in pullulan are water-soluble, linear polysaccharides that consist of three α-1,4-linked glucose molecules polymerized by α-1,6 linkages on the terminal glucose (15). Pullulan is a fermentation product of the yeast *Aureobasidium pullulans*. When made hydrophobic by acetylation, these polymers will self-associate to form nanoparticles with a hydrophobic core that will encapsulate hydrophobic drugs. Pullulan nanoparticles have been prepared by dialysis of an organic solution against water. In one method, a reverse micellar solution of the anionic surfactant, Aerosol OT, in *n*-hexane was prepared and an aqueous solution of the drug and pullulan added (16). The nanoparticles are stabilized by cross-linking with glutaraldehyde. These delivery systems have been used in delivering cytotoxic drugs, genes, and as pH-sensitive delivery systems.

Gliadin
Gliadin is a glycoprotein that, as a component of gluten, is extracted from gluten-rich food such as wheat flour. They are slightly hydrophobic and polar. Bioactive molecules of variable polarity can be encapsulated into gliadin nanoparticles. Gliadin nanoparticles can be prepared by a desolvation method that exploits the insolubility of this polymer in water (17). Briefly, gliadin nanoparticles are precipitated when an ethanolic solution of gliadin is poured into an aqueous solution. Gliadin nanoparticles have been used to deliver *trans*-retinoic acid, α-tocopherol, and vitamin E. Lectins have been conjugated to the surface of gliadin nanoparticles to target the colon and treat *Helicobacter pylori* infections (17).

Synthetic Biodegradable Polymers Used to Prepare Nanoparticles
Polylactide and Polylactide-co-Glycolide
The hydrophobic PLA may be used alone or copolymerized with poly-glycolic acid to form a range of PLGA of widely varying polymeric ratios and hence physico-chemical properties. These FDA-approved polymers have been widely used in drug delivery including nanoparticles. PLA and PLGA polymers degrade by random bulk hydrolysis that is catalyzed in acidic media. The methods used to prepare PLA and PLGA nanoparticles as well as their range of applications, physical properties, biological fate, and targetability have been comprehensively reviewed (2).

Polyanhydrides
Polyanhydrides are biodegradable polymers with a hydrophobic backbone and a hydrolytically labile anhydride linkage. They are synthesized by ring-opening polymerization and degrade by surface hydrolysis (3). The application of polyanhydrides has been limited to film and microsphere formulation for sustained release of a drug or protein at the site.

Poly-ε-Caprolactones
Methods used to prepare nanoparticles using poly-ε-caprolatones have been previously reviewed (18) and include emulsion polymerization, solvent displacement, dialysis, and interfacial polymer deposition. These semicrystalline polymers are chemically stable, possess a low glass transition temperature, and degrade slowly. Hence, they have the potential for long-term drug delivery. Poly-ε-caprolactone nanoparticles have been used as vehicles to deliver a wide range of drugs including tamoxifen, retinoic acid, and griseofulvin.

Polyalkyl-Cyanoacrylates

Polyalkyl-cyanoacrylate (PACA) nanoparticles are prepared by the conventional emulsion-evaporation technique. In addition to sustaining drug release, PACA nanoparticles have the ability to overcome multidrug resistance at both the cellular and subcellular levels (19). The potential for targeted delivery of PACA nanoparticles to cells has been demonstrated by conjugation of polysaccharides to the surface (20).

Nonbiodegradable Polymers Used to Prepare Nanoparticles

Polymethacrylate (PMA) and polymethyl methacrylate (PMMA) have been widely used in a variety of pharmaceutical and medical applications. Specifically, PMMA Eudragit® nanoparticles can be prepared by nanoprecipitation method (21) that involves adding hydroalcoholic solution of the polymer to an organic solvent. Incorporation of poly-acrylic acid into nanoparticles increased the transfection efficiency of DNA. The side chain of PMMA can be modified to make these polymers possess pH-dependent solubility and has been used to prepare pH-sensitive nanoparticles to increase the oral bioavailability.

Thermosensitive Nanoparticles

Polyvinyl caprolactone nanoparticles exist in swollen state when dispersed in water at room temperature. However, they shrink upon increasing temperature above the volume phase transition temperature, expelling water (22). Poly(N-isopropyl acrylamide) (NIPAAM) has been extensively used to prepare thermosensitive hydrogel-based nanoparticles. This polymer has a low critical solution temperature of 32°C to 34°C, above which it shrinks to release the drug.

Solid–Lipid Nanoparticles

Although not polymers, purified triglycerides and waxes that are solid at ambient and body temperatures can also be used as nanoparticulate carriers. These may be prepared by various methods including high-speed homogenization, microemulsions, emulsion-solvent evaporation, and ultrasonication (1). It is possible to prepare lipid nanoparticles with high drug loading, particularly with lipophilic drugs that sustain release due to their hydrophobicity and low drug diffusivity in the matrix.

CHARACTERIZATION OF NANOPARTICLES
Physical Properties of Polymers

The following physicochemical properties of polymers greatly influence the properties, method of preparation, and performance of nanoparticles.

Molecular Weight

The molecular weight of a polymer influences physical properties such as glass transition temperature, viscosity in solutions, solubility, crystallinity, degradation rate, and mechanical strength. In general, polymers with a lower molecular weight exhibit a lower viscosity and tensile strength, and degrade more rapidly. Hence, selection of a polymer with an appropriate molecular weight is important for the intended application. For example, if a polymer degrades by acid-catalyzed, bulk hydrolysis, a low-molecular-weight polymer will degrade faster due to autocatalysis by the greater proportion of oligomers formed. Inefficient polymeric synthesis may form polymers with high polydispersity that degrade more rapidly than homo-polymers of similar molecular weight.

Degree of Crystallinity
The mechanical properties of polymers can be altered by the degree of crystallinity. For example, because of the uniform arrangement of its chains within the lattice structure, a crystalline polymer will degrade slowly than an amorphous form. However, pure crystalline polymers are brittle and usually less suited to drug-delivery applications. Further, amorphous polymers possess poor mechanical toughness. Therefore, the polymers used in drug delivery are usually a mixture of crystalline and amorphous forms.

Hydrophobicity
Factors that influence the hydrophobicity of the polymer include molecular weight, aqueous solubility of the monomers, and the degree of branching. Although increase in molecular weight increases the hydrophobicity, an increase in the degree of branching results in a more water-soluble polymer. Hence, nanoparticles prepared using a hydrophobic polymer exhibit decreased water penetration and wettability, resulting in relatively slower drug release and polymer degradation times than similar hydrophilic forms. However, the incorporation of a hydrophilic polymer or additives into nanoparticles prepared using hydrophobic polymers will form pores in aqueous media to increase the rate of polymer degradation and erosion as well as drug release. It is important to realize that the method used to prepare nanoparticles will be influenced by the relative hydrophilicity and hydrophobicity of both the polymer and the drug.

Copolymer Ratio
The choice of a polymer and the method of polymerization directly affect the type of copolymer as well as its molecular weight, crystallinity, and hydrophobicity. In general, copolymers used to prepare nanoparticles typically contain both hydro-phobic and hydrophilic segments which facilitate greater flexibility in preparation and more predictable physical properties such as release characteristics.

Biodegradability and Biocompatibility
A biodegradable polymer must degrade into physiologically inert products that are eliminated by the body. For example, PLGA polymers hydrolyze to form lactic and glycolic acids that are further degraded into normal constituents of the body. Biocompatible polymers are defined as those that do not elicit immune reaction or inflammation, are stable for the duration of action, and are completely metabolized in the body. Most biodegradable polymers used in drug delivery are specifically intended for parenteral administration, which is not a prerequisite for oral delivery.

Solubility
The solubility spectrum of a polymer influences the method of preparation and in vivo performance of the nanoparticles. In general, if both the drug and the polymer are soluble in organic solvents, a simple o/w emulsion technique or phase separation can be used to prepare the nanoparticles. For protein and peptide drugs, a milder aqueous environment is preferable and therefore, the choice of the polymer is criti-cal and a multiple emulsion technique may be used.

Drug–Polymer Interactions

Chemical and physical interactions that occur depend on the chemical nature of both the polymer and the drug as is well documented in the literature. Drug–polymer interactions are chiefly determined by charge, solubility, and hydrophobicity and may greatly alter the properties of the polymer, for example, glass transition temperature and degree of crystallinity, as well as the properties of the nanoparticles, for example, release characteristics. The interactions that occur between a drug and a polymer can be identified, and in some cases quantified, using differential scanning calorimetry (DSC), thermogravimetric analysis (TGA), solid-state ^{13}C NMR, Fourier transform infrared spectroscopy, Flory Huggins interaction parameters, and comparison of total or partial solubility parameters (23). For example, isothermal calorimetry has been used to determine the binding affinity between alginates and chitosan as well as poly l-lysine (9). Differences in the solubility of the drug in the polymer results in the microphase separation of the drug within the matrix (24). Quantifying the binding affinity using isothermal calorimetry can identify an electrostatic interaction between the polymer and the drugs.

Preparation of Polymeric Nanoparticles

The main methods used to prepare polymeric nanoparticles include emulsion-solvent evaporation, phase separation, and use of supercritical fluid technology. These methods will not be described here as they have been extensively reviewed in the literature (1,2,4,6–14,16,17–22,24,25).

Properties of Nanoparticles that Affect Biological Performance

Route of Administration

Nanoparticles have been administered by the following routes: oral, intravenous, subcutaneous, intrathecal, intraocular, and pulmonary. When selecting a route to administer nanoparticles, it is important to consider the stability of the drug in biological fluids, as well as anatomical and physiological characteristics of the route of administration and at the target site. Oral delivery of nanoparticles may significantly increase the bioavailability of poorly soluble drugs. However, after intravenous administration, the bioavailability of drugs may decrease as macrophages will internalize hydrophobic unmodified nanoparticles. This problem may be circumvented by coating the surface of nanoparticles with hydrophilic polyethylene glycol, which confers "stealth" properties to these particles. It is important to note that, after pulmonary administration, nanoparticles may drain into the lymphatic system and, as with all nebulizers and aerosols, the site of deposition of the particles will depend on the type of the device used. Although not widely employed, intrathecal delivery of nanoparticles may sustain the release of the encapsulated drug.

Particle Size and Particle Size Distribution

The particle size and particle size distribution are critical factors in the performance of nanoparticles, as batches with wide particle size distribution show significant variations in drug loading, drug release, bioavailability, and efficacy. Particle size and particle size distribution can be determined using light scattering techniques and by scanning or transmission electron microscopy (Fig. 1). Formulation of nanoparticles with a narrow size distribution will be a challenge if emulsion cannot be produced with a narrow droplet size distribution. As nanoparticles are internalized into cells by endocytosis, an increase in particle size will decrease uptake and

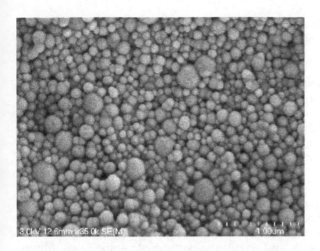

FIGURE 1 Scanning electron microscope image of poly-(lactide-co-glycolide) nanoparticles.

potentially, bioavailability of the drug. The extent of endocytosis is dependent on the type of the target cell.

Zeta Potential
The charge on the surface of the nanospheres will influence their distribution in the body and extent of uptake into the cells. Because cell membranes are negatively charged, there is greater electrostatic affinity for positively charged nanoparticles. Therefore, the surface of cationic or neutral nanoparticles may be modified to confer a positive charge to enhance efficacy. For example, positively charged tripalmitin nanoparticles containing etoposide prolonged residence time in the blood, produced higher blood concentrations, decreased clearance by the liver, and increased distribution into the brain and bone (26).

Drug Loading and Loading Efficiency
Although drug loading expresses the percent weight of active ingredient encapsulated to the weight of nanoparticles, drug loading efficiency is the ratio of the experimentally determined percentage of drug content compared with actual, or theoretical mass of drug used for the preparation of the nanoparticles. The loading efficiency depends on the polymer–drug combination and the method used. Hydrophobic polymers encapsulate larger amounts of hydrophobic drugs, whereas hydrophilic polymers entrap greater amounts of more hydrophilic drugs. Several formulation parameters, such as emulsifier type, weight ratio of polymer to drug, and organic to aqueous phase ratio, will influence the extent of drug loading.

Dissolution Profile
The in vitro release of drugs from nanoparticles may approximate the drug release profile inside the body although the rate is usually faster in vivo due to the presence of enzymes and surfactants in biological fluids. An in vitro dissolution medium mimics the pH and salt concentrations in the body. Particularly for hydrophobic drugs, it is critical during dissolution testing that sink conditions are maintained and pH and salt concentrations of biological fluid are approximated. If solubility of the drug in the media is a limitation, it may be necessary to add surfactants to the dissolution media. The release data must be evaluated using well-known equations

to determine parameters such as the mechanism(s) of release, order of release, dissolution rate constant, extent of release from the nanoparticles, and duration.

Surface Modification
The surface of nanoparticles may be modified to conjugate targeting ligands or alter biodistribution. Coating of nanoparticles with hydrophilic polymers such as polyethylene glycol, heparin, or dextran, protects them from being engulfed by the macrophages or kupffer cells, thereby increasing their circulation time and enhancing drug bioavailability. Surface modification of nanoparticles also involves alteration of the surface charge as discussed previously.

Biocompatibility
Tissue response to polymeric particles occurs in three phases. In phase I, mild inflammation is observed with monocytes, lymphocytes, and leucocytes surrounding the particle. In Phase II, monocytes differentiate into macrophages, which further differentiate into giant body cells and engulf the particles. In some cases, fibrous tissue may be formed. Phase III involves further degradation of the particles. The type of immune response elicited by the nanoparticles will depend on the route of administration, the type of therapeutic agent encapsulated, and the choice of the polymer. Because of dynamic flow, minimal immune responses are generally observed after intravenous administration.

IN VITRO CELL CULTURE
Internalization of Nanoparticles into Cells
The different mechanisms by which the nanoparticles are taken up by the cells include endocytosis, pinocytosis, fluid-phase diffusion, carrier-mediated, and facilitated transport. Although endocytosis and carrier-mediated transport are ATP-dependent, facilitated transport and diffusion are energy-independent. Nanoparticles undergo endolysosomal escape which increases accumulation of particles inside the cell (27). Receptor-mediated transport involves the internalization of nanoparticles through specific cell surface receptors on the cell membrane, and is exploited in the design of nanoparticles to specifically target these receptors (Fig. 2). Nanoparticles are

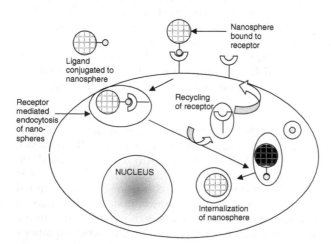

FIGURE 2 (*See color insert.*) Schematic diagram of specific receptor targeting of nanospheres using ligands.

primarily internalized by endocytosis. Once the particles are internalized, they transcytose across cells deeper into the tissue. Recently, it was demonstrated that the drug content in the cells increased with particle size, suggesting that in addition to particle internalization, diffusion of free drug released outside the cells may also play a role in enhancing the total drug content of the cells (28).

Protection from Efflux Pumps
Trans-membrane pumps, such as p-glycoprotein and multidrug-resistance-associated protein, are present on the apical side of the cells and actively efflux foreign substances, including drugs, out of the cell, significantly reducing the drug uptake. Nanoparticles can protect the encapsulated drug from these efflux pumps.

Targeted Delivery
Some limitations of drugs delivered using nanoparticulate vehicles include non-specific uptake into cells, accumulation of particles in nonspecific regions, and inability to differentiate between diseased and normal tissues. Targeted delivery of nanoparticles increases the extent of drug uptake at the site of action while potentially reducing adverse effects. Targeted delivery is based on: (*i*) physiological or externally induced phenomena (pH and thermo-sensitive nanoparticles, ultrasound-triggered nanoparticles, magnetic nanoparticles); (*ii*) cell- or tissue-specific targeting (nanoparticles targeting transferrin, folate, epidermal growth factor); and (*iii*) permeability-enhancing targets [nanoparticles targeting trans-activating transcriptional factor (TAT) peptide, integrin]. Targeted delivery of nanoparticles can significantly improve the therapeutic efficacy and safety of drugs.

REFERENCES
1. Wissing SA, Kayser O, Muller RH. Solid–lipid nanoparticles for parenteral drug delivery. Adv Drug Deliv Rev 2004; 56:1257–1272.
2. Bala I, Hariharan S, Kumar MN. PLGA nanoparticles in drug delivery: the state of the art. Crit Rev Ther Drug Carrier Syst 2004; 21:387–422.
3. Kumar N, Langer RS, Domb AJ. Polyanhydrides: an overview. Adv Drug Deliv Rev 2002; 54:889–910.
4. Tonnesen HH, Karlsen J. Alginate in drug delivery systems. Drug Dev Ind Pharm 2002; 28:621–630.
5. Rajaonarivony M, Vauthier C, Couarraze G, Puisieux F, Couvreur P. Development of a new drug carrier made from alginate. J Pharm Sci 1993; 82:912–917.
6. Gonzalez Ferreiro M, Tillman L, Hardee G, Bodmeier R. Characterization of alginate/poly-l-lysine particles as antisense oligonucleotide carriers. Int J Pharm 2002; 239:47–59.
7. Wee S, Gombotz WR. Protein release from alginate matrices. Adv Drug Deliv Rev 1998; 31:267–285.
8. Zahoor A, Sharma S, Khuller GK. Inhalable alginate nanoparticles as antitubercular drug carriers against experimental tuberculosis. Int J Antimicrob Agents 2005; 26:298–303.
9. De S, Robinson D. Polymer relationships during preparation of chitosan-alginate and poly-l-lysine-alginate nanospheres. J Control Release 2003; 89:101–112.
10. Agnihotri SA, Mallikarjuna NN, Aminabhavi TM. Recent advances on chitosan-based micro- and nanoparticles in drug delivery. J Control Release 2004; 100:5–28.
11. Prabaharan M, Mano JF. Chitosan-based particles as controlled drug delivery systems. Drug Deliv 2005; 12:41–57.
12. Coester CJ, Langer K, van Briesen H, Kreuter J. Gelatin nanoparticles by two step desolvation—a new preparation method, surface modifications and cell uptake. J Microencapsul 2000; 17:187–193.

13. Kaul G, Amiji M. Biodistribution and targeting potential of poly(ethylene glycol)-modified gelatin nanoparticles in subcutaneous murine tumor model. J Drug Target 2004; 12:585–591.
14. Balthasar S, Michaelis K, Dinauer N, von Briesen H, Kreuter J, Langer K. Preparation and characterisation of antibody modified gelatin nanoparticles as drug carrier system for uptake in lymphocytes. Biomaterials 2005; 26:2723–2732.
15. Wolf BW, Garleb KA, Choe YS, Humphrey PM, Maki KC. Pullulan is a slowly digested carbohydrate in humans. J Nutr 2003; 133:1051–1055.
16. Gupta M, Gupta AK. Hydrogel pullulan nanoparticles encapsulating pBUDLacZ plasmid as an efficient gene delivery carrier. J Control Release 2004; 99:157–166.
17. Umamaheshwari RB, Jain NK. Receptor mediated targeting of lectin conjugated gliadin nanoparticles in the treatment of Helicobacter pylori. J Drug Target 2003; 11:415–423; discussion 423–414.
18. Sinha VR, Bansal K, Kaushik R, Kumria R, Trehan A. Poly-epsilon-caprolactone microspheres and nanospheres: an overview. Int J Pharm 2004; 278:1–23.
19. Vauthier C, Dubernet C, Chauvierre C, Brigger I, Couvreur P. Drug delivery to resistant tumors: the potential of poly(alkyl cyanoacrylate) nanoparticles. J Control Release 2003; 93:151–160.
20. Chauvierre C, Labarre D, Couvreur P, Vauthier C. Novel polysaccharide-decorated poly(isobutyl oyanoacrylate) nanoparticles. Pharm Res 2003; 20:1786–1793.
21. Ubrich N, Schmidt C, Bodmeier R, Hoffman M, Maincent P. Oral evaluation in rabbits of cyclosporin-loaded Eudragit RS or RL nanoparticles. Int J Pharm 2005; 288:169–175.
22. Vihola H, Laukkanen A, Hirvonen J, Tenhu H. Binding and release of drugs into and from thermosensitive poly(N-vinyl caprolactam) nanoparticles. Eur J Pharm Sci 2002; 16:69–74.
23. Liu J, Xiao Y, Allen C. Polymer–drug compatibility: a guide to the development of delivery systems for the anticancer agent, ellipticine. J Pharm Sci 2004; 93:132–143.
24. Shen E, Pizsczek R, Dziadul B, Narasimhan B. Microphase separation in bioerodible copolymers for drug delivery. Biomaterials 2001; 22:201–210.
25. Yi YM, Yang TY, Pan WM. Preparation and distribution of 5-fluorouracil (125) I sodium alginate-bovine serum albumin nanoparticles. World J Gastroenterol 1999; 5:57–60.
26. Reddy LH, Sharma RK, Chuttani K, Mishra AK, Murthy RR. Etoposide-incorporated tripalmitin nanoparticles with different surface charge: formulation, characterization, radiolabeling, and biodistribution studies. AAPS J 2004; 6:e23.
27. Panyam J, Zhou WZ, Prabha S, Sahoo SK, Labhasetwar V. Rapid endo-lysosomal escape of poly(dl-lactide-co-glycolide) nanoparticles: implications for drug and gene delivery. FASEB J 2002; 16:1217–1226.
28. De S, Miller DW, Robinson DH. Effect of particle size of nanospheres and microspheres on the cellular-association and cytotoxicity of paclitaxel in 4T1 cells. Pharm Res 2005; 22:766–775.

4 | Nanofiber-Based Drug Delivery

Matthew D. Burke
Department of Pharmaceutical Development, GlaxoSmithKline, Research Triangle Park, North Carolina, U.S.A.

Dmitry Luzhansky
Department of Corporate Technology, Donaldson Company, Inc., Minneapolis, Minnesota, U.S.A.

INTRODUCTION

Electrospinning is a process that was originally developed in the early 1930s, but did not receive much attention until recent decades. Most likely the increased interest is due to the refocusing of more research groups on nanotechnology. Although electrospinning has existed for a significant period of time and is relatively easy to execute, the physics of electrospinning nanofibers is only understood to a limited extent. A typical electrospinning process involves dissolving the drug of interest and a polymer in an appropriate solvent. The solution is then placed in a syringe, and a high voltage is applied. A small amount of the polymer solution is drawn out of the syringe, forming a Taylor cone. Increasing the applied voltage further results in the initiation of a charged fluid jet, which follows a chaotic trajectory of stretching and bending until it reaches the grounded target. A stable jet is formed when the charge is increased above a critical voltage, and there is a balance between the surface tension of the fluid and the repulsive nature of the charge distribution on the surface of the fluid. The presence of molecular entanglements in the polymer solution prevents the jet from breaking into droplets (electrospraying), and when combined with the electrical forces results in a whip-like motion of the jet, known as bending instability. This process typically results in the drawing of a virtually endless fiber with a nanometer-sized to micrometer-sized diameter. The final product is a three-dimensional nonwoven mat of entangled nanofibers with a high surface-area-to-volume ratio (1). Scanning electron microscopy (SEM) is a typical method to evaluate the nanofibers produced through electrospinning, as shown in Figure 1.

Electrospun nanofibers have a very large surface-area-to-volume ratio, as large as 1000 times that of a microfiber. This physical property has generated a significant amount of interest in the biomedical and pharmaceutical industries particularly for drug delivery of poorly soluble drug substances. In the pharmaceutical industry, recent trends in drug discovery have led to the development of a significant number of highly potent compounds with extremely low solubility, thus requiring advanced methods to create efficacious pharmaceutical products that overcome the solubility issues of the drug. Currently, the pharmaceutical industry uses methods such as milling to reduce the particle size of a drug substance, but this is a high-energy method which can lead to stability issues and often cannot produce truly nanosized drug particles. In conventional dry milling, the limit of fineness is reached in the region of 100 μm. Wet grinding or wet bead milling produces further reduction in the particle size, but often not below the micrometer range.

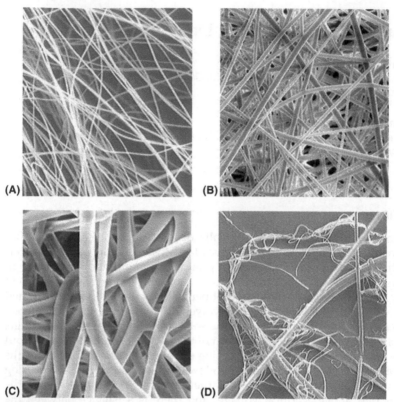

FIGURE 1 Sample SEMs of various types of GRAS polymer nanofibers produced by electrospinning. (**A**) Cellulose acetate, (**B**) PVAc, (**C**) polyethylene oxide, and (**D**) Kollidon® SR (BASF AG, Ludwigshafen, Germany). *Abbreviations*: GRAS, generally regarded as safe; PVAc, polyvinylacetate; SEM, scanning electron microscopy.

The utility of the electrospinning process for pharmaceutical products is the single-step creation of nanosized drug particles with a low-energy process. The selection of the polymer also controls the drug-release properties. Therefore, immediate-release nanofibers can be created by water-soluble polymers, enteric-release nanofibers can be created by enteric polymers such as methacrylic acid copolymers, and sustained-release nanofibers can be created by polylactic acid or polyvinyl acetate polymers. Although the diameter of electrospun fibers is often characterized using SEM as proof that they are nanosized, it is important to note that the size of the drug particles embedded in the nanosized fiber is significantly smaller than the diameter of the fibers themselves.

Further utility may be found with electrospinning by embedding it at the end of the chemical synthesis of the drug substance, which would streamline the transfer of material from chemical development to pharmaceutical development. The last step in the chemical synthesis of a drug is usually a purification/precipitation step to create a drug powder. Then the powder is transferred to pharmaceutical development teams, which often mill the powder to a particular particle size and further granulate/process the material into a tablet. This powder handling and processing, which often requires safety controls, can be avoided if the last step in the chemical synthesis is transformed into a step where the drug and a preferred polymer are in an appropriate solution for electrospinning. Then the drug/polymer solution can be directly electrospun into a final product, thus creating a seamless process from chemical synthesis through creation of an appropriate final pharmaceutical product. This would eliminate powder handling of the drug substance, and possibly reduce variations in the final particle size of the drug substance during manufacturing.

DISSOLUTION ENHANCEMENT FOR IMMEDIATE-RELEASE DOSAGE FORMS

Pharmaceutical tablets or capsules which immediately release their drug cargo when orally ingested are the most common dosage form in the pharmaceutical industry. Creating a product which performs this task is challenging with low-solubility drugs. Inappropriate formulation of low-solubility drugs can result in slow or limited drug dissolution in the gastrointestinal (GI) fluids and subsequently minimal drug being absorbed into systemic circulation. As mentioned above, currently a common technique to overcome this low bioavailability issue is to reduce the particle size of the drug substance to increase the dissolution of the drug into the GI fluids. The particle size of the drug is directly related to the rate that it dissolves. The effect of particle size on the drug dissolution process can be mathematically described by the Nernst and Brunner diffusion layer model (2):

$$\frac{dQ}{dt} = \frac{D}{h} S(C_s - C_g)$$

where Q is the amount of the drug dissolved, t the time, D the diffusion coefficient of the drug in the solubilizing fluids of the GI tract, S the effective surface area of the drug particles, h the thickness of a stationary layer of solvent around the drug particles, C_s the saturation solubility of the drug in the stationary layer h, and C_g the concentration of the drug in the bulk fluids of the GI tract.

Based on the drug dissolution equation described in the previous paragraph, it is clearly evident that the surface area of the drug particle is a key physicochemical property which can be used to increase the rate of drug dissolution. The particle size of the drug substance is often used as a surrogate marker for surface area; therefore, a decrease in the particle size will increase the surface area and thus increase drug dissolution. As mentioned earlier, the current particle size reduction technologies often reach a limit around 1 micron. In contrast, by first intent electrospinning produces nanofibers less than 1 micron, thus electrospinning presents a mechanism to allow further reduction of the particle size beyond the current technologies. The electrospun nanofibers are preferably a homogeneous mixture of polymer and drug, thus the particle size of the drug should be significantly less than the diameter of the nanofiber. Although the exact particle size of the drug in the nanofiber remains challenging to quantify, the dissolution rate can provide indirect evidence that significant particle size reduction has occurred. Reduction of the particle size of the drug substance through electrospinning with a rapidly dissolving polymer causes the drug dissolution rate to be very rapid, as shown in Figure 2.

Another advantage of electrospinning as a dissolution-enhancement tool is the ability to control the morphology of the drug substance (3,4). By selecting a polymer such as hydroxypropylmethylcellulose acetate succinate (HPMC-AS), which has an amorphous character, one can create an amorphous drug substance

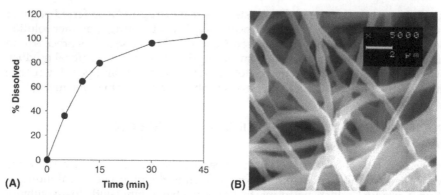

FIGURE 2 (**A**) Dissolution of a model low-solubility drug from polyethylene oxide electrospun fibers in a USP 2 dissolution apparatus. (**B**) Scanning electron microscopy image of the nanofibers.

through electrospinning. Amorphous drug substances are at a higher energy state, therefore, in general have higher solubility and higher dissolution rate compared with crystalline materials. Thus, the creation of an amorphous drug substance represents another technique for dissolution enhancement. Amorphous drugs are generally less stable physically and chemically than corresponding crystalline materials, so appropriate stability assessment needs to be performed (5). Although stability issues can limit the use of amorphous drug substances, there are several marketed oral products such as Vancocin® (Viropharma, USA), Plendil ER® (AstraZeneca Ltd., UK), Cesamet® (Eli Lilly and Co., USA), and Certican® (Novartis AG, Basel, Switzerland) that contain amorphous drug substances.

In addition to increasing the solubility and dissolution by creating an amorphous drug substance with HPMC-AS, it has also been shown to reduce in vivo precipitation of the drug by maintaining the drug as a supersaturated solution in the GI tract. Spray-drying with the drug substance and HPMC-AS has been performed to create amorphous particles to increase the drug exposure for rapid screening of drugs in preclinical models (6). Electrospinning could be used in a similar fashion and it has two additional benefits: first, the ability to create smaller-diameter fibers than the typical particle size of spray-dried material, and second, process collects the product onto a grounded surface, which results in very high efficiencies (99%+) and simplified recovery.

An example of the use of electrospinning to create amorphous materials for dissolution enhancement was performed by Verreck et al. (7). In this case, the researchers used hydroxypropylmethylcellulose as the electrospinning polymer, and itraconazole as the model drug. On the basis of differential scanning calorimetry, they generated data supporting the conclusion that itraconazole was in the amorphous form, and performed dissolution studies to evaluate the rate of release. These data also highlighted the fact that by optimizing the electrospinning conditions to produce fibers with a diameter of 300 to 500 nm versus 1 to 4 μm, the dissolution rate can be further increased (7).

SUSTAINED-RELEASE ELECTROSPUN FIBERS

There is significant interest in the use of electrospinning for dissolution enhancement of poorly water-soluble drugs; however, the majority of the literature on

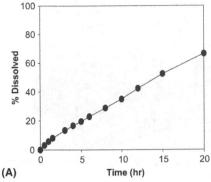
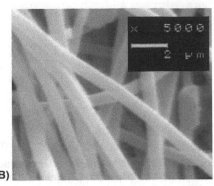

(A)

(B)

FIGURE 3 **(A)** Dissolution of a model low-solubility drug from polyvinylacetate electrospun fibers in a USP 2 dissolution apparatus. **(B)** Scanning electron microscopy image of the nanofibers.

electrospinning of pharmaceutical or biomedical products tends to be for wound dressings or other products which have sustained release of drug substance. This reveals the large range of drug-release profiles which can be obtained by careful selection of the polymer. For release of a drug substance for multiple days to months, a polymer in the biodegradable family, such as polyglycolide, polylactic acid, or polycaprolactone, can be used. A copolymer of ε-caprolactone and ethyl ethylene phosphate was used to sustain the release of human β-nerve growth factor for at least three months (8). However, selection of the polymer needs to be carefully screened because the polymer drug compatibility has been shown to play a critical role in the distribution of drug within the fiber (9).

Polymers which hydrate or swell but are insoluble can also be used to create sustained-release nanofibers. Verreck et al. (10) electrospun segmented polyurethane itraconazole fibers to produce a sustained release of the drug substance. This type of release can be achieved through the use of generally regarded as safe (GRAS) polymers for oral drug delivery such as polyvinylacetate (PVAc) nanofibers. An example of drug release of a poorly water-soluble drug substance from electrospun fibers of PVAc is shown in Figure 3.

As shown by the examples above, various polymer-based methods to control drug release such as enteric polymers, biodegradable polymers, or even polysaccharide can be utilized with electrospinning. The intrinsic properties of the polymer form the basis for the type of drug release that occurs from the nanofibers. Although proof of concept has been achieved with electrospun nanofibers for dissolution enhancement and controlled drug release, the use of electrospinning in the pharmaceutical industry is still in its infancy. More advances such as functionalized nanofibers and nanotube structures through co-axial electrospinning are likely to occur (11,12).

LARGE-SCALE MANUFACTURING

Although electrospinning is still at an early stage in the pharmaceutical industry, commercial use of nanofibers produced by electrospinning in other industries has already been established. Donaldson Company's nanofiber filter media production has increased well beyond 10,000 m2/day during the last 20 years. An SEM example of the filter utilization of a nanofiber web layer on the surface of a spunbond nonwoven is shown in Figure 4.

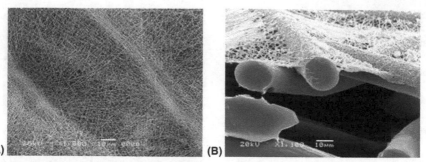

FIGURE 4 Examples of nanofiber composites electrospun by Donaldson. Nanofibers on the surface of (**A**) filter paper and (**B**) spunbond nonwoven.

By utilizing many of the current manufacturing practices used in the filtration industry, the large-scale manufacturing of electrospun nanofibers for pharmaceutical applications can progress at a rapid rate, including the adoption and implementation of appropriate quality control tools for nanofiber production such as automated fiber sizing and mechanical integrity testing (13).

Automated Fiber Sizing

Full process control of the nanofiber production requires measurement and control of fiber size, fiber size distribution, and quantity of fibers. Therefore, there is a need for a tool that can directly measure mean fiber size and fiber size distribution. Routine sampling and measurement of these properties are achieved using an SEM and a developed analysis methodology. Measuring nanofiber diameters usually consists of manually comparing the diameter of fibers in a photomicrograph to a known scale. The process is very time-consuming, and operator consistency and fatigue can reduce the accuracy. Automating the activity of sizing fibers is a natural solution to the problem.

For drug-delivery applications, fiber diameter and fiber diameter distribution will be important parameters to measure. It is expected that fiber diameter is one of the variables that can be controlled to tune the rate of fiber dissolution and control drug release (i.e., a bigger fiber has lower surface area and would lead to a delayed release compared with a smaller fiber). A proprietary algorithm has been developed at Donaldson Company to overcome the limitations of commercially available software. In the automated fiber sizing process, the SEM image is first cropped to a desired size, and unwanted details are eliminated. The calibration bar from the SEM image is used to set the number of pixels per micrometer. Next, the program converts the image to black and white using a gray scale function. The black (nonfiber) areas are sorted according to size. Starting with the largest black area, a straight line is defined on the border pixels and a diameter is drawn from one pixel across the white area at 90°. The diameter drawing stops when another black pixel is intersected. The process is repeated around the black shape at an interval of approximately every five pixels, and then around each black area in order of size (Fig. 5).

All fiber diameter lengths are recorded and a running histogram is generated (Fig. 6). The process that used to take hours of painstaking measurements for an operator can now be completed in seconds. Characterization of fiber size, fiber size distribution, and quantity of fibers is critical to ensure a quality product. In addition,

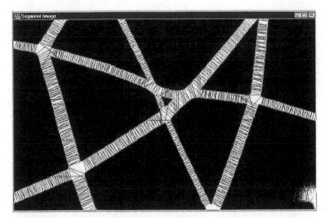

FIGURE 5   Nanofiber scanning electron microscopic photograph with fiber diameter measurement lines shown.

the mechanical integrity of a nanofiber structure can be important for sustained-release drug-delivery applications such as wound dressings, tissue engineering, and regenerative medicine. Knowledge of the strain–stress characteristics is important in understanding the performance of nanofiber composites under dynamic stress such as the gastric compression and peristaltic action of the GI tract. Owing to the small size of fibers and extremely low weight of the layer, traditional measurement methods do not give useful results. It is anticipated that the mechanical integrity of nanofibers should be engineered, measured, and controlled.

Mechanical Integrity Testing
The DL Bending Tester was developed to study the strain properties and failure mechanisms of nanofibers applied to the surface of another material. First, a sample

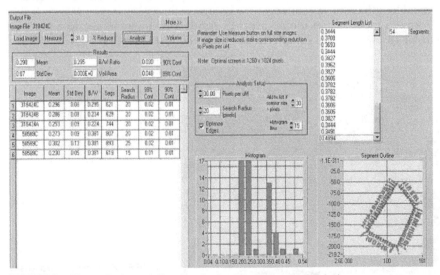

FIGURE 6   (*See color insert.*) Results of automated fiber size analysis.

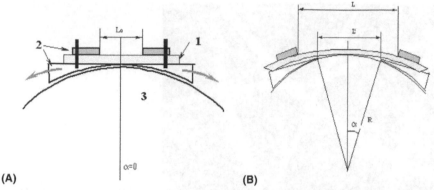

FIGURE 7 (**A**) Specimen before deformation: 1, sample; 2, jaws; 3, cylinder. (**B**) Specimen after deformation.

is secured in the tester and positioned in the optical microscope. A motor then bends and extends the sample around a cylinder with known diameter. The strain condition approximates plane strain because the sample is thin compared with the relatively large radius of the cylinder. Thus, differences in the strain condition between the upper and lower surfaces of the sample are minimal. An area of approximately 6 mm × 4 mm (4 mm in the direction of stretch) is observed and can be varied. An angle of deformation, α, is measured using a scale on the apparatus.

The basic schematic representation of the tester is shown in Figure 7A and B. The general view of the tester is shown in Figure 8.

The strain can be calculated from the measured angle:

$$e = \frac{4p\alpha R}{360L_0}$$

where ε is the calculated strain, α the measured angle, R the cylinder diameter, and L_0 the initial length of the specimen.

A camera mounted on the microscope sends a dynamic image to a monitor that is used to observe the sample throughout the test. The first sign of relative

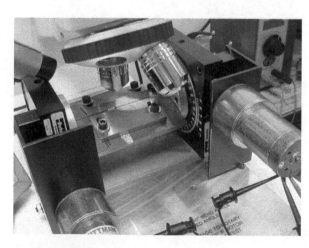

FIGURE 8 Dmitry Luzhansky bending tester.

movement between the components of the composite structure is an indicator of critical strain. An operator records the relative movements and angles of the first destruction in the nanofiber layer and full destruction of nanofiber layer. Comparison of the angles for different composites gives a measure of integrity of the material.

CONCLUSION

Electrospun nanofibers have shown utility in a range of pharmaceutical and medical applications for immediate and controlled drug release, which will increase the need for future process refinement and large-scale manufacturing capabilities to convert these novel concepts into commercial products. Electrospinning represents a nanotechnology that is steadily maturing and its use will grow as companies implement this technology as a platform drug-delivery technique.

REFERENCES

1. McKee MG, Wilkes GL, Colby RH, Long TE. Correlations of solution rheology with electrospun fiber formation of linear and branched polyesters. Macromolecules 2004; 37:1760.
2. Hoener BA, Benet LZ. Factors influencing drug absorption and drug availability. In: Banker GS, Rhodes CT, eds. Modern Pharmaceutics. 4th ed. New York: Marcel Dekker, 2002 (chapter 4).
3. Ignatious F, Baldoni JM. Electrospun pharmaceutical compositions. 2001; WO 01/54667 A1.
4. Ignatious F, Sun L. Electrospun amorphous pharmaceutical compositions. 20041; WO 2004/014304.
5. Yu L. Amorphous pharmaceutical solids: preparation, characterization and stabilization. Adv Drug Del Rev 2001; 48:27.
6. Shanker RM. Drug–polymer systems for the supersaturation of GI luminal fluid. In: Presented at AAPS Annual Meeting, Baltimore, MD, November 7–14, 2004.
7. Verreck G, Chun I, Peeters J, Rosenblatt J, Brewster ME. Preparation and characterization of nanofibers containing amorphous drug dispersion generated by electrostatic spinning. Pharm Res 2003; 20:810.
8. Chew SY, Wen J, Yim EKF, Leong KW. Sustained release of proteins from electrospun biodegradable fibers. Biomacromolecules 2005; 6:2017.
9. Zheng J, Yang L, Liang Q, et al. Influence of the drug compatibility with polymer solution on the release kinetics of electrospun fiber formulation. J Control Release 2005; 105:43.
10. Verreck G, Chun I, Rosenblatt J, et al. Incorporation of drugs in an amorphous state into electrospun nanofibers composed of a water-insoluble, nonbiodegradable polymer. J Control Release 2003; 92:349.
11. Casper CL, Yamaguchi N, Kiick KL, Rabolt JF. Functionalizing electrospun fibers with biologically relevant macromolecules. Biomacromolecules 2005; 6:1998.
12. Huang Z-M, Zhang Y-Z. Micro-structures and mechanical performance of co-axial nanofibers with drug and protein cores and polycaprolactone shells. Gaodeng Xuexiao Huaxue Xuebao 2005; 26:968.
13. Luzhansky D. Quality control in manufacturing of electrospun nanofiber composites. In: Presented at International Nonwovens Technical Conference, Baltimore, MD, September 15–18, 2003.

Drug Nanocrystals—The Universal Formulation Approach for Poorly Soluble Drugs

Jan Möschwitzer and Rainer H. Müller
Department of Pharmaceutical Technology, Biotechnology, and Quality Management, Freie Universität Berlin, Berlin, Germany

INTRODUCTION

During the last two decades, many modern technologies have been established in the pharmaceutical research and development area. The automation of the drug discovery process by technologies such as high-throughput screening, combinatorial chemistry, and computer-aided drug design is leading to a vast number of drug candidates possessing a very good efficacy. Unfortunately, many of these drug candidates are exhibiting poor aqueous solubility. Long before one of these compounds can reach the market, it needs to be formulated for the pharmacological activity tests and for the preclinical studies. The great challenge for the pharmaceutical development is to create new formulation approaches and drug-delivery systems to overcome solubility problems of these drug candidates which are also often associated with poor oral bioavailability (1,2).

The dissolution velocity (low solubility in general is correlated with low dissolution velocity, law by Noyes–Whitney) and intestinal permeability are key determinants for the bioavailability, particularly for perorally administered drugs. To evaluate and characterize pharmaceutical compounds with respect to their aqueous solubility and intestinal permeability, a biopharmaceutics classification system has been developed (3,4). The system divides the drug compounds into four classes. Poorly soluble compounds can belong to either class II or class IV. Class IV means that the drug shows simultaneously poor solubility and low permeability. A solubility enhancement cannot necessarily solve the bioavailability problems of class IV drugs in any case. Drug candidates for a successful improvement of their bioavailability by a solubilization technique belong to class II which means that their bioavailability is only limited by their poor aqueous solubility/dissolution velocity. The term "solubilization techniques" in the present context means technologies which increase the dissolution velocity dc/dt and—ideally—also the saturation solubility c_s.

There are many conventional approaches for the solubilization of poorly soluble drugs. Salt formation and pH adjustment are the first attempts if the molecule is ionizable, because in general the ionized species has a higher aqueous solubility compared to the neutral one. If this approach fails, often cosolvents such as propylene glycol, are used, especially for parenteral or liquid oral dosage forms. Systemic toxicity or pain on injection are typical drawbacks associated with cosolvents (5). Other systems contain a large amount of surfactants to solubilize drugs by an increased wetting of the hydrophobic compound. However, the extended use of surfactants can also cause side effects. A typical example is the hypersensitivity reaction caused by the Cremophor EL® in Taxol® (6). Another example of surfactants is mixed micelles, for example, Valium® MM (7). In case of lipophilic drugs, a low-melting point emulsification system such as microemulsions, self-emulsifying DDSs, or self-microemulsifying DDSs, could be used. The drawbacks of these systems include batch-to-batch variability, chemical instabilities, and high surfactant concentration.

Another approach is the use of liposomes to incorporate hydrophobic drugs in phospho-lipid bilayers of uni- or multilamellar vesicles. One example is the drug Amphotericin B, which is marketed as liposomal formulation Ambisome®.

A specific approach is the formation of inclusion complexes, for example, with cyclodextrins. Cyclodextrines are cyclic oligomers of dextrose or dextrose derivatives, which can form a reversible, noncovalent association with poorly soluble drugs to solubilize them. Especially, the more water soluble and less toxic derivatives, such as sulfobutylether-β-cyclodextrin (Captisol™, CyDex, Inc.) and hydroxy-propyl-β-cyclodextrin (HP-β-cyclodextrin), are used in different pharmaceutical formulations (8). Sporanox® by Johnson and Johnson/Janssen (Itraconazole/HP-β-cyclodextrine) and Zeldox® by Pfizer (Ziprasidone/SBE-β-cyclodextrine; Captisol®) are examples of marketed products. In order to build this complex, it is in general required that the drug molecule fits into the cyclodextrin cavity. For that reason, this promising specific approach can be used only for a limited number of drugs. Another drawback of this technology is the high excipient level of the resulting product.

To sum up, the prementioned technologies are successfully applied for a number of drugs. The marketed products prove their acceptance and applicability. The success of a technology can be rated in two areas:

1. time between developing the technology and first market products and
2. number of products on the market in total (or more precisely, number of products launched per year).

Based on these success criteria, the performance of most specific formulation approaches appears rather poor. Liposomes—rediscovered by Bingham in 1968—needed about 20 years to come to market. The number of products is relatively low, definitely distinctly behind expectations. Similar is the situation for cyclodextrines, currently moving forward with the new, better tolerated derivatives. These technologies are commonly used as primary strategies. However, they are more or less specific approaches for the solubilization of a certain drug candidate. They can be used only in compliance with certain requirements determined by the drug and route of administration; there is no universal formulation approach.

Much smarter are nonspecific formulation approaches applicable to almost any drug molecule (apart from a few exceptions). Particle size reduction has been a nonspecific formulation approach for many years. The micronization of drugs is applied to increase their surface area. Increasing the surface area will proportionally increase the rate of dissolution and the rate of diffusion (absorption). Micronization means transfer of relatively coarse drug powder to micrometer crystals using colloid mills or jet mills. The mean diameter of such micronized drug powders is in the range of approximately 2 to 5 μm, corresponding to a size distribution of approximately 0.1 to 20 μm (9). Owing to their particle size distribution, such formulations in general cannot be used for intravenous (IV) injections. Micronization cannot improve the saturation solubility of a drug substance. In cases of practically insoluble pharmaceutical compounds or compounds of very low solubility, the effect of micronization on the bioavailablity is not sufficient. For that reason, the next consequent step was to go down one further dimension in size, which means to reduce the particle size in the nanometer range.

Since the 1980s, when drug nanoparticles were produced by List and Sucker (10) via precipitation, various techniques for the production of drug nanocrystals have been developed. This chapter will give an overview of the beneficial features of drug nanocrystals, will discuss the most important production techniques, and point out some reasons why drug nanocrystals can be seen as a universal formulation approach for poorly soluble drugs.

DEFINITION

Drug nanocrystals are pure solid drug particles with a mean diameter below 1000 nm. A nanosuspension consists of drug nanocrystals, stabilizing agents such as surfactants and/or polymeric stabilizers, and a liquid dispersion medium. The dispersion media can be water, aqueous solutions, or nonaqueous media. The term "drug nanocrystals" implies a crystalline state of the discrete particles, but depending on the production method they can also be partially or completely amorphous. Drug nanocrystals have to be distinguished from polymeric nanoparticles, which consist of a polymeric matrix and an incorporated drug. Drug nanocrystals do not consist of any matrix material.

PHYSICOCHEMICAL PROPERTIES OF DRUG NANOCRYSTALS

The increased saturation solubility and the accelerated dissolution velocity are the most important differentiating features of drug nanocrystals. In general, the saturation solubility (c_s) is defined as a drug-specific constant depending only on the solvent and the temperature. This definition is only valid for drug particles with a minimum particle size in the micrometer range. A particle size reduction down to the nanometer range can increase the drug solubility.

The saturation solubility of solid particles depends on their particle radius and their lattice structure according to the Ostwald–Freunlich equation and the Kelvin equation:

$$\ln\left(\frac{S}{S_0}\right) = \frac{2v\gamma}{rRT} = \frac{2M\gamma}{\rho rRT} \tag{1}$$

where S is the drug solubility at temperature T, S_0 the solubility if $r = \infty$, M the molecular weight of the compound, v the molar volume, γ the interfacial surface tension, and ρ the density of the compound.

From the Ostwald–Freundlich equation, it can be concluded that a drug shows higher solubility if the particle radius is decreased. This effect is not substantial for larger particles but will be more pronounced for particles below 1 to 2 µm, especially well under 200 nm. Another important factor influencing the solubility is the crystalline structure of the drug. The higher the solid density and the melting point are, the lower the solubility in general is. In contrast, a polymorph form with a lower packaging shows a higher molar volume and lower solid density (11).

The Kelvin equation can also be used to describe the correlation of increased saturation solubility by decreased particle size. The Kelvin equation describes the vapor pressure as a function of the curvature of liquid droplets in a gas phase. The vapor pressure increases with increasing curvature (decreasing particle size).

This can be transferred to solid drug particles in a liquid medium: the dissolution pressure increases with decreasing particle size (12).

$$\frac{dc_x}{dt} = \frac{DA}{h}(c_s - c_x) \tag{2}$$

where dc_x/dt is the dissolution velocity, D the diffusion coefficient, A the surface of the drug particle, h the thickness of diffusional layer, c_s the saturation solubility of the drug, and c_x the concentration in surrounding liquid at time x.

The increased dissolution velocity is the characteristic feature of drug nano-crystals. The Noyes–Whitney equation [Equation (2)] describes now an increase in dissolution velocity is proportional to an increase in surface area. For example, when moving from a spherical 50 µm particle to micronized 5 µm particles, the total surface area enlarges by a factor of 10, moving to 500 nm nanocrystals by a factor of 100. The decrease in the diffusional distance h is an additional factor accelerating the dissolution velocity. According to the Prandtl equation [Equation (3)], the diffusional distance h is reduced with increasing curvature of ultrafine particles. Together with the increased saturation solubility of ultrafine particles, the concentration gradient in the Noyes–Whitney equation is significantly increased. For that reason, nanoni-zation can distinctly increase the dissolution velocity of poorly soluble drugs:

$$h_H = k\left(\frac{L^{1/2}}{V^{1/3}}\right) \tag{3}$$

where h_H is the hydrodynamic boundary layer thickness, V the relative velocity of the flowing liquid against a flat surface, k a constant, and L the length of the surface in the direction of flow.

Drug nanocrystals can be used for a chemical stabilization of chemically labile drugs. The drug paclitaxel can be preserved from degradation when it is formulated as a nanosuspension (13,14). The same result was found for the chemically labile drug omeprazole. When formulated as a nanosuspension, the stability was distinctly increased in comparison to the aqueous solution (15). The increased stability can be explained by a shield effect of the surfactants and the drug protection by a mono-layer made of degraded drug molecules which reduce the accessibility for destruc-tive agents (16).

POTENTIAL CLINICAL ADVANTAGES OF DRUG NANOCRYSTALS
Application for Oral Delivery

The oral route is the most important and preferred route of administration. The formulation of drug nanocrystals can impressively improve the bioavailability of perorally administered poorly soluble drugs. In 1995, Liversidge and Cundy (17) reported an increase in bioavailability for the drug Danazol from $5.1 \pm 1.9\%$ for the conventional suspension to $82.3 \pm 10.1\%$ for the nanosuspension. The increased dissolution velocity and saturation solubility lead to fast and complete drug dissolution, an important prerequisite for drug absorption.

Whenever a rapid onset of a poorly soluble drug is desired, the formulation of drug nanocrystals can be beneficial, for example, in case of analgesics. The analgesic naproxen, formulated as a nanosuspension, has shown a reduced t_{max} but simulta-neously approximately threefold increased AUC in comparison to a normal suspen-sion (Naprosyn®) (18).

Besides the faster onset of action, the naproxen nanosuspension has also shown a reduced gastric irritancy (19,20). If absorption windows limit the drug absorption or by food effects, drug nanocrystals have advantages in comparison to conventional suspensions. Wu et al. have reported reduced fed-fasted ratio and an improved bioavailability for nanocrystalline aprepitant (MK-0869), the active ingredient in Emend®, in beagle dogs.

Another important advantage of drug nanocrystals is their adhesiveness and the increased residence time, which can positively influence the bioavailability. The mucoadhesiveness can be raised by the use of mucoadhesive polymers in the dispersion medium (21,22). Additionally the utilized mucoadhesive polymers can prevent the drug from degradation. The reduced particle size can be also exploited for improved drug targeting, as reported for inflammatory tissues (23) or the lymphatic drug uptake (24).

Parenteral Administration of Drug Nanocrystals

The parenteral application of poorly soluble drugs, particularly intravenous (IV) administration of practically insoluble compounds, using cosolvents, surfactants, liposomes, or cylcodextrines, is often associated with large injection volumes or toxic side effects. Carrier-free nanosuspensions enable potential higher loading capacity compared to other parenteral application systems. Using nanosuspensions, the application volume can be distinctly reduced compared to solutions (15). To fulfil the distinctly higher regulatory hurdles, the drug nanocrystals need to be produced in an aseptic process. Alternatively, nanosuspensions can be sterilized by autoclaving (25) or alternatively by gamma irradiation as well as sterile filtration (26). When a drug is administered as a nanosuspension, the rapid dissolution of the nanocrystals will mimic the plasma concentration profile of a solution. Drug nanosuspensions can be formulated with accepted surfactants and polymeric stabilizers for IV injection. In contrast, solutions of poorly soluble drugs require the use of cosolvents and/or high surfactant contents (e.g., Chremophor EL in Taxol®), which can cause undesired side effects (6). Comparing the toxicity of Taxol® with a paclitaxel nanosuspension, the latter has shown a distinctly reduced toxicity. The nanosuspension was much better tolerated, resulting in an approximately doubled LD50 value (27). The same effect of increased tolerated dose was found for the antifungal drug itraconazole. Itraconazole is marketed as Sporanox IV® by Janssen Pharmaceutica Products, L.P., an inclusion complex of itraconazole and 2-hydroxypropyl-β-cyclodextrine (HP-β-CD). The product exhibits a significant acute toxicity above 10 mg/kg and an LD50 value lower than 40 mg/kg when administered as a bolus in the caudal vein of rats. In contrast, a 1% nanosuspension of itraconazole could be administered up to 320 mg/kg without animal mortality. Besides the decreased acute toxicity, the nanosuspension has also shown a prolonged effect, whereby the administration intervals could be extended almost three times in comparison to the daily administration of Sporanox IV® (11). Comparing a clofazimine nanosuspension with a liposomal formulation, both are similarly effective in the treatment of artificially induced *Mycobacterium avium* infections. The targeting to the reticuloendothelial system, the lung, liver, and spleen was comparable to the liposomal formulation (28). Furthermore, a special targeting can be achieved by a surface modification using the concept of "differential protein adsorption." A surface modification of drug nanocrystals with the surfactant Tween 80 leads to a preferential adsorption of apolipoprotein E. This protein adsorption enables a targeted delivery of drug nanocrystals to the brain. Atovaquone drug nanocrystals modified with Tween 80 have shown an excellent efficacy in the treatment of Toxoplasmosis (29).

Drug Nanocrystals for Pulmonary Drug Delivery

Delivery of water-insoluble drugs to the respiratory tract is very important for the local or systemic treatment of diseases. Many important drugs for pulmonary delivery show poor solubility simultaneously in water and nonaqueous media, for example, important corticosteroids such as budesonide or beclomethasone dipropionate. In the past, most of these drugs were administered as aerosols, but in compliance with the Montreal Protocol of 1987 the use of chlorofluorocarbon (CFC) must be avoided. Therefore, alternatives such as dry powder inhalers or metered dose inhalers without CFC (MDI) were developed. These systems are filled with micronized drug powders produced by jet-milling. The mean particle size in the lower micrometer range (3–25 µm) results in a significant oropharyngeal deposition of larger particles leading to increased occurrence of candidasis. Additionally, the oral deposition of the drug leads to gastrointestinal (GI) drug absorption followed by systemic side effects (30). Nanosuspensions can be successfully applied to overcome these problems. The nebulization of nanosuspensions generates aerosol droplets of the preferred size loaded with a large amount of drug nanocrystals. Using nebulized nanosuspensions, the respirable fraction is distinctly increased in comparison to conventional MDIs (30). The smaller the particle size of the drug nanocrystals, the higher the drug loading of the aerosol droplets (31,32). Therefore, the required nebulization time is distinctly reduced (33). Besides this, drug nanocrystals show an increased mucoadhesiveness, leading to a prolonged residence time at the mucosal surface of the lung.

Other Administration Routes

Dermal nanosuspensions are mainly of interest if conventional formulation approaches fail. The use of drug nanocrystals leads to an increased concentration gradient between the formulation and the skin. The increased saturation solubility leads to "supersaturated" formulations, enhancing the drug absorption through the skin. This effect can further be enhanced by the use of positively charged polymers as stabilizers for the drug nanocrystals. The opposite charge leads to an increased affinity of the drug nanocrystals to the negatively charged stratum corneum (unpublished data).

The ocular delivery of nanoparticles, including drug nanocrystals, is also of high interest. The development of such colloidal delivery systems for ophthalmic use aims at dropable dosage forms with a high drug loading and a long-lasting drug action. The adhesiveness of the small nanoparticles, which can be further increased by the use of mucoadhesive polymers, leads to a more consistent dosing. Blurred vision can be reduced by the use of submicron-sized drug particles (34,35).

PARTICLE SIZE REDUCTION TECHNIQUES

Nanoparticles Produced by Media Milling Processes

The use of media mills for the production of ultrafine particles is very common. From the first half of the twentieth century, ball mills were known for the production of ultrafine particle suspensions (36). In 1991, Liversidge et al. (37) have adapted this technique for the production of surface-modified drug nanoparticles. In order to produce nanocrystalline dispersions by the NanoCrystals® technology, a milling chamber is charged with milling media, dispersion medium (normally water), stabilizer, and the drug. The drug particles are reduced in size by shear forces and forces of impaction generated by a movement of the milling media. Small milling pearls or larger milling balls are used as milling media. With a reduction in the size of grinding media in a media mill, the number of contact points is increased exponentially, resulting in improved grinding and dispersing action (i.e., leading to smaller particles). The pearls or balls consist of ceramics (cerium- or yttrium-stabilized zirconium dioxide), stainless steel, glass, or highly cross-linked polystyrene resin-coated beads. A problem associated with the pearl milling technology is the erosion from the milling material during the milling process. Buchmann et al. (38) reported the formation of glass microparticles when using glass as milling material. In order to reduce the quantity of impurities caused by an erosion of the milling media, the milling beads were coated with highly cross-linked polystyrene resin (39). A perpetual problem is the adherence of product to the large inner surface area of the milling system. The inner surface area is made up of the surface area of the chamber and of all milling beads together. Even in recirculation systems, this product adherence causes a product loss. Of course, this undesirable drug loss can be an issue in very expensive drugs, especially when very small quantities of new chemical entities (NCEs) are processed.

In general, there are two milling principles: either the complete container is moved in a complex movement leading consequently to movement of the milling material or the milling medium is moved by an agitator. Assume that 76% of the milling chamber volume will be filled with milling material (larger batches are difficult to produce in a batch mode). In a 1000-L mill, this corresponds to 760-L milling material, based on the apparent density of zircon oxide pearls being 3.69 kg/L which corresponds to 2.8 tons of milling material. For that reason, agitator bead mills in recirculation mode are preferred for the production of larger batches. Figure 1 shows a cross-section of an agitator bead mill in a horizontal arrangement. The suspension is pumped vertically through the bead mill. In this case, the product is separated from the milling media by a dynamic separator gap. In other cases, separator cartridges are used. The recirculation mode prolongs the required milling time, because the residence time of the drug particles under impaction of shear forces is reduced. The milling time depends on many factors, such as hardness of the drug, surfactant content, temperature, viscosity of the dispersion medium, specific energy input, and size of the milling media. Milling periods from 30 minutes up to several days are reported (18). Milling equipment is now available from the labscale (41) to the large production scale. Besides other factors, this is an important prerequisite for the commercial production of nanocrystalline drugs. In 2000,

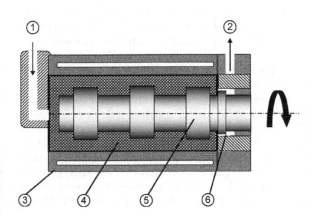

FIGURE 1 Agitator bead mill with dynamic separator gap (continuous mode): 1, product inlet; 2, product outlet; 3, cooling jacket; 4, milling pearls; 5, rotor with grinding disks; 6, dynamic separator gap. *Source:* From Ref. 40.

Rapamune® was launched by Wyeth as the first product containing sirolimus NanoCrystals®. The coated Rapamune® tablets are more convenient and show a 27% increased bioavailability compared to the Rapamune® solution (42). This is an example to compare two formulation strategies. The oral solution shows the principles of cosolvents and surfactants, whereas the tablets shows the nice performance of a particle size reduction technique. Emend® is the second product incorporating the NanoCrystal® technology. It was introduced to the market in 2003 by Merck. Emend® is a capsule containing pellets of nanocrystalline aprepitant, sucrose, microcrystalline cellulose, hyprolose, and sodium dodecylsulfate (43). The third product is TriCor, a nanocrystalline fenofibrate tablet marketed in 2004 by Abott. Megaace ES, an oral suspension containing megestrol acetate for the treatment of HIV-associated anorexia and cachexia, was launched as a fourth product late in the middle of the year 2005.

To sum up, the wet media milling is a viable particle size reduction technology. The performance has been proven by four FDA-approved products. But other nanonization technologies also can benefit from the success of the NanoCrystal® technology by the attraction of the size reduction principle in general.

Precipitation Methods

The classical precipitation process, known as "via humida paratum," is actually a very old pharmaceutical procedure. Later, this basic idea was applied for the production of nanocrystalline drug particles (44). The first application of the precipitation technique was developed by List and Sucker (10). It is known as hydrosol technology, and the IP is owned by Sandoz (now Novartis). A poor water-soluble drug is dissolved in an organic medium, which is water-miscible. A pouring of this solution into a nonsolvent, such as water, will cause a precipitation of finely dispersed drug nanocrystals. As simple as the particle formation process is, the preservation of the nanocrystalline particle size is difficult. The fine particles tend to grow up, driven by a phenomenon called "Ostwald ripening." This is a process where small particles are dissolved in favor of larger particles. Sucker (45) suggested immediate lyophilization to preserve the particle size.

The crystalline state of the particles obtained by the precipitation process can be controlled. Depending on the employed method, amorphous drug nanoparticles can also be generated (46). Beta-carotene is dissolved in a water-miscible organic solvent together with digestible oil. This solution is admixed to an aqueous solution of a protective colloid (gelatine) causing a precipitation of amorphous nanoparticulate beta-carotene. After an annealing step and spray-drying, a stable amorphous product can be obtained. This NanoMorph® technology, invented by Auweter et al., is used by the company Soliqs.

Another approach to preserve the size of the precipitated nanocrystals is the use of polymeric growth inhibitors, which are preferably soluble in the aqueous phase. The increased viscosity of the aqueous phase can reduce particle growing. The resulting suspension is subsequently spray-dried to obtain a dry powder with a relatively high drug loading (47). Using this technique, a tremendous increase in dissolution rate (from 4% to 93% within 20 minutes) was shown for a poor water-soluble drug ECU-01 (48). Although the feasibility of preparing drug nanocrystals by precipitation has been shown by many groups, no commercial drug product using this technology has entered the market. To use the prementioned methods, it is required that the drug is soluble in at least one water-miscible solvent. This is often not the case for NCEs. Many drugs are simultaneously poorly soluble in aqueous and nonaqueous media. Even if there is a suitable solvent available, it is difficult to remove this solvent completely. Solvent residues can be potential risk factors for drug alteration and toxic side effects. In addition, in cases of amorphous drug nanoparticles, it is seen as very critical to preserve the amorphous character throughout the shelf life of a product. Recrystallization would impair the oral bioavailability. This effect is less critical in food products because of less strict regulatory requirements that allow more tolerance.

Nanoparticles Produced by High-Pressure Homogenization

High-pressure homogenization is another universal approach to reduce the particle size of poorly soluble compounds. Considering the homogenization equipment and the homogenization conditions, it has to be divided between three technologies.

Microfluidizer Technology (IDD-P™ Technology)

Particles can be generated by a high shear process using jet-stream homogenizers, such as Microfluidizers (Microfluidizer®, Microfluidics, Inc.). A frontal collision of two fluid streams under pressures up to 1700 bar leads to particle collision, shear forces, and also cavitation forces. To preserve the particle size, stabilization with phospholipids or other surfactants and stabilizers is required. A major disadvantage of this process is the required production time. In many cases, 50 to 100 time-consuming passes are necessary for a sufficient particle size reduction (49,50). SkyePharma Canada, Inc. (previously RTP, Inc.) applies this principle for its IDD-P™ technology to produce submicron particles of poorly soluble drugs (51).

Piston-Gap Homogenization in Water (Dissocubes® Technology)

Drug nanocrystals can also be produced by high-pressure homogenization using piston gap homogenizers. Depending on the homogenization temperature and the dispersion media, there is a difference between the Dissocubes® technology and the Nanopure® technology. The Dissocubes® technology was developed by Müller et al. in 1994 (52) and later acquired by SkyePharma PLC. It involves the production of nanosuspensions in water at room temperature. The trade name Dissocubes® already indicates the improved dissolution behavior and the cubic shape of the resulting drug nanocrystals (53). A drug powder is dispersed in an aqueous surfactant solution. The resulting macrosuspension is subsequently forced by a piston through a tiny homogenization gap applying pressures up to 4000 bar.

Depending on the viscosity of the suspension and the homogenization pressure, the width of the homogenization gap is in the range of 5 to 20 µm (54). Figure 2 shows a cross-section through a piston-gap homogenizer. According to Bernoulli's law, the resulting high streaming velocity of the suspension causes an increase in dynamic pressure that is compensated by a reduction in static pressure below the vapor pressure of the aqueous phase. The water starts boiling and the formation of gas bubbles occurs. These gas bubbles collapse immediately when the liquid leaves the homogenization gap, resulting in cavitation-caused shock waves. The enormous power of these shock waves, turbulent flow, and shear forces break the drug particles (55).

The detailed illustration shows the principle of diminution mechanisms in the homogenization gap (Fig. 3). At the beginning, the particles are broken at crystal imperfections; with continuing the homogenization process, the number of

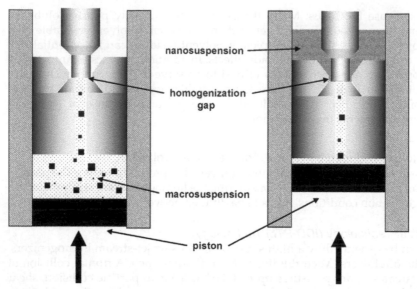

FIGURE 2 Cross-section of a piston-gap homogenizer. A macrosuspension is forced through a very tiny homogenization gap in order to produce drug nanocrystals. *Source*: From Ref. 40.

imperfections decreases and almost perfect small crystals will remain. The required number of cycles is mainly influenced by the hardness of the drug, the finesse of the starting material and the requirements of the application route or the final dosage form, respectively. In general, 10 to 20 homogenization cycles are sufficient to obtain a unimodal size distribution in the nanometer range (56–58).

The use of water as dispersion medium is associated with some disadvantages. Hydrolysis of water-sensitive drugs can occur, as well as problems during drying steps. In cases of thermolabile drugs or drugs possessing a low melting point, a complete water removal requires relatively expensive techniques, such as lyophilization. For these reasons, the Dissocubes® technology is particularly suitable if the resulting nanosuspension is directly used without modifications, such as drying steps.

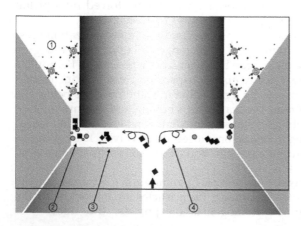

FIGURE 3 Diminution principles during high-pressure homogenization (detailed illustration of a homogenization gap in cross-section): 1, implosion area (cavitation); 2, boiling area and crystal collision; 3, shear forces; 4, turbulent flow. *Source*: From Ref. 40.

Nanopure® Technology
In 1999, Müller et al. (59) found that a similar effective particle diminution can also be obtained in nonaqueous or water-reduced media. The proprietary technique is known as Nanopure® technology developed and owned by PharmaSol GmbH/Berlin. By using dispersion media with a low-vapor pressure and performing the homogenization process at low temperatures (e.g., 0°C), the cavitation in the homogenization gap is distinctly reduced or does not exist at all. It could be shown that even in the absence of cavitation, a sufficient particle size diminution was obtained. The turbulent flow and shear forces during the homogenization process are strong enough to break the drug particles and to produce drug nanocrystals. The high-pressure homogenization in nonaqueous or water-reduced media is particularly beneficial if the nanosuspension has to be transferred into a traditional final dosage form. By reducing the water content in the dispersion medium, the required energy is minimized for drying steps, such as spray-drying, fluidized bed drying, or upon suspension layering onto sugar spheres. The evaporation processes can be performed under milder conditions, which is beneficial for temperature-sensitive drugs. Production of nanosuspensions at 0°C or even below can prevent temperature labile drugs from degradation (15). If the high-pressure homogenization is carried out completely in nonaqueous media, even water-sensitive drugs can be processed without hydrolysis. Nanosuspensions produced in liquid polyethylene glycol (PEG) or hot-melted PEGs can be directly filled into gelatine or hydroxy propyl methyl cellulose (HPMC) capsules (60). Depending on the requirements of the final formulation, the water content can be varied from water-free to isotonic conditions for intravenous suspensions.

Irrespective of the employed technique (Dissocubes® or Nanopure®), the production of drug nanocrystals by high-pressure homogenization is a production-friendly process. Homogenization is a low-cost process; approved production lines are already in use for the production of pharmaceutical products, such as emulsions for parenteral nutrition (12). The process can be easily transferred from the labscale to the large production scale. High-pressure homogenization can be performed starting from 0.5 mL (Avestin EmulsiFlex-B3, Avestin, Inc., Canada) up to large batch sizes of 2000 L/hr (Rannie 118, APV homogenisers, Denmark) (26,61).

When producing nanosuspenions by high-pressure homogenization even at hard homogenization conditions, only a noncritical product contamination below 1 ppm was observed (62). Suspensions with drug concentration up to 30% and more can be easily processed by high-pressure homogenization (63).

Combination Technologies
Nanoedge® Technology
Baxter's NANOEDGE® process relies on the combination of a microprecipitation technique with a subsequent annealing step by applying high shear and/or thermal energy (64). A fine suspension is formed by adding an organic solution of the water-insoluble drug to an antisolvent, for example, aqueous surfactant solution. Depending on the precipitation conditions, either small amorphous or crystalline drug particles in the nanometer range or friable needle-like crystals in the micrometer range are formed. Consequently, the following high-energy input can have two effects on the preformed particles. Small amorphous or crystalline drug particles will be preserved in size by an annealing step without changing the mean diameter. It could be shown that the tendency to crystal growth can be reduced by energy input after the precipitation step. In case long friable needle-like crystals are obtained, they will be reduced in size by the high-energy input using high-pressure

homogenizers. According to the patent (64), particle sizes in the range of 400 to 2000 nm can be obtained. The organic solvent utilized has to be carefully removed from the final nanosuspension without changing the particle size of the drug nanocrystals. Otherwise, crystal growth can be promoted by an increased solubility of the drug. Any content of the organic solvent dissolved in the aqueous phase can act as a "cosolvent," leading to an increased tendency to Ostwald ripening. Also, toxic effects can be caused by potential solvent residues, especially if the nanosuspension is the final product. For these reasons, the NANOEDGE® process is particularly suitable for drugs that are soluble in nonaqueous media possessing low toxicity, such as N-methyl-2-pyrrolidinone.

Nanopure® XP Technology

Considering the commonly used particle size reduction techniques, the production of nanosuspensions is in most cases associated with a high-energy input (high-speed media mills, high-pressure homogenization) and a relatively long period between the drug synthesis and the final product. A micronized drug material (size 10–100 µm) is recommended for milling and high-pressure homogenization processes (37,55). Therefore, the drug often has to be jet-milled before the nanonization. Impurities caused by an abrasion from the milling material or solvent residues from the precipitation process are undesirable. They can causes side effects especially if the drug is administered for the treatment of chronic diseases. The minimal achievable particle size is significantly determined by the hardness of the drug. In cases of very hard drugs, an increasing energy input (by extending the milling time or the number of homogenization cycles) will not lead to a smaller particle size. In general, the smallest achievable size of nanocrystals is around 200 nm; only under special conditions can about 100 nm be produced. However, especially crystals below 100 nm would show an extremely fast dissolution and simultaneously a great increase in saturation solubility (11). Therefore, such particles are of high commercial interest.

In 2005, Möschwitzer (65) developed a new combination method for the production of drug nanosuspensions, which is now owned by PharmaSol GmbH. The Nanopure® XP technologogy (process variant: H42) enables extension of the performance of the Nanopure® technology to very hard and crystalline materials. Modification of the starting material by an evaporation process before the subsequently performed high-pressure homogenization can significantly reduce the number of homogenization cycles (66). Owing to the reason that the solvent will be removed completely before homogenization by the evaporation process, various solvents can be used for the modification process without restrictions due to toxicity reasons. Additionally, excipients can be added to the drug solution to increase the number of crystal imperfections upon drying. Figure 4 makes clear the effectiveness of the new combination method in comparison to the classical high-pressure homogenization. The application of the H42 technology leads to distinctly reduced particle size by a simultaneous reduction of the required number on homogenization cycles. This will consequently reduce the production costs and the wear on the homogenization equipment.

H96 is another technology belonging to the Nanopure® XP platform. The technology, developed in 2005 by Möschwitzer and Lemke (67), is a modified process based on high-pressure homogenization. By using this undisclosed technology, it was shown that drug nanocrystals below 100 nm can be produced by high-pressure homogenization.

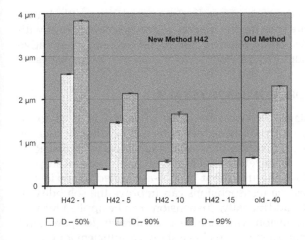

FIGURE 4 Comparison of the new homogenization technology H42 (*left*) with the conventional homogenization in water (*right*), performed in piston-gap homogenizer, influence of cycle numbers, results represent the laser diffractometry diameters (volume-weighted, Coulter Ls 230, Beckman-Coulter, Germany). *Source*: From Ref. 40.

H96 results in a translucent nanosuspension in comparison to another nano-suspension produced using the Dissocubes® technology. Figure 5 shows two nano-suspensions. The left nanosuspension was produced applying the conventional high-pressure homogenization in water; the right nanosuspension was produced by using the H96 technology. Although both formulations are being composed similarly, the right formulation is translucent due to the significantly reduced particle size. The particle size analysis also provides the evidence of the performance of the H96 method. Almost 99% of the particles were smaller than 100 nm [laser diffractometry (LD) D99%, volume size distribution, LS 230, Beckman-Coulter, Germany unpublished data with permission from Ref. 40]. A very small particle size and a narrow range of particle size distribution can be obtained by using the H96 technology.

Other Techniques for the Production of Drug Nanocrystals

Milling, high-pressure homogenization, and precipitation are the main methods employed for the production of drug nanocrystals. The importance for improvement of the bioavailability of poorly soluble drugs by the production of drug nanocrystals is widely accepted. The intensive research for new technologies led to many other

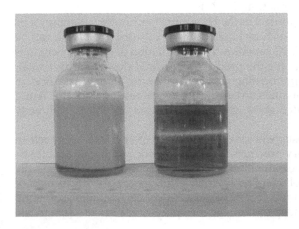

FIGURE 5 (*See color insert.*) Two nanosuspensions composed similarly, produced by high-pressure homogenization, conventional method (*left*) versus translucent nanosuspension (particle size well below 100 nm) resulting from H96 technology. The red laser beam is reflected by the tiny nanocrystals. *Source*: From Ref. 40.

approaches for the production of drug nanocrystals. Even nonpharmaceutical companies, such as Dow Chemical, are entering the market of poorly soluble drugs with solubility-enhancing technologies. Spray-freezing into liquid (68) and evaporative precipitation into aqueous solutions (69) are examples for such new technologies.

FINAL FORMULATIONS FOR DRUG NANOCRYSTALS

In order to show their advantages in vivo, the drug nanocrystals need to be transferred into the right dosage form. Nanosuspensions can be directly used as oral suspensions to overcome the difficulties of swallowing tablets by pediatric or geriatric patients. One example is Megace® (Bristol Meyers Squibb), an oral suspension of megestrol acetate, used for the treatment of HIV-associated anorexia and cachexia. The application of these nanosuspensions can improve the solubility of the drug and the dissolution rate; additionally, suspensions can be applied for reasons of taste-masking. Nanosuspensions can also be used directly for parenteral drug administration. Although nanosuspensions have shown a sufficient long-term stability without Ostwald ripening, for intravenous products a lyophilization step is recommended in order to avoid aggregation or caking of settled drug nanocrystals. The lyophilized product can be easily reconstituted before use by adding isotonic water, aqueous glucose solution, or other reconstitution media (27,70).

Without question, both the patients and the marketing experts prefer the oral administration of traditional dosage forms. Hence, to enter the pharmaceutical market successfully in most cases drug nanocrystals have to be formulated as traditional products, such as tablets or capsules. A perfect solid dosage form should preserve the in vivo performance of drug nanocrystals. When reaching the target part of the GI tract, the dosage form should release the drug nanocrystals as a fine, nonaggregated suspension. Otherwise, self-agglomeration or aggregation can impair the drug release (71).

Using nanosuspensions as granulation fluid for a further tablet production is a very simple approach. The nanosuspension is admixed to binders and other excipients, and the granules are finely compressed to tablets. This dosage form is limited in the maximum achievable drug content. A maximum drug content of about 50% or less is suggested in order to ensure a complete disintegration into a finely dispersed suspension (72). Nanosuspensions can also be used for the production of matrix pellets (Fig. 6) or as layering dispersions in a fluidized bed process. After the pellet preparation, the cores can be coated with several polymers in order to modify the release profile of the final formulation (73–75).

A very smart formulation approach is the Nanopure® technology. Nanocrystals produced in nonaqueous media, such as liquid PEG or oils (e.g., Miglyol), can be directly filled into gelatine or HPMC capsules. The production of drug nanocrystals in melted PEGs is a new strategy for the production of final dosage forms containing drug nanocrystals. After performing the high-pressure homogenization in melted PEG at about 60°C, the mixture can be solidified. The resulting matrix, fixing the drug nanocrystals in separated state, can be compressed to tablets or directly filled into capsules (76).

Spray-drying of the nanosuspensions is another cost-effective approach to transfer nanosuspensions into dry products. The drug nanocrystals can directly be produced by high-pressure homogenization in aqueous solutions of water-soluble matrix materials, for example, polymers [polyvinylpyrrolidone, polyvinylalcohol or long-chained PEG, sugars (saccharose, lactose) or sugar alcohols (mannitol, sorbitol)]. Afterwards, the resulting nanosuspension can be spray-dried under appropriate

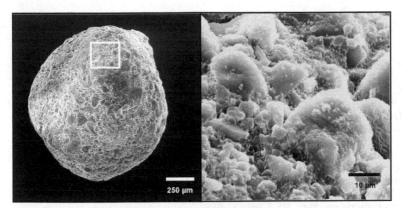

FIGURE 6 SEM photograph of uncoated matrix core containing drug nanocrystals: (*left*) overview (magnification 60×), (*right*) detailed magnification (1000×) showing drug nanocrystals combined with the binder material.

conditions. The dry powder, composed of drug nanocrystals embedded in a water-soluble matrix, can be filled in hard gelatine capsules for oral administration (77).

Another attractive approach using the spray-drying principle is described as "direct compress technology" (78). Lactose and other matrix-forming materials, such as micronized polymer powders or lipids, are admixed to the prior-produced nanosuspension. The resulting suspension is transferred into a drug–matrix–compound by spray-drying. Subsequently, the free-flowable powder can be used for direct compression of fast dissolving or prolonged release tablets. Alternatively, the powder can also be filled into hard gelatine capsules.

CONCLUSION

Poor aqueous solubility is clearly recognized by the pharmaceutical industry as a major problem. The use of drug nanocrystals is a universal formulation approach to increase the therapeutic performance of these drugs in any route of administration. Almost any drug can be reduced in size to the nanometer range. Owing to their great formulation versatility drug nanocrystals are no longer only the last chance rescue for a few drugs. Many insoluble drug candidates are in clinical trials formulated as drug nanocrystals (at present about 10).

Various nanonization techniques are available. Production facilities are available to produce tons of nanosuspensions. Currently, attention is turned to improving the diminution performance to produce drug nanocrystals well below 100 nm, also in cases of very hard drugs. First approaches were already successful. New technologies are in development to produce final dosage forms with higher drug loadings, better redispersability at their site of action, and an improved drug targeting.

REFERENCES

1. Merisko-Liversidge E. Nanocrystals: resolving pharmaceutical formulation issues associated with poorly water-soluble compounds in particles. Orlando: Marcel Dekker, 2002.
2. Lipinski C. Poor aqueous solubility—an industry wide problem in drug delivery. Am Pharm Rev 2002; 5:82–85.
3. FDA. Waiver of in vivo bioavailability and bioequivalence studies for immediate-release solid oral dosage forms based on a biopharmaceutics classification system. FDA, 2000.

4. Kanfer I. Report on the international workshop on the biopharmaceutics classification system (BCS): scientific and regulatory aspects in practice. J Pharm Pharm Sci 2002; 5(1):1–4.
5. Gupta PK, Patel JP, Hahn KR. Evaluation of pain and irritation following local administration of parenteral formulations using the rat paw lick model. J Pharm Sci Technol 1994; 48(3):159–166.
6. Singla AK, Garg A, Aggarwal D. Paclitaxel and its formulations. Int J Pharm 2002; 235(1–2):179–192.
7. Mattila MA, Suistomaa M. Intravenous premedication with diazepam: a comparison between two vehicles. Anaesthesia 1984; 39(9):879–882.
8. Uekama K. Design and evaluation of cyclodextrin-based drug formulation. Chem Pharm Bull (Tokyo) 2004; 52(8):900–915.
9. Müller RH, Peters K, Becker R, Kruss B. Nanosuspensions: a novel formulation for the i.v. administration of poorly soluble drugs. First World Meeting APGI/APV, Budapest, 1995.
10. List M, Sucker H. Hydrosols of pharmacologically active agents and their pharmaceutical compositions comprising them. US 5,389,382, 1991.
11. Kipp JE. The role of solid nanoparticle technology in the parenteral delivery of poorly water-soluble drugs. Int J Pharm 2004; 284(1–2):109–122.
12. Müller RH, Böhm BHL. Nanosuspensions. In: Müller RH, Benita S, Böhm B, eds. Emulsions and Nanosuspensions for the Formulation of Poorly Soluble Drugs. Stuttgart: Medpharm, 1998:149–174.
13. Troester F. Cremophor-free aqueous paclitaxel nanosuspension—production and chemical stability. Controlled Release Society 31st annual meeting, Honolulu, HI, 2004.
14. Liversidge E, Wei L. Stabilization of chemical compounds using nanoparticulate formulations. US 2001;952032 20010914. CAN 138:243327, US 2003054042 A1, 2003.
15. Möschwitzer J, Achleitner G, Pomper H, Muller RH. Development of an intravenously injectable chemically stable aqueous omeprazole formulation using nanosuspension technology. Eur J Pharm Biopharm 2004; 58(3):615–619.
16. Müller RH, Keck CM. Challenges and solutions for the delivery of biotech drugs—a review of drug nanocrystal technology and lipid nanoparticles. J Biotechnol 2004; 113(1–3):151–170.
17. Liversidge GG, Cundy KC. Particle size reduction for improvement of oral bioavailability of hydrophobic drugs. I Absolute oral bioavailability of nanocrystalline danazol in beagle dogs. Int J Pharm 1995; 125:91–97.
18. Merisko-Liversidge E, Liversidge GG, Cooper ER. Nanosizing: a formulation approach for poorly water-soluble compounds. Eur J Pharm Sci 2003; 18(2):113–120.
19. Liversidge GG, Conzentino, Phil. Drug particle size reduction for decreasing gastric irritancy and enhancing absorption of naproxen in rats. Int J Pharm 1995; 125:309–313.
20. Eickhoff WM, Engers DA, Mueller KR. Nanoparticulate NSAID compositions, Application. US 95-385614, 5518738, 1996.
21. Jacobs C, Kayser O, Müller RH. Production and characterisation of mucoadhesive nanosuspensions for the formulation of bupravaquone. Int J Pharm 2001; 214(1–2):3–7.
22. Müller RH, Jacobs C. Buparvaquone mucoadhesive nanosuspension: preparation, optimisation and long-term stability. Int J Pharm 2002; 237(1–2):151–161.
23. Lamprecht A, Ubrich N, Yamamoto H, et al. Biodegradable nanoparticles for targeted drug delivery in treatment of inflammatory bowel disease. J Pharmacol Exp Ther 2001; 299(2):775–781.
24. Hussain N, Jaitley V, Florence AT. Recent advances in the understanding of uptake of microparticulates across the gastrointestinal lymphatics. Adv Drug Deliv Rev 2001; 50(1–2):107–142.
25. Na GC, Stevens Jr J, Yuan BO, Rajagopalan N. Physical stability of ethyl diatrizoate nanocrystalline suspension in steam sterilization. Pharm Res 1999; 16(4):569–574.
26. Müller RH, Jacobs C, Kayser O. Nanosuspensions for the formulation of poorly soluble drugs. In: Nielloud F, Marti-Mestres G, eds. Pharmaceutical Emulsions and Suspensions. New York: Marcel Dekker, 2000:383–407.
27. Böhm B. Production and characterisation of nanosuspensions as novel delivery system for drugs with low bioavailability. In: Pharmaceutical Technology. Berlin: Free University of Berlin, 1999.
28. Peters K et al. Preparation of a clofazimine nanosuspension for intravenous use and evaluation of its therapeutic efficacy in murine Mycobacterium avium infection. J Antimicrob Chemother 2000; 45(1):77–83.

29. Scholer N et al. Atovaquone nanosuspensions show excellent therapeutic effect in a new murine model of reactivated toxoplasmosis. Antimicrob Agents Chemother 2001; 45(6):1771–1779.

30. Ostrander KD, Bosch HW, Bondanza DM. An in vitro assessment of a NanoCrystal beclomethasone dipropionate colloidal dispersion via ultrasonic nebulization. Eur J Pharm Biopharm 1999; 48(3): 207–215.

31. Jacobs C, Müller RH. Production and characterization of a budesonide nanosuspension for pulmonary administration. Pharm Res 2002; 19(2):189–194.

32. Wiedmann TS, DeCastro L, Wood RW. Nebulization of NanoCrystals: production of a respirable solid-in-liquid-in-air colloidal dispersion. Pharm Res 1997; 14(1):112–116.

33. Kraft WK et al. The pharmacokinetics of nebulized nanocrystal budesonide suspension in healthy volunteers. J Clin Pharmacol 2004; 44(1):67–72.

34. Mainardes RM et al. Colloidal carriers for ophthalmic drug delivery. Curr Drug Targets 2005; 6(3):363–371.

35. Keipert S. Ophtalmika: etablierte Arzneiformen und neue Konzepte. In: Müller RH, Hildebrand GE, eds. Pharmazeutische Technologie: Moderne Arzneiformen. Stuttgart: Wissenschaftliche Verlagsgesellschaft mbH, 1998:77–98.

36. Pahl MH. Zerkleinerungstechnik. Praxiswissen Verfahrenstechnik. Köln: TÜV Rheinland GmbH, 1991.

37. Liversidge GG, Cundy KC, Bishop JF, Czekai DA. Surface Modified Drug Nanoparticles. USA, 1992.

38. Buchmann S, Fischli W, Thiel FP, Alex R. Aqueous microsuspension, an alternative intra-venous formulation for animal studies. In: 42nd annual congress of the International Association for Pharmaceutical Technology (APV), Mainz, 1996.

39. Bruno JAD, Brian D. Gustow Evan, Illig, Kathleen J, Rajagopalan, Nats, Sarpotdar. Method of grinding pharmaceutical substances. US 5,518,187, 1992.

40. Möschwitzer J. Pharmaceutical Technology. Ph.D. Thesis. Berlin, Free University of Berlin. In preparation.

41. Cunningham JL, Elaine, Cooper, Eugene R, Liversidge, Gary G. Milling microgram quantities of nanoparticulate candidate compounds. US 20040173696, 2004.

42. Wyeth Research Drug Information, Rapamune (Sirolumus) Oral Solutions and Tablets. Company Communications, 2004.

43. Merck, Drug Information Emend. 2004.

44. Violanto MR. Method for making uniformly sized particles from water-insoluble organic compounds. US 4,826,689, 1989.

45. Sucker H. Hydrosole, eine Alternative für die parenterale Anwendung von schwer was-serlöslichen Wirkstoffen. In: Müller RH, Hildebrand GE, eds. Pharmazeutische Technologie: Moderne Arzneiformen. Stuttgart: Wissenschaftliche Verlagsgesellschaft mbH, 1998:383–391.

46. Auweter H, Bohn H. Luddecke E. Stable, aqueous dispersions and stable, water-disper-sible dry powders of xanthophylls, their production and their use, Application. WO 2000-EP3467, 2000066665, 2000.

47. Mueller BW, Rasenack, Norbert. Method for the production and the use of microparticles and nano-particles by constructive micronisation. WO 002003080034A3, 2003.

48. Rasenack N, Hartenhauer H, Müller BW. Microcrystals for dissolution rate enhancement of poorly water-soluble drugs. Int J Pharm 2003; 254(2):137–145.

49. Parikh IS, Ulagaraj. Composition and method of preparing microparticles of water-insoluble substances. 93969997, 1997.

50. Dearn AR. Atovaquone pharmaceutical compositions. US, 974248, 6,018,080, 2000.

51. Haynes DH. Phospholipid-coated microcrystals: injectable formulations of water-insoluble drugs. US 5,091,187, 1992.

52. Müller RHB, Robert, Kruss, Bernd, Peters, Katrin. Pharmazeutische Nanosuspensionen zur Arzneistoffapplikation als Systeme mit erhöhter Sättigungslöslichkeit und Lösungsgeschwindigkeit.

53. Müller RHJCK O. DissoCubes—a novel formulation for poorly soluble and poorly bioavailable drugs, In: Roberts MJRJHMS, ed. Modified-Release Drug Delivery Technology. New York: Marcel Dekker, 2003:135–149.

54. Müller RH, Möschwitzer J, Bushrab FN. Manufacturing of nanoparticles by milling and homogenisation techniques. In: Kompella G, ed. Nanoparticle Technology for Drug Delivery. New York: Marcel Dekker. Submitted.

55. Müller RH, Jacobs C, Kayser O. Nanosuspensions as particulate drug formulations in therapy: rationale for development and what we can expect for the future. Adv Drug Deliv Rev 2001; 47(1):3–19.
56. Grau MJ, Kayser O, Müller RH. Nanosuspensions of poorly soluble drugs—reproducibility of small scale production. Int J Pharm 2000; 196(2):155–159.
57. Müller RH, Peters K. Nanosuspensions for the formulation of poorly soluble drugs. I. Preparation by a size-reduction technique. Int J Pharm 1998; 160(2):229–237.
58. Müller RH, Böhm BHL, Grau MJ. Nanosuspensions—a formulation approach for poorly soluble and poorly bioavailable drugs. In: Wise DL, ed. Handbook of Pharmaceutical Controlled Release. New York: Marcel Dekker, 2000:345–357.
59. Müller RH, Krause K, Mader K. Method for controlled production of ultrafine microparticles and nanoparticles, Application. WO 2000-EP6535, 2001003670, 2001.
60. Bushrab FN, Müller RH. Drug nanocrystals: Amphotericin B-containing capsules for oral delivery. Philadelphia: AAPS, 2004.
61. Liedtke S et al. Influence of high pressure homogenisation equipment on nanodispersions characteristics. Int J Pharm 2000; 196(2):183–185.
62. Krause KP et al. Heavy metal contamination of nanosuspensions produced by high-pressure homogenisation. Int J Pharm 2000; 196(2):169–172.
63. Krause KP, Müller RH. Production and characterisation of highly concentrated nanosuspensions by high pressure homogenisation. Int J Pharm 2001; 214(1–2):21–24.
64. Kipp JEW, Joseph Chung Tak, Doty, Mark J, Rebbeck, Christine L. Microprecipitation method for preparing submicron suspensions. US 6,869,617, 2001.
65. Möschwitzer. Method for the production of ultra-fine submicron suspensions. DE 10 2005 011 786.4, 2005.
66. Müller RH, Möschwitzer J. Oral drug nanocrystal fomulations based on non-aqueous/water-reduced homogenization technology. In: Annual meeting of the Controlled Release Society, Miami, 2005.
67. Möschwitzer JP, Lemke A. Method for the gentle production of ultrafine particle suspensions, Germany. DE 10 2005 017 777.8, 2005.
68. Hu J, Johnston KP, Williams RO III. Spray freezing into liquid (SFL) particle engineering technology to enhance dissolution of poorly water soluble drugs: organic solvent versus organic/aqueous co-solvent systems. Eur J Pharm Sci 2003; 20(3):295–303.
69. Chen X et al. Preparation of cyclosporine as nanoparticles by evaporative precipitation into aqueous solution. Int J Pharm 2002; 242(1–2):3–14.
70. Grau M. Investigation of dissolution velocity, saturation solubility and stability of ultrafine drug suspensions. Dissertation. Pharmazeutische Technologie. Berlin: Free University of Berlin, 2000.
71. Stewart PJ, Zhao FY. Understanding agglomeration of indomethacin during the dissolution of micronised indomethacin mixtures through dissolution and de-agglomeration modeling approaches. Eur J Pharm Biopharm 2005; 59(2):315–323.
72. Kirkof N. Creation and characterization of Nanoparticles. In: 32nd annual meeting and exposition of the Controlled Release Society, Miami, 2005.
73. Möschwitzer J, Müller RH. From the drug nanocrystal to the final mucoadhesive oral dosage form, 2004.
74. Möschwitzer J, Müller RH. Spray coated pellets as carrier system for mucoadhesive drug nanocrystals. Eur J Pharm Biopharm. Submitted.
75. Möschwitzer J, Müller RH. Controlled drug delivery system for oral application of drug nanocrystals. In: 2004 AAPS annual meeting and exposition, Baltimore, MD, 2004.
76. Bushrab NF, Müller RH. Nanocrystals of poorly soluble drugs for oral administration. NewDrugs 2003; 5:20–22.
77. Bushrab FN, Müller RH. Drug nanocrystals for oral delivery—compounds by spray drying. Philadelphia: AAPS, 2004.
78. Müller RH. Preparation of a matrix material—excipient compound containing a drug. WO 1997-EP6893, WO 9825590, 1998.

6 Lipid-Based Nanoparticulate Drug Delivery Systems

Jun Wu and Xiaobin Zhao
Division of Pharmaceutics, College of Pharmacy, The Ohio State University, Columbus, Ohio, U.S.A.

Robert J. Lee
Division of Pharmaceutics, College of Pharmacy, NCI Comprehensive Cancer Center, NSF Nanoscale Science Engineering Center for Affordable Nanoengineering of Polymeric Biomedical Devices, The Ohio State University, Columbus, Ohio, U.S.A.

INTRODUCTION

Phospholipids, upon hydration, spontaneously form bilayer membrane vesicles (liposomes) or may act as surfactants in forming micro- or nanoemulsions or solid–lipid nanoparticles. Phospholipids, triglycerides, and cholesterol are the main ingredients of liposomes and lipid nanoparticles. They are natural components of biological membranes and lipoproteins and are, therefore, presumed to be highly biocompatible (1). Drugs and cell-targeting ligands can be incorporated into these structures by encapsulation (for hydrophilic molecules), lipid-phase solubilization (for lipophilic molecules), conjugation to a lipid anchor (as a lipid-derivatized pro-drug), or electrostatic complexation (for poly-anionic molecules such as nucleic acids), depending on their specific physicochemical properties. Liposomes and lipid nanoparticles smaller than 300 nm are potentially suitable for systemic administration. In this chapter, various aspects of these nanoparticulate systems are discussed in the context of drug delivery.

LIPOSOMES

Liposomes are phospholipid bilayers with an entrapped aqueous volume. On the basis of the number of layers (lamellarity) and diameter, liposomes are classified into multilamellar vesicles (MLVs, diameter >200 nm), large unilamellar vesicles (diameter 100–400 nm), and small unilamellar vesicles (diameter <100 nm). On the basis of surface charge (zeta potential), they are classified into cationic, neutral, and anionic liposomes. In addition, liposomes can be deliberately engineered to possess unique properties, such as long systemic circulation time, target cell specificity, pH and reductive environmental sensitivity, and temperature sensitivity. These are achieved by selecting the appropriate lipid composition and surface modification for the liposomes.

METHODS OF LIPOSOME PREPARATION AND CHARACTERIZATION

Liposomes form spontaneously when phospholipids are hydrated. Additional steps are often necessary to modify the size distribution and lamellarity of liposomes. Several methods have been established for liposome preparation based on the scale of the preparation and other considerations, such as drug encapsulation efficiency. The first step in liposome preparation is to dissolve lipid ingredients in a suitable solvent; this is then followed by lipid hydration and particle size reduction. For example, lipids are first dissolved in chloroform/methanol and dried into a thin film on a rotary evaporator and are then hydrated in an aqueous buffer above the phase-transition temperature (2). This process will result in the formation of heterogeneous MLVs. The lamellarity of the MLVs can be reduced by repeated cycles of freezing and thawing. If phospholipids are dissolved in a water-miscible solvent such as ethanol and rapidly diluted into an aqueous buffer, liposomes with relative small particle sizes can be generated directly. This is then followed by removal of the solvent from the liposome preparation and/or further size-modifying steps (3).

Particle size can then be reduced by a number of methods, including sonication, extrusion, and homogenization. Sonication, typically using an ultrasonic probe sonicator, can reduce liposome particle size by inducing cavitation (4). Extrusion is performed using a high-pressure filter unit, such as the Lipex™ extruder by Northern Lipids, Inc., containing a track-etched polycarbonate membrane at a temperature above the phase-transition temperature of the liposomal bilayer (5). The polycarbonate membrane has straight through cylindrical pores of precise diameters and can withstand pressure of 3000 psi with proper support. Liposomes extruded through the polycarbonate membranes typically have narrow particle size distribution. Large-scale production of liposomes is possible using the extrusion method employing high-surface-area extrusion filter units. Another potentially scalable method for liposome particle size reduction is high-pressure homogenization usually at pressures above 5000 psi (2). This method can be used for continuous production of liposomes or nanoparticles at large scale. In the labscale, liposomes can be synthesized by detergent dialysis in which lipids are first solubilized in a dialyzable detergent, such as octylglucoside and then dialyzed against a buffer (6). Alternatively, reversed-phase evaporation method may be used to form a water-in-oil emulsion in a volatile organic solvent followed by phase inversion upon solvent removal. This method was designed to maximize entrapment efficiency of water-soluble agents (7).

Methods suitable for drug loading into liposomes depend on the properties of the drug. Lipophilic drugs can be codissolved with the lipids during liposome preparation. Hydrophilic drugs can be passively entrapped into liposomes during liposome formation. Alternatively, drugs can be incorporated into liposomes by a pH gradient-driven remote loading procedure. For example, an inward-directed pH gradient could be established by entrapment of a low pH buffer (e.g., pH 4 sodium citrate) or by entrapping ammonium sulfate followed by external buffer exchange resulting in reduction of intraliposomal pH. Addition of a weakly basic drug, such as doxorubicin and vincristine, results in near-quantitative loading of the drug into the liposomes due to intraliposomal protonation of the drug molecules and complexation with entrapped counterion (8,9). For polyelectrolytes such as DNA, loading into liposomes can be achieved by electrostatic complexation with incorporation of cationic lipids into the liposome composition (10,11). Structure of DNA complexes of cationic liposomes may not be similar to the structure of typical liposomes and is highly dependent on lipid head group structure, cationic-to-anionic charge ratio, and kinetics of complex formation (12).

Liposomes can be purified by a number of methods. At the labscale, liposomes can be purified based on their size by high-speed centrifugation, size exclusion chromatography, or dialysis (3). At a larger scale, liposomes can be purified by tangential flow diafiltration (13). Liposomes can also be lyophilized in the presence of a cryoprotectant, typically a disaccharide such as sucrose, lactose, or trehalose, which can prevent vesicle fusion and particle size increase, although significant leakage of aqueous content may occur upon rehydration of the liposomes (14).

A liposomal formulation can be characterized by a number of established methods. First, particle size distribution can be measured by dynamic light scattering, by cryo- or negative-staining electron microscopy, or by atomic force microscopy. Surface electrical property of liposomes can be measured by zeta potential measurement. Other useful analyses include colloidal stability and rate of drug release in storage and in plasma by dialysis, kinetics of uptake, and internalization of fluorescence labeled liposomes in cultured cells by fluorescence microscopy and flow cytometry. Cytotoxicity of drug-carrying and empty liposomes can be studied in tissue culture. Furthermore, plasma clearance kinetics, tissue biodistribution, toxicity, and therapeutic efficacy of drug-carrying liposomes can be assessed in appropriate animal models.

LIPOSOMES AS DRUG CARRIERS

The application of liposomes as a drug-delivery system has become more popular over the last decades, because of their biocompatibility and versatility in carrying systemically administered drugs such as chemotherapeutics and antibiotics with narrow therapeutic windows. A variety of therapeutic agents have been incorporated into liposomes. Several have reached clinical use. These include liposomal doxorubicin (15) (Doxil™), daunorubicin (16) (Daunoxome™), amphotericin B (17) (Amphotec™, Ambisome™, and Abelcet™), cytarabine (18) (Depocyte™), and verteporfin (19) (Visudyne™). Numerous liposomal formulations are in clinical trial, including those for vincristine, all-*trans* retinoic acid, topotecan, and cationic liposome-based therapeutic gene transfer vectors. Many more are in preclinical evaluation including liposomal formulations of chemotherapeutics, neutron capture agents, oligonucleotides, plasmid DNA, photosensitizers, antibiotics, and vaccines (20). Besides potential use in systemic gene delivery, cationic liposomes are routinely used as transfection reagents for plasmid DNA and oligonucleotides in the laboratory.

Liposomal delivery of anticancer drugs has been shown to greatly extend their systemic circulation time, reduce toxicity by lowering plasma free drug concentration, and facilitate preferential localization of drugs in solid tumors based on increased endothelial permeability and reduced lymphatic drainage, or enhanced permeability and retention (EPR) effect (21–23). For example, liposomal entrapment of doxorubicin greatly reduces its dose-limiting cardiotoxicity. Clearance of drugs in a liposomal formulation is mediated by phagocytic cells of the reticuloendothelial system (RES), primarily located in liver and spleen. Liposomal entrapment can protect drugs such as nucleic acids from rapid metabolism by plasma enzymes (24). In addition, liposomal delivery of drugs appears to mediate bypassing of P glycoprotein (Pgp)-related multidrug resistance in tumor cells. Liposomes also present a platform for delivery of drug combinations. For example, Wang et al. (25) coencapsulated doxorubicin and verapamil (a Pgp inhibitor) into liposomes and studied their in vitro cytotoxicity. The result demonstrated effective reversal of multidrug resistance in doxorubicin-resistant cell lines.

FORMULATION STRATEGIES FOR LIPOSOMES
Lipid Composition for Increased Stability In Vivo

As drug permeability over the lipid bilayer is reduced in the "gel" state compared to "fluid" state, stability of liposomal entrapment can be maximized by selecting high-phase-transition phospholipids, for example, phosphatidylcholines (PCs) with long and saturated fatty acyl chains, such as distearoyl PC and hydrogenated soy PC, which remain in a gel state at physiological temperature. Addition of 30 to 50 mol% of cholesterol can further improve stability of the lipid bilayers by filling in gaps between PC molecules. Having a tight bilayer also reduces insertion of plasma proteins and reduces RES clearance of the liposomes.

Sterically Stabilized Liposomes

RES clearance of liposomes is mediated by adsorption of plasma proteins to the bilayer surface. Incorporation of 3 to 10 mol% of polyethylene glycol (PEG)-conjugated lipid, such as monomethoxy-PEG (molecular weight 2000)–distearoyl phosphatidylethanolamine (mPEG$_{2000}$–DSPE) has been shown to greatly extend the circulation time of liposomes by providing steric hindrance on the bilayer surface (21,22). PEGylated liposomes exhibit circulation half-life of up to two days compared to several hours for non-PEGylated liposomes. The prolongation in mean residence time of PEGylated liposomes is due to slower clearance of these liposomes by RES organs (26). This can, in addition, increase EPR effect-mediated tumor localization and antitumor therapeutic efficacy.

pH-Sensitive Liposomes

Although high stability of liposomes prior to reaching the cellular target is generally desirable, efficient release of liposomal drug in the target tissue and/or cell is essential for its therapeutic activity. Environmentally sensitive liposomes are designed to take advantage of the differences in the microenvironment of a solid tumor or inside the cell and to undergo destabilization on reaching their target. pH-sensitive liposomes are designed to destabilize at mildly acidic pH found in solid tumors and in endosomal compartments. These are typically composed of dioleoyl phosphatidylethanolamine (DOPE), which has a cone-shaped geometry that favors transition from bilayer to H$_{II}$ phase, and a weakly acidic amphiphile, such as oleic acid or cholesteryl hemisuccinate, which stabilizes the bilayer structure at neutral pH but not at mildly acidic pH (27–29). pH-sensitive liposomes have been shown to be much more effective in facilitating endosomal release of membrane-impermeable drugs from internalized liposomes in cells. Other nonbilayer-favoring lipids, such as oleyl alcohol and diolein, are also effective in forming pH-sensitive liposomes (30,31). Alternatively, a pH-sensitive oligopeptide that undergoes coil to α-helix conformational transition, such as glutamic acid-alanine-leucine-alanine (GALA), influenza fusion peptides, and pH-responsive polymer poly-2-ethyl-acrylic acid linked to a lipid anchor, can also mediate intracellular disruption of the endosomal membrane (32–34).

Fusogenic and Endosomolytic Liposomes

These liposomes can be constructed by reconstitution of envelope proteins of viruses into liposomes or encapsulation of hemolysins from bacteria with varying degrees of pH dependence (35). In addition to pH, the reducing and enzymatic environment inside the endosomal compartment can be utilized to trigger the cleavage of disulfide or enzyme-sensitive linker that may be incorporated into a bilayer-stabilizing lipid (36,37). For example, gelonin, a type I plant toxin, was coencapsulated inside pH-sensitive liposomes with listeriolysin O (LLO), the pore-forming protein that mediates escape of the intracellular pathogen listeria monocytogens from the endosome into the cytosol (38). Such a strategy resulted in a dramatic improvement on the cytotoxicity of encapsulated gelonin against the murine B16 melanoma cell line, over free gelonin or gelonin encapsulated in non-LLO-containing pH-sensitive liposomes. In another study, Mastrobattista et al. (35) have demonstrated that coencapsulation of a pH-dependent fusogenic peptide (diINF-7) and diphtheria toxin A chain (DTA) in non-pH-sensitive immunoliposomes promotes efficient cytosolic delivery of DTA.

Temperature-Sensitive Liposomes

Local release of liposomal drug can also be triggered by hyperthermia by adopting a bilayer composition with phase-transition temperature slightly above 37°C, such as dipalmitoyl phosphatidylcholine or conjugation to a thermosensitive polymer (39,40). Temperature-sensitive liposomes that show phase transition at 40°C can be synthesized by incorporating lipid-conjugated copolymers of N-isopropylacryl-amide and N-acryloylpyrrolidine (41). A thermosensitive liposome formulation entrapping doxorubicin (ThermoDox™) is currently undergoing clinical evaluation.

Cationic Liposomes

These liposomes can form electrostatic complexes with plasmid DNA and facilitate gene transfer (42). A wide variety of cationic lipids have been synthesized including those with a monovalent headgroup, such as 1,2-dioleoyl-3-trimethylammonium-propane, N-[2,3-(dioleyloxy)propyl]-N,N,N-trimethylammonium chloride, and 3-β-[N-(N',N'-dimethylaminoethyl)carbamoyl]-cholesterol, and those with a multi-valent headgroup, such as 2,3-dioleyloxy-N-[2(spermine-carboxamido)ethyl]-N,N-dimethyl-1-propanaminium trifluoroacetate. DOPE is often used as a helper lipid in these liposomes to enhance their fusogenicity (43). Cationic liposomes with multivalent cationic lipids form particles with condensed structure with plasmid DNA, whereas those with monovalent cationic lipids have been shown to form extended spaghetti-like structures. Although cationic liposomes exhibit efficient gene transfer activity in tissue culture and are currently commonly used reagents for in vitro transfection, only low-level transfection in select tissues, typically the lung, can be obtained upon systemic administration of cationic liposome/DNA complexes in murine models (44,45). This might be due to the trapping of the cationic complexes in the capillary blood vessels in the lung, which is the first-pass organ encountered by intravenously administered liposome complexes. In addition to plasmid DNA, cationic liposomes have been used in the delivery of antisense oligo-deoxyribonucleotides (ODNs) and siRNA into cells. Liposomes with a weakly basic cationic lipid, such as 1,2-dioleyl-3-dimethylammonium-propane, can efficiently incorporate plasmid DNA or ODNs at acidic pH, where the lipids are largely cat-ionic and return to a mostly neutral zeta potential at pH 7.4, where the lipids are mostly deprotonated (46). These liposomes have longer circulation time than cationic liposomes carrying permanently charged cationic lipids and may be useful for systemic delivery of DNA to solid tumors. Cationic liposome complexes with plasmid DNA, ODNs, or siRNA can also activate the innate immune system and may play a role in immunotherapy (47). In addition to nucleic acid delivery, cationic liposomes carrying chemotherapy agent paclitaxel have been shown to preferentially target tumor endothelium, suggesting a possible role for these liposomes in tumor-targeted drug delivery. Schmitt-Sody et al. (48) showed that cationic liposomal paclitaxel exhibits high selectivity for tumor endothelium and is highly efficacious in tumor growth inhibition.

Targeted Liposomes

Liposomes can be targeted to specific cell populations via incorporation of a targeting moiety. The targeting ligand can consist of a lipid-anchored antibody or antibody fragment, transferrin, folate, or carbohydrate. Immunoliposomes are synthesized by conjugation of the liposome to an antibody [e.g., anti-HER2 (49), antitransferrin receptor (50,51), anti-CD20 (52), and anti-CD19 (53)] or an antibody fragment such as F_{ab} (54) and scF$_v$ (55). HER2 is a receptor tyrosine kinase, a product of the HER2 (c-erbB2) proto-oncogene, which has been shown to play an important role in the development and progression of breast and other cancers. Park et al. (56,57) reported that anti-HER2 immunoliposomes, with encapsulated doxorubicin, displayed significantly enhanced therapeutic efficacy in four different breast cancer xenograft models when compared to nontargeted liposomes, free drug, or free antibody. For targeting PEGylated liposomes, it is helpful to incorporate a long PEG-based linker between the targeting ligand and the lipid anchor. Incorporation of the targeting moiety can be accomplished during liposome formation by detergent dialysis, or postliposome formation by conjugation to reactive lipids or postinsertion of ligands from micelles of lipid-derivatized antibodies (58,59). The last method seems highly promising for future clinical development. In addition to antibodies, other targeting moieties such as transferrin (51,60) and folic acid (61–63) have been frequently evaluated in targeting liposomes to tumor cells that overexpress the transferrin or the folate receptor. Targeted liposomes are specifically taken up by target cells and have been shown to be highly efficient in drug delivery and to bypass multidrug resistance in cell lines (64). Tumor localization of targeted liposomes often does not greatly exceed that of nontargeted liposomes because biodistribution of liposomes is dictated by vascular permeability and the associated EPR effect. Furthermore, there is concern that liposomes, due to their size, cannot penetrate into solid tumors, which typically have high interstitial pressure. Nevertheless, targeted liposomes such as anti-HER2 immunoliposomes and folate receptor-targeted liposomes have shown improved antitumor efficacy in murine models over nontargeted control liposomes (51,63). Leukemias, which have greater accessibility from circulation, are also potentially good targets for targeted liposomes, as suggested by recent reports. The advantage of using immunoliposome for MAb-based targeted therapy in leukemia exists in: (*i*) liposomes containing high payload of cytotoxic agents have unrestricted access to malignant cells and (*ii*) application of a chemotherapeutic agent that has already shown clinical efficacy can potentially bring synergistic effect with therapeutic MAb, based on a different killing mechanism. Pan et al. (65) studied the therapeutic efficacy of folate receptor-targeted liposomes in combination with upregulation of FR-β expression in an ascitic xenograft model of acute myelogenous leukemia using all-*trans* retinoic acid. In vivo antitumor activity of folate receptor-targeted liposomal daunorubicin in the L1210-JF ascitic murine leukemia model has also been reported by Pan and Lee (66). The result showed that folate receptor-targeted liposomes could effectively target receptor-positive leukemia cells in vivo.

Lipid Nanoparticles

Lipid nanoparticles are nanoscale spherical particles composed of lipids with a lipidic core. These are suitable for delivery of lipophilic therapeutic agents. The molecule of interest can be formulated to lipid nanoparticle matrix through lipid-phase dissolution. They have considerable utility as controlled delivery system for drugs and vaccines. Lipid nanoparticles can be synthesized by combining an oil phase (e.g., triolein) with phospholipids as emulsifiers. The oily core can be used to incorporate lipid-soluble drugs such as paclitaxel (67,68), hematoporphyrin (69), and lipid-conjugated prodrugs (70). They can be synthesized by similar methods as those used in liposomes, such as high-pressure homogenization. Like liposomes, these particles are cleared by RES, localized in tumors via EPR effect, and can be made long circulating by incorporation of PEGylated lipid.

CONCLUSIONS

Lipid-based nanoparticulates are versatile drug carriers with significant potential for clinical applications. Technological advances such as introduction of remote loading methods, PEGylated liposomes, and targeted liposomes provided additional advantages. In addition to modulating toxicity, pharmacokinetics, and biodistribution, liposomal delivery has shown promise as a mechanism to overcome multidrug resistance. Furthermore, liposomes are promising delivery vehicles for novel therapeutic agents such as siRNA and drugs that lack aqueous solubility. Particularly promising for future development are targeted liposomes, which have yet to be thoroughly evaluated in clinical studies. Given current trends, lipid-based nanoparticulates are likely to have an expanding role in drug delivery in the clinical setting.

REFERENCES

1. Allen TM. Liposomal drug formulations: rationale for development and what we can expect for the future. Drugs 1998; 56:747.
2. Chaterjee S, Banerjee DK. Preparation, isolation, and characterization of liposomes containing natural and synthetic lipids. In: Basu SC, Basu M, eds. Liposome Methods and Protocols. Totowa: Humana Press, 2002 (chapter 1).
3. Martin FJ. Pharmaceutical manufacturing of liposomes. In: Tyle P, ed. Specialized Drug Delivery System Manufacturing and Production Technology. New York: Marcel Dekker, 1990 (chapter 6).
4. Huang H. Studies on phosphatidylcholine vesicles: formulation and physical characteristics. Biochemistry 1969; 8:344.
5. Hope MJ, Bally MB, Webb G, Cullis PR. Production of large unilamellar vesicles by a rapid extrusion procedure characterization of size distribution, trapped volume, and ability to maintain a membrane potential. Biochim Biophys Acta 1985; 55:812.
6. Hauser H, Grains N. Spontaneous vesiculation of phospholipids: a simple and quick method of forming unilamellar vesicles. Proc Natl Acad Sci USA 1982; 79:1683.
7. Szoka F, Papahadjopoulos D. Procedure for preparation of liposomes with large internal aqueous space and high capture by reverse-phase evaporation. Proc Natl Acad Sci USA 1978; 75:4194.
8. Bolotin EM, Cohen R, Bar LK, et al. Ammonium sulfate gradients for efficient and stable remote loading of amphipathic weak bases into liposomes and ligandoliposomes. J Liposome Res 1994; 4:455.
9. Boman NL, Masin D, Mayer LD, Cullis PR, Bally MB. Liposomal vincristine which exhibits increased drug retention and increased circulation longevity cures mice bearing P388 tumors. Cancer Res 1994; 54:2830.
10. Gao X, Huang L. Cationic liposome-mediated gene transfer. Gene Ther 1995; 2:710.
11. Meyer O, Kirpotin D, Hong K, Sternberg B, Park JW, Woodle MC. Cationic liposomes coated with polyethylene glycol as carrier for oligonucleotides. J Biol Chem 1998; 273:15621.

12. Wrobell I, Collins D. Fusion of cationic liposomes with mammalian cells occurs after endocytosis. Biochim Biophys Acta 1995; 1235:296.
13. Martin FJ, Morano JK. US Patent 4,752,425, 1988.
14. Thomas DM, Nancy B. Lyophilization of liposomes. In: Andrew SJ, ed. Liposomes Rational Design. New York: Marcel Dekker, 1999:261.
15. Tardi PG, Boman NL, Cullis PR. Liposomal doxorubicin. J Drug Target 1996; 4:129.
16. Bellott R, Auvrignon A, Leblanc T, et al. Pharmacokinetics of liposomal daunorubicin (DaunoXome) during a phase I to II study in children with relapsed acute lymphoblastic leukaemia. Cancer Chemother Pharmacol 2001; 47:15.
17. Gregoriadis G, Florence AT. Liposomes in drug delivery: clinical, diagnostic and ophthalmic potential. Drugs 1993; 45:15.
18. Hamada A, Kawaguchi T, Nakano M. Clinical pharmacokinetics of cytarabine formulations. Clin Pharmacokinet 2002; 41:705.
19. Konan YN, Gurny R, Allemann E. State of art in the delivery of photosensitizers for photodynamic therapy. J Photochem Photobiol B 2002; 66:89.
20. Florence AT. Liposomes as pharmaceuticals. In: Andrew SJ, ed. Liposomes Rational Design: Introduction. New York: Marcel Dekker, 1999.
21. Gabizon A, Papahadjopoulos D. Liposome formulations with prolonged circulation time in blood and enhanced uptake by tumors. Proc Natl Acad Sci USA 1988; 85:6949.
22. Klibanov AL, Maruyama K, Torchilin VP, Huang L. Amphipathic polyethyleneglycols effectively prolong the circulation time of liposomes. FEBS Lett 1990; 268:235.
23. Uster PS, Allen TM, Daniel BE, Mendez CJ, Newman MS, Zhu GZ. Insertion of poly(ethylene glycol) derivatized phospholipids into pre-formed liposomes results in prolonged in vivo circulation time. FEBS Lett 1996; 386:243.
24. Lee RJ, Wang S, Turk MJ, Low PS. The effects of pH and intraliposomal buffer strength on the rate of liposome content release and intracellular drug delivery. Biosci Rep 1998; 18:69.
25. Wang J, Goh B, Lu WL, et al. In vitro cytotoxicity of stealth liposomes co-encapsulating doxorubicin and verapamil on doxorubicin-resistant tumor cells. Biol Pharm Bull 2005; 28:822.
26. Bradley AJ, Devine DV, Ansell SM, Janzen J, Brooks DE. Inhibition of liposome-induced complement activation by incorporated poly(ethylene glycol)-lipids. Arch Biochem Biophys 1998; 357:185.
27. Simões S, Slepushkin V, Duzgunes N, Pedroso de Lima MC. On the mechanisms of internalization and intracellular delivery mediated by pH-sensitive liposomes. Biochim Biophys Acta 2001; 1515:23.
28. Slepushkin VA, Simoes S, Dazin P, et al. Sterically stabilized pH-sensitive liposomes: intracellular delivery of aqueous contents and prolonged circulation in vivo. J Biol Chem 1997; 272:2382.
29. Düzgünes N, Straubinger RM, Baldwin PA, Friend DS, Papahadjopoulos D. Proton-induced fusion of oleic acid-phosphatidylethanolamine liposomes. Biochemistry 1985; 24:3091.
30. Guo W, Gosselin MA, Lee RJ. Characterization of a novel diolein-based LPDII vector for gene delivery. J Control Release 2002; 83:121.
31. Sudimack JJ, Guo W, Tjarks W, Lee RJ. A novel pH-sensitive liposome formulation containing oleyl alcohol. Biochim Biophys Acta 2002; 1546:31.
32. Chung JC, Gross DJ, Thomas JL, Tirrell DA, Opsahl-Ong LR. pH-sensitive, cation-selective channels formed by a simple synthetic polyelectrolyte in artificial bilayer membranes. Macromolecules 1996; 29:4636.
33. Chen T, Choi LS, Einstein S, Klippenstein MA, Scherrer P, Cullis PR. Proton-induced permeability and fusion of large unilamellar vesicles by covalently conjugated poly(2-ethylacrylic acid). J Liposome Res 1999; 9:387.
34. Li WJ, Nicol F, Szoka FC Jr. GALA: a designed synthetic pH-responsive amphipathic peptide with applications in drug and gene delivery. Adv Drug Deliv Rev 2004; 56:967.
35. Mastrobattista E, Koning GA, van Bloois L, Filipe AS, Jiskoot W, Storm G. Functional characterization of an endosome-disruptive peptide and its application in cytosolic delivery of immunoliposome-entrapped proteins. J Biol Chem 2002; 277:27135.

36. Simoes S, Slepushkin V, Gaspar R, de Lima MC, Duzgunes N. Gene delivery by negative charged ternary complexes of DNA, cationic liposomes, and transferrin or fusigenic peptides. Gene Ther 1998; 5:955.
37. Aronsohn AI, Hughes JA. Nuclear localization signal peptides enhance cationic liposome-mediated gene therapy. J Drug Target 1998; 5:163.
38. Provoda CJ, Stier EM, Lee KD. Tumor cell killing enabled by listeriolysin O-liposome-mediated delivery of the protein toxin gelonin. J Biol Chem 2003; 278:35102.
39. Needham D, Dewhirst MW. The development and testing of a new temperature-sensitive drug delivery system for the treatment of solid tumors. Adv Drug Deliv Rev 2001; 53:285.
40. Kong G, Dewhirst MW. Review hyperthermia and liposomes. Int J Hyperther 1999; 15:345.
41. Kono K, Nakai R, Morimoto K, Takagishi T. Thermosensitive polymer-modified liposomes that release contents around physiological temperature. Biochim Biophys Acta 1999; 1416:239.
42. Brigham KL, Meyrick B, Christman B, Magnuson M, King G, Berry LC Jr. In vivo transfection of murine lungs with a functioning prokaryotic gene using a liposome vehicle. Am J Med Sci 1989; 298:278.
43. Sandrine AL, de Leij LF, Hoekstra D, Molema G. In vivo characteristics of cationic liposomes as delivery vectors for gene therapy. Pharm Res 2002; 19:1559.
44. Zhu N, Liggitt D, Liu Y, Debs R. Systemic gene expression after intravenous DNA delivery into adult mice. Science 1993; 298:278.
45. McLean JW, Fox EA, Baluk P, et al. Organ-specific endothelial cell uptake of cationic liposome–DNA complexes in mice. Am J Physiol 1997; 273:H387–H440.
46. Reddy JA, Dean D, Kennedy MD, Low PS. Optimization of folate-conjugated liposomal vectors for folate-receptor-mediated gene therapy. J Pharm Sci 1999; 88:1112.
47. Sioud M, Sorensen DR. Cationic liposome-mediated delivery of siRNAs in adult mice. Biochem Biophys Res Commun 2003; 312:1220.
48. Schmitt-Sody M, Strieth S, Krasnici S, Sauer B. Neovascular targeting therapy: paclitaxel encapsulated in cationic liposomes improves antitumoral efficacy. Clin Cancer Res 2003; 9:2335.
49. Baselga J, Norton L, Albanell J, Kim YM, Mendelsohn J. Recombinant humanized anti-HER2 antibody (Herceptin) enhances the antitumor activity of paclitaxel and doxorubicin against HER2/neu overexpressing human breast cancer xenografts. J Cancer Res 1998; 58:2825.
50. Li H, Qian Z. Transferrin/transferrin receptor-mediated drug delivery. Med Res Rev 2002; 22:225.
51. Ishida O, Maruyama K, Tanahashi H, Iwatsuru M. Liposomes bearing polyethyleneglycol-coupled transferrin with intracellular targeting property to the solid tumors in vivo. Pharm Res 2001; 18:1042.
52. Sapra P, Allen TM. Internalizing antibodies are necessary for improved therapeutic efficacy of antibody-targeted liposomal drugs. Cancer Res 2002; 62:7190.
53. Ishida T, Kirchmeier MJ, Moase EH, Zalipsky S, Allen TM. Targeted delivery and triggered release of liposomal doxorubicin enhances cytotoxicity against human B lymphoma cells. Biochim Biophys Acta 2001; 1515:144.
54. Pastorino F, Brignole C, Marimpietri D, et al. Doxorubicin-loaded Fab' fragments of anti-disialoganglioside immunoliposomes selectively inhibit the growth and dissemination of human neuroblastoma in nude mice. Cancer Res 2003; 63:86.
55. Marty C, Odermatt B, Schott H, et al. Cytotoxic targeting of F9 teratocarcinoma tumours with anti-ED-B fibronectin scFv antibody modified liposomes. Br J Cancer 2002; 87:106.
56. Park JW, Hong K, Kirpotin DB, Colbern G. Anti-HER2 immunoliposomes: enhanced efficacy attributable to targeted delivery. Clin Cancer Res 2002; 8:1172.
57. Park JW, Kirpotin DB, Hong K, et al. Tumor targeting using anti-her2 immunoliposomes. J Control Release 2001; 74:95.
58. Schiffelers RM, Koning GA, ten Hagen TL, et al. Anti-tumor efficacy of tumor vasculature-targeted liposomal doxorubicin. J Control Release 2003; 91:115.

59. Hood JD, Bednarski, MF, Ricardo G, et al. Tumor regression by targeted gene delivery to the neovasculature. Science 2002; 296:2404.
60. Iinuma H, Maruyama K, Okinaga K, et al. Intracellular targeting therapy of cisplatin-encapsulated transferrin-polyethylene glycol liposome on peritoneal dissemination of gastric cancer. Int J Cancer 2002; 99:130.
61. Sudimack J, Lee RJ. Drug targeting via the folate receptor. Adv Drug Deliv Rev 2000; 41:147.
62. Zhao X, Lee RJ. Tumor-selective targeted delivery of genes and antisense oligodeoxyribonucleotides via the folate receptor. Adv Drug Deliv Rev 2004; 56:1193.
63. Pan XQ, Wang H, Lee RJ. Antitumor activity of folate receptor-targeted liposomal doxorubicin in a KB oral carcinoma murine xenograft model. Pharm Res 2003; 20:417.
64. Goren D, Horowitz AT, Tzemach D, Tarshish M, Zalipsky S, Gabizon A. Nuclear delivery of doxorubicin via folate-targeted liposomes with bypass of multidrug-resistance efflux pump. Clin Cancer Res 2000; 6:1949.
65. Pan XQ, Zheng X, Shi G, Wang H, Ratnam M, Lee RJ. A strategy for the treatment of acute myelogenous leukemia based on folate receptor type-β targeted liposomal doxorubicin combined with receptor induction using all-*trans*-retinoic acid. Blood 2002; 100:594.
66. Pan XQ, Lee RJ. In vivo antitumor activity of folate receptor-targeted liposomal daunorubicin in a murine leukemia model. Anticancer Res 2005; 25:343.
67. Mo Y, Lim L. Nanoparticles of poly(lactide)/vitamin E TPGS copolymer for cancer chemotherapy: synthesis, formulation, characterization and in vitro drug release. J Control Release 2005; 107:30.
68. Yeh TK, Lu Z, Wientjes MG, Au JL-S. Formulating paclitaxel in nanoparticles alters its disposition. Pharm Res 2005; 22:867.
69. Stevens PJ, Sekido M, Lee RJ. Synthesis and evaluation of a hematoporphyrin derivative in a folate receptor-targeted solid–lipid nanoparticle formulation. Anticancer Res 2004; 24:161.
70. Stevens PJ, Sekido M, Lee RJ. A folate receptor-targeted lipid nanoparticle formulation for a lipophilic paclitaxel prodrug. Pharm Res 2004; 21:2153.

7 Nanoengineering of Drug Delivery Systems

Ashwath Jayagopal and V. Prasad Shastri
Biomaterials, Drug Delivery, and Tissue Engineering Laboratory, Department of Biomedical Engineering, Vanderbilt University, Nashville, Tennessee, U.S.A.

INTRODUCTION

Challenges in drug delivery include the attainment of tunable release profiles, drug solubility and structural stability, biocompatibility, and the confinement of therapeutic action to diseased sites. Increased attention has been directed toward the nanoscale manipulation or nanoengineering of drug-delivery systems (DDSs) for conferring unique properties on the drug or drug vehicle often not achievable by either conventional- (e.g., free-form) or microscale-drug carriers. Nanoengineering may be achieved at various levels during formulation of a drug within a carrier. Examples include modulation of the drug environment at the molecular level, alteration of the physicochemical characteristics of the drug (e.g., solubility and structural integrity), control of drug-diffusive mobility, and modification of the bulk and surface chemistry of the drug nanocarrier. These approaches have potential in the achievement of favorable therapeutic endpoints, such as enhanced drug efficacy for prolonged intervals, minimal drug toxicity, reduced dosage and cost burden, and improved patient compliance. In this chapter, we discuss recent significant advances in DDSs in which nanoengineering is the enabling technology for such objectives, with an emphasis on the application of nanoengineering principles to the design of controlled- and triggered-release DDSs, enhancement of drug activity and stability, and smart tissue-targeted therapies. Specific attention is given to the unique effects of nanoscale modifications on critical drug-delivery parameters. We evaluate the promise of such approaches in drug-delivery technology, and discuss future considerations relevant to their clinical implementation.

CONTROLLED- AND TRIGGERED-RELEASE SYSTEMS

To develop suitable therapies for a diverse range of diseases, a host of natural and/or synthetic biomaterials have been selected based on their physicochemical characteristics which enable the development of sustained- and triggered-release DDSs. Sustained-release systems are administered for the maintenance of drug concentration within optimal therapeutic windows over extended periods ranging from hours to months. In other cases, for instance where instant drug activity is required, DDSs can be tuned for pulsatile release in response to varying physiological stimuli or external triggers, such as acidic pH and acoustic pulses. Nanoscale modulation of drug-transport characteristics, with or without entrapment within a nanocarrier, can be achieved by formulation with novel drug-complexation agents for enhancement of both controlled- and triggered-release applications.

Polymeric Drug Delivery Systems for Sustained and Triggered Release

The engineering of drug carriers to bear one or more polymeric agents, with each block having a specific role in the solubility and degradative susceptibility of the resulting vehicle, allows for nanoscale design of controlled-release DDSs. Biodegradable polymer-based DDSs feature labile groups, the presence of which can be tuned to control the extent of degradation and hence drug release over time. The well-characterized and biocompatible poly(D,L-lactide-co-glycolide) (PLGA) drug carriers are an example of a system which undergoes bulk erosion by hydrolysis, enabling its utilization in controlled-release applications. The PLGA block copolymer is composed of poly(lactic acid) and poly(glycolic acid), the former of which is slower to degrade due to increased crystallinity and steric hindrance to scission by water. Both are safely eliminated by the body. Varying the relative composition of the two blocks on a PLGA nanoparticle surface provides a means of tailoring drug-release rates via modulation of the hydrophilic–lipophilic balance. PLGA can also be incorporated into nanoparticulate DDSs for sustained intracellular drug delivery. This is a beneficial consequence of two events: first, the nonspecific endocytic internalization of PLGA nanoparticles into subcellular compartments and second, the escape of PLGA nanoparticles into the cytoplasm made possible by surface cationization within acidic endolysosomal compartments (1). These features suggest the versatility of PLGA nanoparticles as intracellular sustained-release depots for gene or drug delivery, which bypass previous challenges such as nucleic acid degradation in the cytoplasm, or drug efflux pumps which can be a barrier to passive drug diffusion. A more recent DDS utilizing polyester-based hydrolytic degradation has been reported by Ahmed and Discher (2). In this application, an amphipathic polymersome composed of a water-soluble polyethylene glycol (PEG) and hydrolytically labile polylactic acid or poly(caprolactone) block is synthesized by self-assembly and can be utilized to encapsulate hydrophobic or hydrophilic therapeutics, or imaging agents. Release is tunable from hours to weeks by adjustment of the hydrophilic–lipophilic balance, which controls hydrolytic-dependent poration of the membrane. Although encapsulation efficiencies are similar to well-characterized drug-delivery carriers such as liposomes, polymersomes exhibit enhanced mechanical strength due to increased membrane thickness and extended circulation half-life, suggesting the utility of this carrier for applications requiring prolonged circulation in vivo with a resistance to destabilization mechanisms. In a fundamentally different approach, therapeutics can be directly incorporated into a polymer backbone (trade name PolymerDrug, Polymerix Corp.) (3). Adjustment of the physical properties of the resulting polymer offers a pharmacokinetic tuning mechanism, and biodegradation products are inert. This technology offers a platform for the low-risk incorporation of therapeutics with known safety profiles that can be implemented in implantable or degradable DDSs.

Polymeric DDSs have also been applied as ad hoc triggered-release systems. One route to this goal is the blending of polymers to create polymer chain compositions which are more susceptible to rapid degradation. By this approach, sustained-release polymers can be modified for rapid release of encapsulated contents when needed. For example, although PLGA is a well-characterized copolymer for biodegradable sustained-release systems, its intracellular release profile may not be rapid or efficient enough for some gene-delivery applications. Little et al. addressed this challenge by coblending PLGA with a pH-sensitive poly(β-amino ester) which is insoluble at physiologic pH, with a solubility transition occurring within the acidic pH range of lysosomes (4). Taking advantage of the rapid solubility of the polymer below pH 6.5, poly(β-amino ester) blends with PLGA in microparticle-containing genetic vaccines rapidly released their contents within dendritic cells (5), and were also noted to have higher plasmid DNA-loading efficiencies (6). The same polymer was also incorporated within poly(ethylene oxide) (PEO)-engineered nanoparticles for the enhanced, pH-selective delivery of Taxol within tumors (7). In another triggered-release strategy, micelles consisting of a hydrophilic PEO and a hydrophobic polypropylene oxide (PPO) in a triblock copolymer formulation (PEO–PPO–PEO) were observed to rapidly release doxorubicin and ruboxyl upon nanoparticle perturbation induced by ultrasonic cavitation (8). In addition, upon removal of the ultrasonic pulse, released drug was observed to become reencapsulated within micelles, and intracellular presence of 10% Pluronic micelles expedited the sealing of ultrasound-induced cell membrane poration, resulting in minimal drug efflux (9,10). Together, these data indicate that Pluronic micelles can tightly bear their cargoes (in this case, due to PPO–hydrophobic interactions with drug) with a spatially and temporally controlled acoustic-release mechanism. Taking advantage of reencapsulation upon removal of acoustic pulses, therapeutic action can be confined solely within the sonophoretic range, and due to the micelle-induced membrane "sealing" effect, which increases intracellular drug retention, a lower dosage may be used. These findings reinforce the concept that nanoscale delegation of polymer block roles in drug release, solubility of the nanocarrier, and interactions with the surrounding environment and external stimuli can be harnessed for diverse and powerful drug-delivery approaches.

Lipid-Based Drug Delivery Systems for Sustained and Triggered Release

Controlled-release DDSs have also been formulated using the unique properties conferred by lipid-based materials. The fluidity of lipid domains on the nanoscale is a parameter which, when tuned, allows for a mechanism controlling water influx. Palm oil, a biocompatible vegetable oil, was used as a hydrophobic excipient along with the phospholipid dipalmitoyl phosphatidylcholine for entrapment and controlled release of the highly hydrophilic drug terbutaline sulfate for pulmonary administration (11). Hydrogenation of palm oil excipient was utilized to tightly pack hydrophobic domains together for a tighter microsphere barrier. Degradation of the spray-dried hydrophobic coat resulted in the sustained release of drug nanoparticles without burst effects observed with free-drug nanoparticles. This approach may serve as a potential high-compliance method of delivering drugs of varying solubility through the pulmonary route featured by noninvasive circulatory access as spray-dried microspheres with near-optimal aerodynamic diameters, as suggested by Edwards et al. (12) for improved deep-lung deposition with reduced clearance by alveolar macrophages.

Using a judicious selection of components with appropriate physicochemical characteristics, lipid-based DDSs can also be formulated for instant trigger-based release applications. By altering the phase transition of the lipid chains from closely packed arrangements (crystalline) to loose, disordered fluid chains, ideally at an achievable, clinically relevant temperature, diffusion of drug from internal lipid nanocarrier compartments can be achieved. Such phase transitions can occur within sharp, predictable temperature ranges on the order of a few degrees celsius, and are primarily a function of hydrocarbon length, extent of saturation, charge, and the presence of other structures which affect lipid packing, such as cholesterol or double bonds. In low-temperature thermosensitive liposomes (LTSLs), for example, the gel phase rapidly transitions to the liquid crystalline phase at 42°C upon mixture formulation of a conventional phospholipid combination with lysolecithin, at which temperature excessive efflux of drug is observed, with full release of doxorubicin within 20 seconds (13). The rapid release of high quantities of drug from LTSLs has important consequences on triggered chemotherapeutic applications. Peak intratumoral doxorubicin concentrations upon hyperthermia of LTSLs were measured to be 30-fold higher than free-drug and twofold higher than previous thermosensitive liposome designs. Manganese-guided loading of LTSLs with doxorubicin has been carried out to achieve similar loading concentrations as nontemperature-sensitive liposomes (14), suggesting that hyperthermia-based chemotherapy may be a viable clinical option to conventional liposomes for delivering more toxic payloads to the tumor space. Given the current clinical usage of liposomal formulations such as Doxil, similar liposomal formulations triggered by hyperthermia may be readily accepted if thermal dosimetry protocols can be standardized. Novel nanoengineering approaches involving the incorporation of transition-temperature-lowering components as well as metallic drug-loading schemes to achieve high encapsulation efficiencies are helpful in facilitating the implementation of liposomes with enhanced trigger functionality in the clinic.

Modulation of Drug Environment and Physicochemical Properties for Sustained and Triggered Release

In many cases, nanoscale modulation of the actual drug structure is needed to enhance its solubility or otherwise increase its efficiency of transport. In alternative administration routes, such as the transdermal pathway, this type of modification is gaining increased attention. The benefits of transdermal administration are several fold: (*i*) first-pass liver metabolism associated with oral and systemic therapy is avoided, (*ii*) there is generally increased patient compliance (e.g., wearing a patch vs. repeated injections), and (*iii*) adverse reactions associated with conventional administrations of drug may be avoided in this form. However, the skin has low permeability to most therapeutics, especially high-molecular-weight compounds, and thus is not by itself an efficient administration site for most therapies. Several approaches have been reported to address this challenge, and include physical skin barrier perturbation and/or the promotion of drug penetration using ultrasound (sonophoresis), electroporation, drug molecule electrophoresis (iontophoresis), and chemically assisted cotransport (15). The latter involves the nanoscale modulation of drug-diffusive mobility by the transient induction of skin permeability, and/or the improvement of drug portioning within the skin. Known permeation enhancers include fatty acids, ethanol, and other skin-permeable solvents (15). Lee et al. (16,17) reported the synergistic effect of *n*-methyl pyrrolidone and oleic acid in the enhancement of hydrophobic and hydrophilic drug flux (Fig. 1).

N-Methyl pyrrolidone is perfectly miscible with water for comixing in aqueous transdermal formulations, and is thought to exert its effects by promotion of hydrogen bonding with the therapeutic, as well as the transient disruption of lipid bilayers, enabling drug partitioning in the stratum corneum for enhanced flux (16,17). Given enhancements in drug transport observed with physical perturbation methods, the combination of chemical permeation enhancers with ultrasound, a widely available technology, is likely to have a significant impact on the transport of a wide spectrum of drugs for sustained release.

The alteration of drug solubility is often critical to its therapeutic efficacy. A technique of modulating drug solubility and thus its partitioning dynamics is supramolecular complexation. In this approach, the therapeutic is combined with a

Drug (2% w/v)	Flux$_{ss}$ from H$_2$O(μg/cm^2/h $\pm$ SD)	Flux$_{ss}$ from H$_2$O/NMP(μg/cm^2/h $\pm$ SD)	Enhancement
Lidocaine HCl	1.00 $\pm$ 0.22	4.35 $\pm$ 1.84	4.3 $\pm$ 2.1
Prilocaine HCl	2.44 $\pm$ 0.98	6.31 $\pm$ 0.14	2.6 $\pm$ 1.0

$N = 3$.

% NMP	Lidocaine Flux$_{ss}$(μg/cm^2/h $\pm$ SD)	NMP Flux$_{ss}$(mg/cm^2/h $\pm$ SD)
40	2.25 $\pm$ 0.67	0.058 $\pm$ 0.041
50	1.69 $\pm$ 0.20	0.095 $\pm$ 0.047
60	4.57 $\pm$ 5.28	0.47 $\pm$ 0.23
80	35.1 $\pm$ 9.1	7.6 $\pm$ 1.9
90	37.6 $\pm$ 7.9	17.6 $\pm$ 1.9
100	290 $\pm$ 103	18.0 $\pm$ 0.4

$N = 3$.

FIGURE 1 *Top*: Flux enhancement of hydrophilic HCl salt drugs from 1:1 H$_2$O/*n*-methyl pyrrolidone cosolvent through stripped human cadaver skin. *Bottom*: Transport of lidocaine and *n*-methyl pyrrolidone from H$_2$O/*n*-methyl pyrrolidone 1% oleic acid systems. *Abbreviation*: NMP, *N*-methyl pyrrolidone. *Source*: From Ref. 17.

stabilizing agent to form an inclusion complex, with the overall structure then inheriting the physicochemical properties of the complexing agent. Cyclodextrins (CDs), cyclic polysugars, have been known to perform this task very efficiently in oral-dosage formulations, enabling powerful sustained-release applications which are not achievable with the free-drug alone. For example, the poorly water-soluble antimicrobial agent chlorhexidine was complexed with β-CDs of varying lipophilicity (18). The CD–drug complex was loaded into PLGA-implantable DDSs, creating a concentration gradient. Enhanced solubility conferred by the complex allowed for improved drug diffusivity, whereas the lipophilicity of the drug–CD inclusion complex could be altered to modulate sustained-release kinetics. Furthermore, the antimicrobial activity of the chlorhexidine was enhanced by complexation with CD, through a plausible mechanism that involves enhancement of the interaction of the drug with the glycocalyx (polysaccharide coat) on the bacteria (US Patent 6,699,505). Thus, the direct alteration of drug physicochemical properties is a powerful approach in extending the scope of drugs that can be administered by DDSs with high efficacy.

ENHANCEMENT OF DRUG STRUCTURAL STABILITY AND DURATION OF ACTIVITY

Several diverse approaches have been reported for the preservation of drug structural integrity and enhancement of therapeutic activity. Therapeutics such as proteins and peptides are especially prone to in vivo degradation and clearance, which are barriers to their bioavailability and duration of action. Other therapies may be poorly soluble, or degrade within harsh nanocarrier environments over time in circulation or in storage prior to administration. Approaches to address these challenges on the nanoscale include the maintenance of controlled drug microenvironments within the vehicle, polymeric surface engineering to modulate drug interactions with the surrounding environment, and the development processing techniques which utilize suitable temperatures, solvents, and/or complexation agents which confer stability upon labile drugs, thus enhancing their efficacy and applications.

Formulation Processing Strategies for Enhanced Drug Stability and Activity

Many promising therapeutics are limited in clinical applications by poor solubility. Such drugs also have low dissolution rates which hinder bioavailability even in cases of rapid drug uptake. Previous approaches focused on increasing dissolution rates by increasing the surface area of the drug powder using milling of the drug to create microparticles. However, for low-solubility drugs, this is often not a sufficient surface area enhancement to promote adequate dissolution. Nanoengineering of the drug particle formulation itself has been performed to improve drug solubility and dissolution. For example, a "nanonization" process utilizing high-pressure homogenization techniques was developed by Keck and Muller (19), which avoids undesirable effects associated with solvent precipitation and pearl milling (trade name: DissoCubes). The decrease in particle size and diffusion distance afforded by DissoCubes provides for an enhanced drug dissolution rate and solubility. The latter is strictly a consequence of the fact that the drug is less than 1 μm in diameter (above which size, temperature and solvent characteristics are primary determinants of particle solubility), and increased curvature of the drug particle increases its dissolution pressure, which thus enhances solubility. Owing to the homogeneity of the particles within the nanosuspension, which may include electrostatic and steric stabilizing agents, potentially degradative processes such as Ostwald ripening are not observed, providing drug stability in storage.

To attain suitable intracarrier environments for drug stability within DDSs such as PLGA nanoparticles, antacid salts have been introduced during encapsulation to neutralize the acidic internal microclimate, reducing protein aggregation and degradation (20). Saccharides such as trehalose have been used as a cryoprotectant in drugs encapsulated within solid–lipid nanoparticles (21). The CDs previously discussed are known to protect labile drugs against hydrolysis, oxidation, and photodegradation (22). The utility of CD complexation for the protection of a thermally labile drug, rhodium (II) citrate, was reported by Sinisterra et al. (23), highlighting the potential of CD complexation to stabilize drugs from high-temperature compression and injection molding processes used to manufacture polymeric DDSs (Fig. 2).

Hydrophilic CDs with hydrophobic cavities, such as HPβCD, can serve as nanoscale shields which protect hydrophobic residues on proteins, for reduced denaturation and aggregation, and reduce unwanted polymer–drug interactions within the carrier. These are examples of nanoscale-drug-stabilization strategies which can be utilized to enhance solubility and structural conformation of drugs for incorporation into nanoscale DDSs, or simply for improved transport parameters of the drug itself.

Polymeric Strategies for Prolongation of Drug Action

Polymeric surface functionalization of DDSs is now commonly used to modulate the interaction of DDSs with the surrounding environment, for enhanced drug activity through enhanced half-life in the body, and reduced biodegradation. PEG is well known for its ability to diminish carrier clearance by the reticuloendothelial

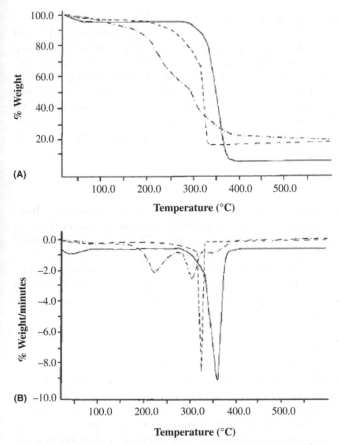

FIGURE 2 **(A)** Thermogravimetric curves of hydroxypropyl-β-cyclodextrin (HPβCD) (—), Rh(II) citrate (·· ··), and association complex between Rh(II) citrate and HPβCD (- - -). **(B)** Differential thermogravimetric (DTG) curves of HPβCD (—), Rh(II) citrate (·· ··), and association complex between Rh(II) citrate and HPβCD (- - -). The thermogravimetric and DTG curves of the Rh(II) citrate–HPβCD complex indicate only one thermal transition at higher temperature, around 310°C, which was accompanied by an 80% mass loss. This data suggests that HPβCD complexation with Rh(II) citrate results in enhanced thermal stability. *Source*: From Ref. 23.

system and inhibit protein surface adsorption. This is a consequence of the exclusion volume exerted by the freely mobile polymer chain of the carrier surface. The biocompatible PEG imparts water solubility to the conjugated (PEGylated) therapeutic. This strategy has been recently utilized for the protection of therapeutic proteins, as reinforced by the increasing number of PEGylated drugs in the clinic, such as PEGASYS (interferon alfa-2b, Roche) and Exubera (inhaled insulin, Pfizer). Strategies for utilizing PEGylation for future protein-based therapies are dependent on the development of PEGylation chemistries which confer the advantages of PEG without significant losses in protein functionality. This goal is being achieved with therapeutic monoclonal antibodies. Random PEGylation of protein amine groups using PEG coupled with NHS esters was implicated in the loss of monoclonal antibody-binding affinities in several cases. However, attachment of PEG to Fab' fragments using cysteine cross-linking in the hinge region (i.e., through thiol-maleimide chemistry) reduced or eliminated most affinity problems while conferring enhanced circulation half-life (24). To expand this idea, conjugation of branched and linear bifunctional PEGs to single-chain antibodies (scFvs) with an engineered unpaired cysteine to create multivalent conjugates was also carried out with success (25,26). Although the problem is more difficult for proteins other than antibodies which have the unique benefit of unpaired cysteines not needed for biological activity, site-specific PEGylation has also been reported using enzymatic or site-directed muta-genetic approaches (27,28). The technology for site-specific PEGylate therapeutic proteins is an area of active research and that is likely to expand the library of available protein-based therapies.

TARGETED THERAPIES

Several approaches for the specific targeting of therapeutics to disease sites have been developed, for the purposes of maximizing the effective dose delivered to the site while lowering the total dose needed, and sparing healthy tissue from potential adverse drug effects via confinement of therapeutic activity. Generally, these strategies involve optimization of geometry of the nanocarrier to optimize tissue uptake of DDSs, a generally passive route, and the bioconjugation of ligands such as peptides to the nanocarrier surface to promote interactions with diseased tissue, an active targeting mechanism.

Strategies for Passive Tissue Targeting

The geometry and mechanical properties of a carrier has a profound influence on its therapeutic efficacy in that the ability for DDSs to target tissue can be dependent on them. For example, spherical and inflexible carriers have been suggested to have reduced transport in tumor interstitial models compared to flexible and extended structures, and due to tumor vessel pore size restrictions, extravasation of nanospheres in cancerous tissue may be a highly size-dependent event (29). Gastrointestinal mucosa has size-dependent uptake phenomena affecting oral dosage of biodegrad-able nanoparticles (30,31). It follows that the physical characteristics of DDSs must be optimized for the intrinsic properties of the specific targeting site. The leaky vasculature of tumors has been exploited by the well-known enhanced permeability and retention effect, whereby long-circulating PEGylated "stealth" liposomes are capable of accu-mulating in the tumor space due to a lack of rapid clearance conferred by PEG, com-bined with the accessibility of the tumor pores to passive liposomal uptake.

Strategies for Actively Targeted Therapies

The bioconjugation of ligands, such as monoclonal antibodies, proteins, or peptides to the nanocarrier surface, has been exploited on many nanoparticulate DDSs for the purpose of concentrating therapeutic action to specific sites. Nonspecific peptide-based internalization systems, such as those based on cell-penetrating peptides, have been shown to be efficient in preliminary in vitro studies, and may internalize in an energy-independent mechanism depending on the cargo involved (32,33), but their use for in vivo targeting may not be clinically relevant due to the ability of these peptides to nonspecifically target many cell types irrespective of pathology. Cancerous cells have been targeted by nanoparticles toward unique surface antigens inherent to the tumor type (e.g., HER2 in breast cancer) (34) or radiation area (35). Other targets exploited by nanoparticulate systems with promising therapeutic outcomes include folate receptors (36) and cell-adhesion molecules (37–39), both prominent examples of ligand-mediated internalization processes that are clinically relevant in a number of pathologies.

Strategies for Drug Delivery System Transport Across Tight Endothelial Junctions

Tight endothelial barriers, such as the blood–brain barrier (BBB) and blood–retinal barrier, pose significant challenges to the transport of therapies, most of which traverse such barriers only under extreme pathological conditions. Methods to traverse these tight junctions would enable the clinical usage of multiple therapies and imaging modalities using contrast agents. Nanoparticulate delivery across the BBB for the transport has been achieved with numerous approaches. Transport of ligand-coated PEGylated polylactide–PLGA nanoparticles across the BBB has been demonstrated (40). A novel strategy was recently reported for PLGA nanoparticle transport across the BBB with the surface engineering of peptides similar to synthetic opioids (41). Our laboratory is currently investigating the potential of functionalized solid–lipid nanoparticles to transport magnetic resonance contrast agents, proteins, and fluorescent probes across the BBB. Thus, one can retain the desirable properties of nanocarriers with the added feature of BBB penetration, for the delivery of therapeutic or diagnostic agents which are not lipid-soluble enough or do not meet the physical criteria to normally cross the BBB.

FUTURE DIRECTIONS

The potential of nanoengineering strategies in the development of controlled- and triggered-release DDSs, preservation of drug activity, and disease-specific targeting has been presented. Many of these studies are preliminary in nature, and various systems require further toxicity and efficacy data to facilitate their transition to clinical trials. However, the synthetic and natural basic units which form the basis of these strategies, such as the therapeutics, PLGA, and solid lipids, have entered these phases. The success of these initial nanodelivery systems will usher in the clinical application of combinatorial, integrative strategies which constitute "smart" delivery systems, such as the multimodal "nanocell," a PLGA, PEG, and phospholipid-based nanoparticle which delivers both antiangiogenic and chemotherapeutic agents with temporally controlled kinetics (42). Other considerations, such as the ability to scale-up laboratory techniques for mass production of DDSs and the ability to upgrade existing, approved systems with stepwise functional additions, will also expedite their clinical usage. Nanoengineering offers the unique ability to manipulate the smallest interactions at the most fundamental scales, which is certain to provide a series of major advancements in drug delivery technology.

ACKNOWLEDGMENTS

This chapter was made possible by generous funding from the Vanderbilt University Institute for Integrative Biosystems Research and Education (VIIBRE), and the Vanderbilt Vision Research Center Training Grant (NEI T32 EYO7135).

REFERENCES

1. Panyam J, Labhasetwar V. Biodegradable nanoparticles for drug and gene delivery to cells and tissue. Adv Drug Deliv Rev 2003; 55(3):329–347.

2. Ahmed F, Discher DE. Self-porating polymersomes of PEG–PLA and PEG–PCL: hydroly-sis-triggered controlled release vesicles. J Control Release 2004; 96(1):37–53.
3. Schmeltzer RC, Schmalenberg KE, Uhrich E. Synthesis and cytotoxicity of salicylate-based poly(anhydride esters). Biomacromolecules 2005; 6(1):359–367.
4. Lynn DM, Amiji MM, Langer R. pH-responsive polymer microspheres: rapid release of encapsulated material within the range of intracellular pH. Angew Chem Int Ed Engl 2001; 40(9):1707–1710.
5. Little SR, Lynn DM, Ge Q, et al. Poly-beta amino ester-containing microparticles enhance the activity of nonviral genetic vaccines. Proc Natl Acad Sci USA 2004; 101(26): 9534–9539.
6. Little SR, Lynn DM, Puram SV, Langer R. Formulation and characterization of poly(beta amino ester) microparticles for genetic vaccine delivery. J Control Release 2005; 107(3): 449–462.
7. Potineni A, Lynn DM, Langer R, Amiji M. Poly(ethylene oxide)-modified poly(beta-amino ester) nanoparticles as a pH-sensitive biodegradable system for paclitaxel delivery. J Control Release 2003; 86(2–3):223–234.
8. Husseini GA, Myrup GD, Pitt WG, Christensen DA, Rapoport NY. Factors affecting acoustically triggered release of drugs from polymeric micelles. J Control Release 2000; 69(1):43–52.
9. Marin A, Muniruzzaman M, Rapoport N. Mechanism of the ultrasonic activation of micellar drug delivery. J Control Release 2001; 75(1–2):69–81.
10. Rapoport N, Marin A, Luo Y, Prestwich GD, Muniruzzaman MD. Intracellular uptake and trafficking of Pluronic micelles in drug-sensitive and MDR cells: effect on the intrac-ellular drug localization. J Pharm Sci 2002; 91(1):157–170.
11. Cook RO, Pannu RK, Kellaway IW. Novel sustained release microspheres for pulmonary drug delivery. J Control Release 2005; 104(1):79–90.
12. Edwards DA, Ben-Jebria A, Langer R. Recent advances in pulmonary drug delivery using large, porous inhaled particles. J Appl Physiol 1998; 85(2):379–385.
13. Chen Q, Tong S, Dewhirst MW, Yuan F. Targeting tumor microvessels using doxorubicin encapsulated in a novel thermosensitive liposome. Mol Cancer Ther 2004; 3(10): 1311–1317.
14. Chiu GN, Abraham SA, Ickenstein LM, et al. Encapsulation of doxorubicin into thermo-sensitive liposomes via complexation with the transition metal manganese. J Control Release 2005; 104(2): 271–288.
15. Mitragotri S, Langer R, Kost J. Enhancement of transdermal transport using ultrasound in combination with other enhancers. Handbook of Pharmaceutical Controlled-Release Technology. New York: Marcel Dekker, 2000.
16. Lee PJ, Langer R, Shastri VP. Novel microemulsion enhancer formulation for simultane-ous transdermal delivery of hydrophilic and hydrophobic drugs. Pharm Res 2003; 20(2):264–269.
17. Lee PJ, Langer R, Shastri VP. Role of n-methyl pyrrolidone in the enhancement of aque-ous phase transdermal transport. J Pharm Sci 2005; 94(4):912–917.
18. Yue IC, Poff J, Cortes ME, et al. A novel polymeric chlorhexidine delivery device for the treatment of periodontal disease. Biomaterials 2004; 25(17):3743–3750.
19. Keck CM, Muller RH. Drug nanocrystals of poorly soluble drugs produced by high pressure homogenisation. Eur J Pharm Biopharm 2006; 62:3–16.
20. Zhu G, Mallery SR, Schwendeman SP. Stabilization of proteins encapsulated in injectable poly(lactide-co-glycolide). Nat Biotechnol 2000; 18(1):52–57.
21. Heiati H, Tawashi R, Phillips NC. Drug retention and stability of solid lipid nanoparti-cles containing azidothymidine palmitate after autoclaving, storage and lyophilization. J Microencapsul 1998; 15(2):173–184.
22. Loftsson T, Brewster ME. Pharmaceutical applications of cyclodextrins 1: drug solubili-zation and stabilization. J Pharm Sci 1996; 85(10):1017–1025.
23. Sinisterra RD, Shastri VP, Najjar R, Langer R. Encapsulation and release of rhodium(II) citrate and its association complex with hydroxypropyl-beta-cyclodextrin from biode-gradable polymer microspheres. J Pharm Sci 1999; 88(5):574–576.
24. Chapman AP, Antoniw P, Spitali M, West S, Stephens S, King DJ. Therapeutic antibody fragments with prolonged in vivo half-lives. Nat Biotechnol 1999; 17(8):780–783.

25. Albrecht H, Burke PA, Natarajan A, et al. Production of soluble ScFvs with C-terminal-free thiol for site-specific conjugation or stable dimeric ScFvs on demand. Bioconjug Chem 2004; 15(1):16–26.

26. Natarajan A, Xiong CY, Albrecht H, DeNardo GL, DeNardo SJ. Characterization of site-specific ScFv PEGylation for tumor-targeting pharmaceuticals. Bioconjug Chem 2005; 16(1):113–121.

27. Cazalis CS, Haller CA, Sease-Cargo L, Chaikof EL. C-terminal site-specific PEGylation of a truncated thrombomodulin mutant with retention of full bioactivity. Bioconjug Chem 2004; 15(5):1005–1009.

28. Sato H. Enzymatic procedure for site-specific pegylation of proteins. Adv Drug Deliv Rev 2002; 54(4):487–504.

29. Stroh M, Zimmer JP, Duda DG, et al. Quantum dots spectrally distinguish multiple species within the tumor milieu in vivo. Nat Med 2005; 11(6):678–682.

30. Desai MP, Labhasetwar V, Amidon GL, Levy RJ. Gastrointestinal uptake of biodegradable microparticles: effect of particle size. Pharm Res 1996; 13(12):1838–1845.

31. Desai MP, Labhasetwar V, Walter E, Levy RJ, Amidon GL. The mechanism of uptake of biodegradable microparticles in Caco-2 cells is size dependent. Pharm Res 1997; 14(11):1568–1573.

32. Hallbrink M, Floren A, lmquist A, Pooga M, Bartfai T, Langel U. Cargo delivery kinetics of cell-penetrating peptides. Biochim Biophys Acta 2005; 15(2):101–109.

33. Padari K, Saalik P, Hansen M, et al. Cell transduction pathways of transportans. Bioconjug Chem 2005; 16(6):1399–1410.

34. Kirpotin D, Park JW, Hong K, et al. Sterically stabilized anti-HER2 immunoliposomes: design and targeting to human breast cancer cells in vitro. Biochemistry 1997; 36(1):66–75.

35. Hallahan D, Geng L, Qu S, et al. Integrin-mediated targeting of drug delivery to irradiated tumor blood vessels. Cancer Cell 2003; 3(1):63–74.

36. Hilgenbrink AR, Low PS. Folate receptor-mediated drug targeting: from therapeutics to diagnostics. J Pharm Sci 2005; 94(10):2135–2146.

37. Kelly KA, Allport JR, Tsourkas A, Shinde-Patil VR, Josephson L, Weissleder R. Detection of vascular adhesion molecule-1 expression using a novel multimodal nanoparticle. Circ Res 2005; 96(3):327–336.

38. Muro S, Gajewski C, Koval M, Muzykantov VR. ICAM-1 recycling in endothelial cells: a novel pathway for sustained intracellular delivery and prolonged effects of drugs. Blood 2005; 105(2):650–658.

39. Muro S, Koval M, Muzykantov V. Endothelial endocytic pathways: gates for vascular drug delivery. Curr Vasc Pharmacol 2004; 2(3):281–299.

40. Olivier JC. Drug transport to brain with targeted nanoparticles. NeuroRx 2005; 2(1):108–119.

41. Costantino L, Gandolfi F, Tosi G, Rivasi F, Vandelli MA, Forni F. Peptide-derivatized biodegradable nanoparticles able to cross the blood–brain barrier. J Control Release 2005; 108(1):84–96.

42. Sengupta S, Eavarone D, Capila I, et al. Temporal targeting of tumour cells and neovasculature with a nanoscale delivery system. Nature 2005; 436(7050):568–572.

Aerosol Flow Reactor Method for the Synthesis of Multicomponent Drug Nano- and Microparticles

Janne Raula
NanoMaterials Group, Laboratory of Physics and Center for New Materials, Helsinki University of Technology, Helsinki, Finland

Hannele Eerikäinen
Pharmaceutical Product Development, Orion Corporation Orion Pharma, Espoo, Finland

Anna Lähde
NanoMaterials Group, Laboratory of Physics and Center for New Materials, Helsinki University of Technology, Helsinki, Finland

Esko I. Kauppinen
NanoMaterials Group, Laboratory of Physics and Center for New Materials, Helsinki University of Technology, and VTT Biotechnology, Helsinki, Finland

INTRODUCTION

Nano- and microparticle drug carriers have potential applications for administration of therapeutic molecules (1,2). Targeted drug delivery can be achieved by small particles due to their tendency to accumulate in targeted areas of the body. Moreover, the solubility of material from the nanoscale objects is notably enhanced due to the increased surface-to-volume ratio of small particles. As well, the systemic side effects in drug targeting, for example, into a cancerous tumor, can be minimized by the decrease a particle size (3). Sub-micron, solid-state drug particles that tend to be unstable for many drug molecules can be stabilized by specific polymers. In these composite particles, the polymer may act, in addition to stabilizer, as functional material that controls the release and diffusion of a drug depending on the environmental conditions such as pH, temperature, ionic strength, humidity, and so on (4,5).

Several methods have been studied for the preparation of the drug nano- and microparticles. A common liquid route method to prepare the drug nano- and microparticles is the use of an emulsion. Probably, the most used method is an oil-in-water emulsion consisting of two immiscible solvents such as chloroform and water (6). As the drug particles show a large tendency towards agglomeration and growth, surfactants have to be added to stabilize the droplets and particles. Other related methods include salting-out (7), nanoprecipitation (interfacial precipitation) (8), phase separation (9), and evaporative precipitation into aqueous solution (10). In general, the production of particles including two or more drug molecules is difficult.

Size-reduction techniques, such as wet milling and high-pressure homogenization, have also been used to prepare nano- and microparticles (11). High-shear forces and thus high energies used in milling processes can create uncontrollable changes in the product, such as chemical degradation, changes in surface energetics, and damage in crystal structure. Furthermore, long processing times increase the risk of microbiological contamination. Surfactants are needed to reduce particle agglomeration and sintering during wet milling. Multicomponent particles with controlled morphology and surface characteristics (composition and morphology) cannot be produced.

Small particles have also been prepared using supercritical fluids either as solvents or antisolvents for the drug and the polymer (12). The preparation of uniform multicomponent particles consisting of a drug and a polymer has been shown to be difficult due to different crystallization and precipitation kinetics of the drug and the polymer molecules and due to partitioning of the drug into super-critical fluid.

Spray-drying has been widely used for the production of micrometer-sized particles (13). Spray-drying involves the conversion of a solution droplet into a dry particle by evaporation of the solvent in a one-step process. Both water-soluble and -insoluble compounds can be prepared. Thus, the recovery of the drug in the particles is almost quantitative. Also temperature-labile compounds such as proteins and enzymes have been successfully spray-dried. The solvent properties and the spray-drying variables can control the particle properties, especially morphology. Multicomponent particles with spherical morphology can be produced. However, particles are typically amorphous, and surface structure as well composition cannot be controlled in detail.

This chapter presents the novel aerosol flow reactor method for the synthesis of single- and multicomponent nanoparticles as well as nanostructured, micron-sized particles (14–21). We demonstrate the production of powders made from different drug and/or excipient materials. Besides the drug molecules, the polymeric drug nanoparticles contained methacrylic polymers, which are pharmaceutically acceptable (22,23). It was observed that the solubility of a drug within the polymer matrix depends not only on the amount of the drug, but also on the polymer itself. The drug dissolution form of the nanoparticles, interactions between the drug and the polymer, and drug crystallinity within the polymer particles will be discussed. This chapter also discusses the formation of the polymeric nano-particles from several solvents. The studied subjects were polymer solubility in a solvent medium and the influence of solvent vapor pressure.

Chemical and physical stability of dry powders in storage is crucial. Amorphous materials tend to crystallize in time, thus building bridges between individual particles. This in turn affects the powder flowability and handling. A part of this work presents the attempts to crystallize the drug within the aerosol reactor in different conditions. This chapter discusses the reactor conditions affecting the drug crystallization.

Adding leucine derivatives to drug particles has been shown to reduce the adhesion between particles (24,25). Furthermore, a α-amino acid L-leucine is a surface-active compound in aqueous solutions. It is also important that L-leucine is generally regarded as safe material for the human body. This chapter discusses the preparation of the composite powders using L-leucine to increase the stability of powders. Main materials were sodium chloride, which is a representative inorganic material that crystallizes with ease, and lactose that forms amorphous particles. The incorporation of L-leucine modifies particle surface structure and changes, for instance, spherical particles to wrinkled ones depending on the L-leucine content.

Moreover, L-leucine has been shown to reinforce the structure of particles where material is in a rubbery state.

AEROSOL FLOW REACTOR METHOD

In the aerosol flow reactor method, the solution containing solute(s) is atomized to produce droplets that are transferred with the aid of a carrier gas to a heated flow reactor (part I in Fig. 1). The inert carrier gas is either dry or saturated with a solvent. In the latter, the droplets remain wet in the reactor until the aerosol is heated (part II

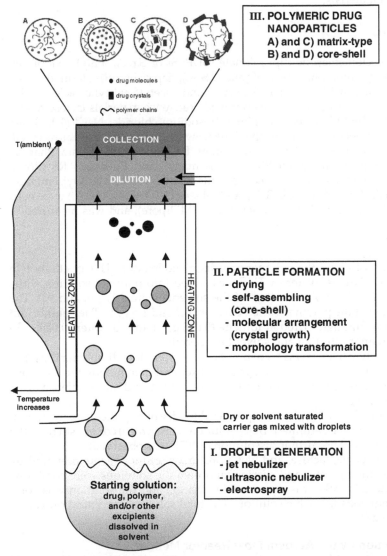

FIGURE 1 Schematical presentation of the novel aerosol flow reactor method for the production of nano and micronsized drug powders.

in Fig. 1). The fast drying promotes the formation of amorphous particles. Allowing time for droplet drying provides also time for molecular arrangements such as crystal growth to occur. Varying flow rate and the residence time, drying rate of particles and accordingly particle morphology can be manipulated in the process. Downstream from the heated section, the dry aerosol is diluted with dry inert gas to avoid solvent condensation onto dry particles. Polymeric drug nanoparticles of several types, that is, matrix and core shell as shown in part III in Figure 1 have been produced. Moreover, this aerosol method produces dry partocles directly without a need for further purification, and no additives are required. In the following, we describe the production of nano- and micron-sized dry particles containing the drugs, polymers, and some model materials.

EXPERIMENTAL
Materials
Drug materials beclomethasone dipropionate (BDP; Sicor S.p.A., Italy), ketoprofen (2-(3-benzoylphenyl) propionic acid) (Sigma, U.S.A.), naproxen [(S)-2-(6-methoxy-2-naphthyl) propionic acid] (Sigma, U.S.A.), and acetyl salicylic acid (ASA; Sigma-Aldrich, Germany) were used as received. Reference materials lactose monohydrate (provided by Orion Pharma, Finland), sodium chloride, NaCl (J.T. Baker, Holland), and excipient material L-leucine (Fluka, Switzerland) were used as received. Pharmaceutically accepted methacrylic polymers Eudragit® L100 (Röhm Pharma, Germany), Eudragit® E100 (Röhm Pharma, Germany), and Eudragit® RS (Röhm Pharma, Germany) were used as received. Solvents ethanol (99.6%, Alko Oyj, Finland), tetrahydrofuran (THF; J.T. Bakers, U.S.A.), and toluene (J.T. Bakers, U.S.A.) were used as received. Water was purified by ion-exchange (Millipore), and was measured to have pH 6.

Precursor Solutions
For pure polymer solutions, the polymer was dissolved in either THF or ethanol. In a case of solvent mixtures, water or THF was added into polymer solution while stirring the mixture. The volume ratios of the solvents were 0.1, 1.0, and 9.0. The total concentration of the polymer varied between 0.2 and 1.5 g/L. The equilibrium concentrations for Eudragit® L100 in toluene (0.058 g/L) and in water (0.029 g/L) were determined after filtration and solvent evaporation.

The drug–polymer solutions were prepared by separately dissolving the polymer and the drug in ethanol using a magnetic stirrer and then mixing the solutions in respective amounts. The total concentration of a drug and an excipient varied between 0.25 and 2.0 g/L.

BDP solutions 5 and 25 g/L were prepared by dissolving the drug in ethanol at room temperature. A saturated BDP solution was prepared by stirring the solution for 1 hour until no further dissolution of BDP was observed.

Aqueous L-leucine, lactose, and NaCl precursor solutions were prepared by separately dissolving in water and stirring, and then the solutions were combined in respective amounts. ASA was dissolved in ethanol, and the solution was combined with the aqueous L-leucine solution. The total solution concentration varied from 0.25 to 30.0 g/L.

Particle Production by the Aerosol Flow Reactor Method
The set-up of the aerosol flow reactor is presented in Figure 2. All the experimental conditions for the preparation of nano- and microparticles are given in Table 1. The

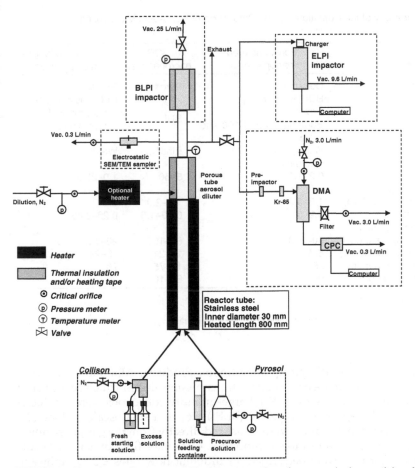

FIGURE 2 Experimental set-up used in the preparation of nano and microparticles. N_2=clean, dry pressurized nitrogen. *Abbreviations*: Vac., vacuum; L/min, liters per minute; Kr-85, aerosol neutralizer using ^{85}Kr β-source; BLPI, berner-type low pressure impactor; CPC, condensation particle counter; DMA, differential mobility analyzer; ELPI, electrical low-pressure impactor; SEM, scanning electron microscope; TEM, transmission electron microscope.

solutions to produce nanoparticles were atomized using a Collison-type air jet atomizer (TSI 3076, TSI, Inc., Particle Instruments, St. Paul, U.S.A.). The atomizer produces a lognormal droplet size distribution with a geometric number mean droplet size of approximately 300 nm and a geometric standard deviation between 1.6 and 2.0. The microparticle droplets were generated with an ultrasonic nebulizer (RBI Pyrosol 7901, Meylan, France). The droplets were carried in dry nitrogen gas into a heated reactor where aerosol flow was laminar. Depending on the flow rate, the residence time for droplet/particles in the reactor can be modified. The temperature of the stainless steel reactor was controlled with four separate heaters. Downstream from the heated section of the reactor, the aerosol was diluted by dry nitrogen in a porous diluter to avoid solvent condensation onto particle surface as well as particle deposition to reactor walls via thermophoresis. After fully mixing the reactor and dilution gas flows, a sample of particles was collected by

TABLE 1 Summary of the Conditions for the Production of Nano- and Micronsized Dry Powders

Type of powder	Polymeric drug nanoparticles	BDP microparticles	Composite L-leucine microparticles
Droplet generation	Collison[a]	Pyrosol[b]	Pyrosol[b]
Materials	BDP, ketoprofen, naproxen Eudragit® L100, E100 and RS100	BDP	NaCl, lactose, acetyl salicylic acid, L-leucine
Solvents	Water, ethanol, THF, toluene	Ethanol	Water
Precursor solution concentration (g/L)	0.2–1.5	5–50	1.0–27.5
Carrier gas flow rate (L/min)	1.5–3.5	1.5–2.0	1.4
Precursor solution consumption (mL/min)	0.2–0.4	0.09–1.6	0.28–0.45
Reactor wall temperature (°C)	40–200	50–150	20–100
Residence time in reactor (s)	6–21	16–21	19–24
Flow rate in dilution (L/min)	25	10–75	76
Dilution gas temperature (°C)	20	50–100	20

[a]Collison-type air jet atomizer.
[b]Ultrasonic nebulizer.
Abbreviations: BDP, beclomethasone dipropionate; THF, tetrahydrofuran.

a point-to-plane electrostatic precipitator (InTox Products, Albuquerque, U.S.A.) onto either a plain or carbon-coated copper transmission electron microscope (TEM) grid (Agar Scientific Ltd., Essex, U.K.). Large-quantity collections were conducted by a Berner-type low-pressure impactor (BLPI) (26) or a small-scale cyclone (27). Particle size and size distribution were measured directly from the gas phase downstream from the dilution and mixing processes. Computer fluid dynamics calculations of the reactor tube were performed for different flow rates ≤ 3.5 L/min with temperatures covering the temperature range used in the experiments. The calculations showed that in the heated zone a fully developed laminar flow was achieved, and the wall temperature was reached for all the particles (28).

Instrumentation and Characterization

The particle size (geometric number mean diameter, GNMD) and polydispersity (geometric standard deviation, GSD) of the nanoparticles in the gas phase, that is, at the reactor outlet, were determined with a TSI scanning mobility particle sizer equipped with a differential mobility analyzer (DMA, model 3081) (TSI, Inc., Particle Instruments, St. Paul, U.S.A.) and a condensation particle counter (CPC, model 3027) (TSI, Inc., Particle Instruments, St. Paul, U.S.A.). The average values of GNMD and GSD were determined from three to six measurements. The maximum standard errors were 5% and 0.5% for GNMD and GSD, respectively.

The GNMD and GSD of the produced microparticles were determined with an electrical low-pressure impactor (ELPI; Dekati Ltd., Tampere, Finland) (29,30). Oiled porous collection stages (Dekati Ltd., Tampere, Finland) were used to avoid the bouncing of the particles from upper stages to lower ones. The GNMD and GSD of the particles were calculated using equations GNMD $= \exp(\Sigma \ (n_i \ln D_i)/N)$ and GSD $= \exp((\Sigma n_i (\ln D_i - \ln GNMD)^2)/(N-1))^{1/2}$, respectively. Here n_i is the number of particles in the ith group, D_i the aerodynamic diameter of the ith group, and N the total number of particles, that is, Σn_i.

Mass median aerodynamic diameter (MMAD) and GSD of the dispersed particles were determined with the BLPI and using equations MMAD = $\exp(\Sigma (m_i \ln D_i))/M$ and GSD = $\exp((\Sigma (m_i D^3_i (\ln D_i - \ln MMAD)^2))/(\Sigma (m_i D^3_i) - 1))^{1/2}$, respectively. Here m_i is the mass fraction of the particles on the collection stage and M the sum of mass fractions and is unity. In all the experiments, the density of the particle is assumed to be 1 g/cm^3.

The morphology of the particles was analyzed with a field emission scanning electron microscope (SEM; Leo DSM982 Gemini, LEO Electron Microscopy, Inc., Oberkochen, Germany). Internal structure of the particles was studied using a TEM (TEM; Philips CM200 FEG, FEI Company, Eindhoven, The Netherlands). Some of the samples were coated with platinum sputtering in order to stabilize the particle under electron beam and to enhance image contrast.

The crystallinity of nanoparticles was studied using X-ray diffraction (XRD; Philips PW 1710, Eindhoven and Almelo, The Netherlands) with Cu Kα radiation. Diffraction angles (2θ) (goniometer PW 1820) used in the recording of the XRD patterns were 3° to 40°. The crystallinity of individual microparticles was investigated with TEM as well. The thermal properties of the nanoparticles were studied using a differential scanning calorimeter (DSC; Mettler Toledo DSC 822e, Mettler Toledo AG, Greifensee, Switzerland) where the samples were heated from 25°C to 300°C or from −50°C to 200°C using a heating rate of 10°C/min. A nitrogen purge of 50 mL/min was used in the oven.

RESULTS AND DISCUSSION
Polymer Nanoparticles
This section discusses the control of the polymer Eudragit® L100 nanoparticle morphology when produced from different solvent media (21). The morphology of nanoparticles depends on both the droplet drying rate and the polymer solubility in solvent medium. Vapor pressure of the solvent is essential because it mainly determines the solvent evaporation rate. Vapor pressures for THF, ethanol, toluene, and water at 25°C are 21.6, 7.87, 3.79, and 3.17 kPa, respectively. Also, a concept of solvent quality for a polymer is noteworthy (31). The solubility of Eudragit® L100 in used solvents was experimentally observed, and found to decrease in the following order: ethanol > THF > toluene > water. The first two solvents are good solvents for Eudragit® L100. The size of the dry Eudragit® L100 particles from ethanol and THF solutions increased, respectively, from 75 to 130 and 65 to 95 nm within the concentration range from 0.2 to 1.5 g/L. Accordingly, the GSD of the particles, that is, the spread of the size distribution of the particles from THF increased from 1.9 to 2.2 but that from ethanol remained the same, ~1.9. With added water, the solvent quality for the polymer worsens, that is, the polymer coil shrinks in the solution prior to atomization. As a result, the size of dry nanoparticles prepared from ethanol/water = 1:1 solution decreased approximately to two-thirds of the particles from pure ethanol. Moreover, the sizes from THF/water = 1:1 solutions at 0.2 and 1.0 g/L decreased, respectively, to four-fifths and two-thirds of the particles from pure THF. Polymer particles from toluene and water were small with the particle size around 35 nm and the GSD less than 1.9.

Figure 3 shows exemplary SEM images of the particles prepared from different solvent media. The figure summarizes the factors influencing the particle formation. Three main routes are discussed: (A) Non-hollow solid particles can be obtained

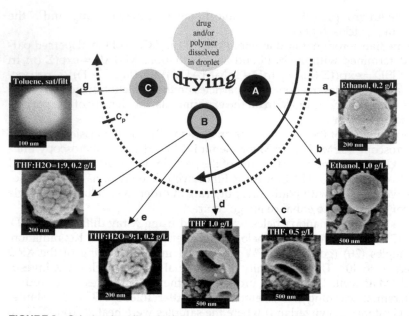

FIGURE 3 Scheme describes the influence of the experimental parameters on the particle formation and resulting particle morphology. A droplet containing drug and/or polymer dries in the reactor mainly in three ways: A, solidifying, B, film formation, and C, early precipitation. Along the solid arrow is the solvent vapor pressure, solvent evaporation rate , and polymer concentration increase. Along the dashed arrow is the solvent quality for the polymer (Eudragit® L100) decreases.

when solvent(s) evaporates slowly. The particles are often spherical. (B) If solvent evaporation is fast, the solute(s) forms a crust or film on the droplet surface. If the crust is impermeable to solvent, the particle will form a hollow interior due to pressure build-up on further solvent evaporation, which expands the particle (32–36). Hollow spherical particles can also collapse to raisin- or lens-shaped particles (SEM images **c** and **d** in Fig. 3) (34,37–39). (C) Polymer being close to its solubility limit in solvent prior to atomization precipitates at very early stages of solvent evaporation. For clarification, the solvent evaporation rate and polymer concentration increase along a curved solid arrow. When following the curved dashed arrow, the solvent quality for the polymer worsens. At some point of droplet drying, the polymer reaches its solubility limit (C_p^*) and precipitates (image **g** in Fig. 3). These particles have often very irregular shape. In between these two extremes, the particles may have very unusual morphologies, such as blistered (image **f** in Fig. 3) and wrinkled (image **e** in Fig. 3) structures (21).

Polymeric Drug Nanoparticles

This section discusses the production of polymeric drug nanoparticles where the drug and the polymer form a solid solution (18,19). The morphological stability of the nanoparticles, that is, whether the state of matter of the drug will change during storage, depends on the polymer used and will be discussed. Table 2 lists the experimental conditions as well as the physical properties of some of the polymeric drug nanoparticles. The solvent was ethanol in every solution. Nanoparticles prepared

TABLE 2 Summary of the Conditions and Physical Characteristics of Some of the Drug Nanoparticles Produced

Drug material	Eudragit®	C_{drug} (g/L)	$T_{reactor}$ (°C)	GNMD (nm)	GSD
Ketoprofen 0%	L100 100%	2	80	120	1,8
Ketoprofen 10%	L100 90%	2	80	120	1,8
Ketoprofen 25%	L100 75%	2	80	116	1,8
Ketoprofen 33%	L100 67%	2	80	112	1,9
Ketoprofen 50%	L100 50%	2	80	108	1,9
Ketoprofen 67%	L100 33%	2	80	107	1,9
Ketoprofen 33%	E100 67%	2	80	106	1,7
Ketoprofen 33%	RS 67%	2	80	96	1,7
Naproxen 50%	L100 50%	1	80	94	1,8
Naproxen 50%	L100 50%	2.5	80	124	1,8
Naproxen 50%	L100 50%	5	80	136	1,8
Naproxen 50%	L100 50%	10	80	160	1,7
Naproxen 50%	L100 50%	25	80	201	1,6

Drug concentration in precursor solution (C_{DRUG}) and reactor wall temperature ($T_{REACTOR}$) when producing drug-polymer composite nanoparticles are shown. Also geometric number mean diameter and geometric standard deviation of the particle size distribution as determined with the differential electrical mobility method are shown. *Abbreviations*: GNMD, geometric number mean diameter; GSD, geometric standard deviation.

with various proportions of ketoprofen and Eudragit® L100 at the reactor wall temperature of 80°C showed a decreasing particle size as a function of the amount of ketoprofen. With the same amount, 33% (w/w) of ketoprofen but a different polymer, the particle size decreased in order Eudragit® L100 > Eudragit® E100 > Eudragit® RS. The effect of solution concentration on particle size is also shown in Table 2.

The amorphous form of the drug has a tendency to spontaneously convert to a crystalline form (40,41). The structural stabilization, however, can be achieved by incorporating the drug into the polymer matrix. Polymer-drug nanoparticles were prepared from the drug materials BDP (18), naproxen (19), and ketoprofen (19). For naproxen and ketoprofen, it was observed that there is a limit to how much drug can be incorporated in an amorphous form into nanoparticles. When the amount of the drug in the nanoparticles was for ketoprofen ≤ 33% (w/w) and for naproxen ≤ 10%, the nanospheres were amorphous, proved by XRD, DSC, and TEM. No crystallinity or grain boundaries were found; instead, the nanoparticles were smooth with a uniform interior. The formation of an amorphous, polymer–drug structure has previously been observed for spray-dried particles containing methacrylic polymers and ketoprofen drug (42,43). When the amount of the drug in the nanoparticles was increased to 50% (w/w) ketoprofen and 25% naproxen, an endothermic transition corresponding to melting of the drug crystals was detected with DSC (Fig. 4). Moreover, in the XRD analyses, the broad background diffraction pattern of the amorphous structure became overlapped by peaks corresponding to the diffraction from the drug crystal lattice. However, the drug molecules on the particle surface crystallized, thus forming large crystalline bridges between neighboring nanoparticles, that is, phase-transition-induced sintering of the nanoparticles occurred.

Molecular size was assumed to affect drug crystallization during particle formation. BDP (*Mw* 521 g/mol) is a larger molecule than ketoprofen (254 g/mol) or naproxen (230 g/mol) molecules. The molecular mobility of BDP was expected to be slow due to its large size and high glass transition temperature ($T_g \sim 66°C$) (44,45).

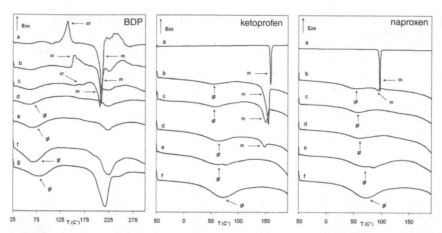

FIGURE 4 DSC thermograms of the Eudragit® L100 nanoparticles with drugs beclomethasone dipropionate (BDP), ketoprofen, and naproxen (marked in the figures). The content of BDP (a) 100% (w/w), (b) 80%, (c) 60%, (d) 50%, (e) 40%, (f) 20%, and (g) 0%. The content of ketoprofen (a) 100%, (b) 50%, (c) 33%, (d) 25%, (e) 10%, (f) 0%. The content of naproxen (a) 100%, (b) 50%, (c) 33%, (d) 25%, (e) 10%, (f) 0%. *Abbreviations:* cr, crystallization; m, melting; gt, glass transition.

The glass transition temperature, T_g, was calculated using the relation $T_g \sim 0.7\, T_m$ where temperatures were in Kelvin (46,47), a melting temperature, T_m, measured by DSC (18). Thus, the amorphous state of pure BDP nanoparticles, that is, no added polymer, is kinetically preserved even though it is not thermodynamically stable. The nanoparticles containing BDP both with and without polymer showed single, separate nanoparticles. Crystallization of BDP in the nanoparticles could be induced by heating, which can be seen as an exotherm in DSC measurements (Fig. 4).

In the amorphous structure, the drug is solubilized by the polymer, and the two components form an amorphous solid solution (48). The interactions between the drug and the polymer molecules determine the solubility of these materials in each other (49). When the drug–polymer molecular interactions are comparable to the drug–drug and the polymer–polymer interactions, the drug is well solubilized by the polymer and large amounts of drug can be incorporated in the polymer matrix without drug crystallization (50). However, when the drug–polymer interactions are weaker than the drug–drug or the polymer–polymer interactions, the drug and the polymer have a preference to interact with the molecules of their own kind, leading to a potential for drug crystallization. The amount of drug below the solubility limit of the drug in the polymer can be solubilized by the polymer matrix (51,52). On increasing the amount of the drug over this limit, the drug is no longer soluble in the amorphous polymer, but can form separate crystallites (53). An analogy to the solubility of the drug in the polymer can be found from plasticization, where flexible small molecules are mixed with the polymer to lower the T_g (53–55). Also in plasticization, it is essential that the plasticizing material forms a uniform mixture with the polymer, and is solubilized by the polymer. Consequently, from this point of view, ketoprofen was a more effective plasticizing agent for the Eudragit® L100 polymer than naproxen (53). Thus, the choice of the polymer is important for controlling the amorphous–crystalline transition. The nanoparticles were stored at three different conditions to study the influence of temperature and relative humidity on the morphology of particles. The nanoparticles containing 33%

(w/w) of ketoprofen and 67% of Eudragit® L100 polymer were stored for three months in a refrigerator, at 25°C and 0% of relative humidity, and at 25°C and 75% of relative humidity (sat. NaCl). After storage for three months, no changes in the morphology of the nanoparticles were observed, that is, still spheres were observed. As well, no crystallization of the drug within the nanoparticle occurred. To conclude, these nanoparticles were physically stable in all the conditions; however, chemical stability was not studied during this period of time.

Nanostructured Drug Microparticles
Drug Crystallization in the Reactor
Amorphous materials tend to crystallize over storage causing problems in instability but also in powder handling. Therefore, the crystalline form of the drug is preferred. The experimental conditions to crystallize beclomethasone dipropionate particles while producing them will be discussed in this section (56). Two solutions, 5 and 25 g/L, were atomized in the heated reactor at different temperatures. Table 3 summarizes the physical characteristics of the particles. The saturated precursor solutions prior to atomization included crystal seeds that were expected to induce the particle crystallization. The sizes of the powders were in a respirable size range (1–5 μm) and the size distributions were relatively narrow (i.e., GSD <2.1).

The main issue of this work was to explore the reactor conditions affecting the particle crystallization while producing them. Table 3 also lists the state of matter (crystalline and/or amorphous) in the final powders. Low solution concentration as well as low reactor temperature resulted in smooth-surfaced spheres that were amorphous. However, the increase in reactor temperature seemed to promote the crystallization process in the reactor. Appearance of roughness on the particle surface was indicative of crystals (Fig. 5A), and it was, in fact, proved by the XRD analysis. For comparison, fully amorphous, smooth-surfaced BDP powder is shown in Figure 5B. The evaporation of ethanol from the droplets is kinetically faster than the organization of the drug molecules to crystals. Therefore, the BDP powders were often amorphous. However, the diffusion of the BDP molecules in the amorphous solid state depends on T_g and the overall rate of crystallization. The latter is at its maximum at the mid-temperature between T_g and T_m (41). As the T_g and T_m were,

TABLE 3 Summary of the Production Conditions and Physical Characteristics of the Beclomethasone Dipropionate Powders Prepared from Ethanolic Solutions

C_{BDP} (g/L)	$T_{reactor}$ (°C)	MMAD (μm)	GSD	State of matter[c]
5[a]	150	1.4	1.8	Amorphous
25[a]	50	2.5	2.0	Amorphous
25[b]	100	1.7	2.0	Some crystallites
25[a]	150	2.2	2.0	Crystalline
Saturated[b]	100	2.1	2.1	Crystalline core

The concentration of BDP in precursor solution (C_{BDP}) and reactor wall temperature ($T_{reactor}$) when producing drug microparticles are shown. Also mass median aerodynamic diameter and geometric standard deviation of the particle size distribution as determined with the Berner-type low pressure impactor are shown.
[a]Flow rate 1.5 L/min through pyrosol.
[b]Flow rate 10 L/min through pyrosol, then divided into 5 tubes where 2 L/min.
[c]Directly from the production.
Abbreviations: BDP, beclomethasone dipropionate; GSD, geometric standard deviation; MMAD, mass median aerodynamic diameter.

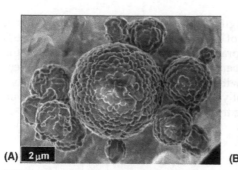 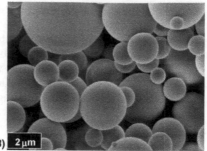

FIGURE 5 SEM images of the beclomethasone dipropionate powders in different state of matter: (**A**) rough and crystalline and (**B**) smooth and amorphous.

respectively, ~66°C (see the relation above) and ~212°C, the maximum crystallization rate was expected to be around 139°C. This explains the significance of reactor temperature for the particle crystallization. Thermal treatment accelerated crystal growth in the sites of crystal nucleation. The slurry solution with crystal nuclei was expected to promote heterogeneous nucleation and directing the crystal growth (57). The particles produced at 100°C were spheres with smooth particle surface that is a strong indication of amorphous state. However, the XRD analysis showed that the powder was crystalline. The particles contained crystalline core of the original crystal seeds. The crystals were covered by amorphous drug material.

Postannealing of the collected amorphous particles at various temperatures initiated and/or accelerated crystallization. The crystallization unfortunately extended between neighboring particles forming crystalline bridges between them. As powders tend to agglomerate and form clusters, the crystal bridge formation was inevitable. However, the agglomerates can be broken easily to individual particles by mild milling.

Coating of Particles by a Peptide

The morphology as well as stability of the particles can be modified with a surface-active peptide such as L-leucine (58). This is analog to the stabilization of drug nanoparticles by polymers as discussed earlier. The materials chosen for the preparation of the composite L-leucine powders have different physical and chemical properties. NaCl crystallizes with ease, whereas large lactose molecules are not able to organize during the droplet drying and the powders are amorphous in the collection. Moreover, using the relation $T_g \sim 0.7\, T_m$, the T_g of ASA was estimated to be rather low, around 13°C. Accordingly, pure ASA microparticles should have poor physical stability when collected.

Leucine derivatives are surface-active materials in aqueous solutions. Besides the surface tension measurements, the surface activity of a compound can be determined by surface accumulation parameters that reflect the degree of hydrophobicity of the compound. This is calculated by the equation $-(\Delta\sigma/\Delta c)$, where a change in surface tension $\Delta\sigma$ is measured as a function of solution concentration Δc (59). On the flat surface, the $-(\Delta\sigma/\Delta c)$ values for glycine, S-, L-, di-, and tri-leucine are −0.9 (σ values from Ref. 59), 40 (σ values from Ref. 59), 20 (σ values from Ref. 60), 870 (σ values from Ref. 24), and 1414 (σ values from Ref. 24), respectively. The accumulation of the surface-active molecules on droplet surface is most probably enhanced

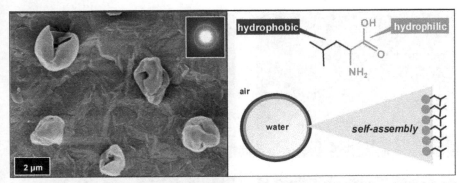

FIGURE 6 SEM image (*left*) of the pure L-leucine particles prepared from aqueous 15 g/L solution. The scheme on the right presents the self-assembling of L-leucine molecules on the surface of the droplet at the interface of water and air.

due to a high surface-to-volume ratio of the droplet. Pure L-leucine particles had spherical but strongly wrinkled structure (see an SEM image in Fig. 6). L-Leucine molecules gathered at the air–water interface on the droplet thus form a film. This film increasingly prevents the evaporative removal of water as it thickens. A drying particle expands while water molecules penetrate through the L-leucine film and after complete removal of water the film collapses to give wrinkled morphology (see the scheme in Fig. 6). During the surface organization, the L-leucine molecules crystallize to some extent giving partly polycrystalline structure (see diffraction patterns in the inset of Fig. 6).

Table 4 summarizes the physical characteristics of the produced composite powders. The size of saline composite particles increased slightly with the added L-leucine and the spread of size distribution did not vary, with GSD being around 2.5. With the added L-leucine from 0 to 7.5 g/L, however, the size of lactose particles decreased notably from 0.9 to below 0.5 µm, whereas the size distribution broadened and GSD increased from 1.9 to 3.8.

TABLE 4 Summary of the Production Conditions and Physical Characteristics of the L-leucine Composite Powders

Material	$C_{\text{L-leucine}}$ (g/L)	GNMD (µm)	GSD	State of matter
L-leucine	15	0.67	2.1	Partly polycrystalline[a]
NaCl 20 g/L	0	0.54	2.7	Crystalline[a,b]
NaCl 20 g/L	2.5	0.64	2.6	Crystalline[b]
NaCl 20 g/L	7.5	0.66	2.5	Crystalline[b]
Lactose 20 g/L	0	0.91	1.9	Amorphous[a,b]
Lactose 20 g/L	2.5	0.52	3.5	Amorphous[b]
Lactose 20 g/L	7.5	0.51	3.8	Amorphous[b]
ASA 15 g/L	7.5	0.43	1.9	Amorphous[b]

The concentrations of L-leucine in aqueous precursor solutions ($C_{\text{L-leucine}}$) when producing drug microparticles at the reactor wall temperature of 100 °C are shown. Also geometric number mean diameter and geometric standard deviation of the particle size distribution as determined with the electrical low pressure impactor (ELPI) are shown.
[a]TEM.
[b]XRD.
Abbreviations: GNMD, geometric number mean diameter; GSD, geometric standard deviation.

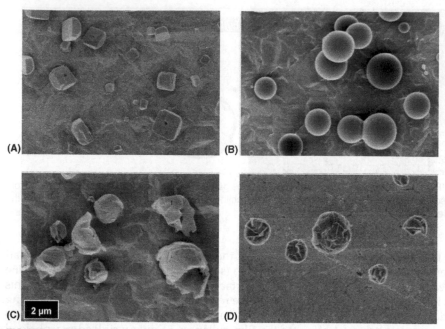

FIGURE 7   SEM images of (**A**) NaCl, (**B**) NaCl/L-leucine, (**C**) lactose, and (**D**) lactose/L-leucine particles. In the precursor solutions the concentration of NaCl and lactose was 20 g/L, and that of L-leucine was 7.5 g/L.

The morphology of the composite particles was controlled by the amount of L-leucine. The surface of lactose particles changed from smooth to wrinkled, whereas cubic crystalline salt particles changed from spheroidal to leafy ones with increasing L-leucine content (Fig. 7A–D). The XRD studies showed that the produced powders were amorphous except saline composite particles that have the strong diffraction peaks of NaCl at 31.7° and 45.5° (2θ). The structure of the NaCl composite particles was studied by the evaporative removal of L-leucine in the oven at 200°C for 10 minutes (Tsub of L-leucine is ~145–148°C) (61). After the thermal treatment, the remaining particle was a salt cube with holes on the surface. This showed that the L-leucine molecules formed the shell around the salt core, partly mixing with salt core. The structure of lactose composite powder could not studied because the T_g of lactose monohydrate (~101°C) was lower than the temperature for L-leucine removal.

The materials that have T_g below the collection temperature and do not crystallize in the reactor cannot be collected as compact individual particles. Above T_g, the material is in rubbery state, and is soft and even fluidly. Pure ASA particles produced from an ethanolic solution (15 g/L) were found flat and crystalline—a rough particle surface is indicative of crystallinity—on the collector surface. They flatten during collection with the formation of rubbery film that subsequently crystallizes after collection. Thus, L-leucine has been used to stabilize the structure of the ASA particles. The aqueous L-leucine solution was mixed with the ethanolic ASA solution and then droplets were produced. At low L-leucine concentration (2.5 g/L), some flat particles were still observed (Fig. 8A) but at the concentration of 7.5 g/L all the particles were spherical and compact with porous structure (Fig. 8B).

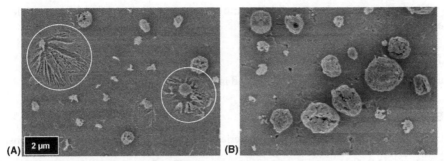

FIGURE 8 SEM images of acetyl salicylic acid composite particles prepared from aqueous ethanol solution. The concentration of ASA was 15 g/L and that of L-leucine was (**A**) 2.5 g/L and (**B**) 7.5 g/L in ethanol/water solution. Flat and crystalline particles where L-leucine content is low (2.5 g/L) are circled in the image.

The physical stability, that is, morphological changes of the powders were examined in two conditions: at 25°C and 0% relative humidity, and at 25°C and 44% relative humidity (sat. K_2CO_3) for three months. After three months, pure L-leucine as well as all saline particles showed no changes in morphology. However, pure lactose powder showed neck formation between particles even at 0% relative humidity but this did not occur with L-leucine-containing lactose particles. The surface of lactose particles was hardened by an L-leucine layer and such bridges between neighboring particles were not observed.

CONCLUSIONS

The aerosol flow reactor method is a novel method to produce drug particles from atomized solutions. The reactor can be modified to produce particles of different sizes, that is, nano- or microparticles. This method has been used to prepare spherical and amorphous matrix-type drug–polymer nanoparticles as well as micrometer-sized dry powders for dry powder inhalation. Experimental conditions influenced drastically the particle formation and morphology. Solvent vapor pressure as well as the crust formation on the droplet surface mainly determined the resulting morphology of the polymer nanoparticles. Moreover, the solute solubility in the starting solution also affected the particle shape. The state of drug in the polymer nanoparticles depends on the drug molecule itself, that is, size and chemical structure. With increasing size of the molecule, the diffusion within the polymer matrix decreased. As it was shown, large drug molecule BDP was amorphous in all particles, whereas smaller molecules ketoprofen and naproxen were amorphous to some extent. As the number of these latter molecules increased, they crystallized and the nanoparticles coalesced. The difference in the interaction between the drug and the polymer was observed as the change of the glass transition temperature of the particles. The drug crystallization depended on the thermal history experienced in the reactor. The molecular mobility increased with increasing reactor temperature that in some cases produced fully or partly crystalline drug particles.

Particle morphology and surface properties of the microparticles can be modified by the peptide L-leucine. Owing to the surface activity of the peptide in aqueous solutions, it is also possible to stabilize the structure of the drug particles that are otherwise structurally unstable.

ACKNOWLEDGMENT

Financial support from the Academy of Finland is gratefully acknowledged.

REFERENCES

1. Edelstein AS, Cammarata RC. Nanomaterials: Synthesis, Properties and Applications. Bristol: JW Arrowsmith Ltd., 1996:1.
2. Ravi Kumar MNV. Nano and microparticles as controlled drug delivery devices. J Pharm Pharmaceut Sci 2000; 3:234, and references therein.
3. Brigger I, Dubernet C, Couvreur P. Nanoparticles in cancer therapy and diagnosis. Adv Drug Deliv Rev 2002; 54:631.
4. Galaev IYu, Mattiasson B. Thermoreactive water-soluble polymers, nonionic surfactants, and hydrogels as reagents in biotechnology. Enzyme Microb Technol 1993; 15:354.
5. Yuk SH, Bae YH. Phase-transition polymers for drug delivery. Crit Rev Ther Drug Carrier Syst 1999;16:385.
6. Allémann E, Curny R, Doelker E. Drug-loaded nanoparticles—preparation methods and drug targeting issues. Eur J Pharm Biopharm 1993; 39:173.
7. Allémann E, Doelker E, Curny R. Drug loaded poly(lactic acid) nanoparticles produced by a reversible salting-out process: purification of an injectable dosage form. Eur J Pharm Biopharm 1993; 39:13.
8. Fessi H, Puisieux F, Devissaguet JP, Ammoury N, Benita S. Nanocapsule formation by interfacial polymer deposition following solvent displacement. Int J Pharm 1989; 55:R1.
9. Niwa T, Takeuchi H, Hino T, Nohara M, Kawashima Y. Biodegradable submicron carriers for peptide drugs: preparation of d,l-lactide/glycolide copolymer (PLGA) nanospheres with nafarelin acetate by a novel emulsion-phase separation method in an oil system. Int J Pharm 1995; 121:45.
10. Chen X, Young TJ, Sarkari M, Williams RO, Johnston KP. Preparation of cyclosporine A nanoparticles by evaporative precipitation into aqueous solution. Int J Pharm 2002; 242:3.
11. Liversidge GG, Cundy KC. Particle size reduction for improvement of oral bioavailability of hydrophobic drugs. I. Absolute oral bioavailability of nanocrystalline danazol in beagle dogs. Int J Pharm1995; 125:91.
12. Bodmeier R. Polymeric microspheres prepared by spraying into compressed carbon dioxide. Pharm Res 1995; 12:1211.
13. Broadhead J, Pouan SKE, Rhodes CT. The spray drying of pharmaceuticals. Drug Dev Ind Pharm 1992; 18:1169.
14. Watanabe W, Kauppinen EI, Ahonen P, Brown DP, Muttonen E. Combination drugs for the treatment of asthma. Patent Application FI 20002216, 2000.
15. Watanabe W, Kauppinen EI, Ahonen P, Brown DP, Muttonen E. Combination particles. Patent Application FI 20002215, 2000.
16. Watanabe W, Ahonen P, Kauppinen EI, et al. Inhalation particles. Patent Application WO World IPO 0149263, 2001.
17. Eerikäinen H, Watanabe W, Kauppinen EI, Ahonen PP. Aerosol flow reactor method for synthesis of drug nanoparticles. Eur J Pharm Biopharm 2003; 55:357.
18. Eerikäinen H, Kauppinen EI. Preparation of polymeric nanoparticles containing corticosteroids by a novel aerosol flow reactor method. Int J Pharm 2003; 263:69.
19. Eerikäinen H, Kauppinen EI, Kansikas J. Polymeric drug nanoparticles prepared by an aerosol flow reactor method. Pharm Res 2004; 21:136.
20. Kauppinen EI, Eerikäinen H, Brown DP, Raula J, Hua J. Nanoparticles and a method for the preparation of nanoparticles. Patent FI20031183, 2003.
21. Raula J, Eerikäinen H, Kauppinen EI. Influence of the solvent composition on the morphology of polymer drug composite nanoparticles. Int J Pharm 2003; 284:13.
22. Shukla AJ. Polymethacrylates. In: Wade A, Weller PJ, eds. Handbook of Pharmaceutical Excipients. Washington, DC: Pharmaceutical Press, 1994:362–366.

23. Dittgen M, Durrani M, Lehmann K. Acrylic polymers: a review of pharmaceutical applications. STP Pharma Sci 1997; 7:403.
24. Lechuga-Ballesteros D, Kuo M-C. Dry powder compositions having improved dispersivity. WO World IPO 01/32144, 2001.
25. Chew NYK, Chan H-K. Effect of humidity on the dispersion of dry powders. In: Dalby RN, Byron PR, Farr SJ, Peart J, eds. Respiratory Drug Delivery VII. Raleigh: Serentec Press, 2000:615.
26. Hillamo R, Kauppinen EI. On the performance of the Berner low pressure impactor. Aerosol Sci Technol 1991; 14:33.
27. Zhu Y, Lee KW. Experimental study on small cyclones operating at high flow rates. J Aerosol Sci 1999; 30:1303.
28. Brown DP. Development of a three-dimensional coupled flow, species and aerosol model: applications to particle deposition in gas turbines and aerosol formation and growth in jet engine exhausts. Ph.D. Thesis. University of Cincinnati, Cincinnati, USA, 1996.
29. Keskinen J, Pietarinen K, Lehtimäki M. Electrical low pressure impactor. J Aerosol Sci 1992; 23:353.
30. Moisio M. Real time size distribution measurement of combustion aerosols. Ph.D. Thesis. Tampere University of Technology, Tampere, Finland, 1999.
31. Grosberg AYu, Khokhlov AR. Giant Molecules, Here, There, and Everywhere. USA: Academic Press, 1997; 117:109–125.
32. Che S, Sakurai O, Shinozaki K, Mizutani N. Particle structure control through intraparticle reactions by spray pyrolysis. J Aerosol Sci 1998; 29:271.
33. Zhou XD, Zhang SC, Huebner W, Ownby PD, Hongchen Gu. Effect of the solvent on the particle morphology of spray dried PMMA. J Mater Sci 2001; 36:3759.
34. Esposito E, Roncarati R, Cortesi R, Cervellati F, Nastruzzi C. Production of Eudragit microparticles by spray-drying technique: influence of experimental parameters on morphological and dimensional characteristics. Pharm Dev Technol 2000; 5:267.
35. Wang F-J, Wang C-H. Sustained release of etanidazole from spray dried microspheres prepared by non-halogenated solvents. J Control Release 2002; 81:263.
36. Gurav A, Kodas T, Pluym T, Xiong Y. Aerosol processing of materials. Aerosol Sci Technol 1993; 19:411.
37. Maa Y-F, Nguyen P-AT, Hsu SW. Spray-drying of air–liquid interface sensitive recombinant human growth hormone. J Pharm Sci 1998; 87:152.
38. Leong KH. Morphological control of particles generated from the evaporation of solution droplets: experiment. J Aerosol Sci 1987; 18:525.
39. Giunchedi P, Torre ML, Maggi L, Conti B, Conte U. Cellulose acetate trimetillate ethylcellulose blends for non-steroidal anti-inflammatory drug (NSAID) microspheres. J Microencapsul 1996; 13:89.
40. Yu L. Amorphous pharmaceutical solids: preparation, characterization and stabilization. Adv Drug Deliv Rev 2001; 48:27.
41. Hancock BC, Zografi G. Characteristics and significance of the amorphous state in pharmaceutical systems. J Pharm Sci 1997; 86:1.
42. Palmieri GF, Bonacucina G, Di Martino P, Martelli S. Gastro-resistant microspheres containing ketoprofen. J Microencapsul 2002; 19:111.
43. Palmieri GF, Elisei I, Di Martino P, Martelli S. Formulation of microparticulate systems for modified release containing ketoprofen.In: 19th Pharmaceutical Technology Conference, Italy, 2000.
44. Morimoto Y, Kokubo T, Sugibayashi K. Diffusion of drugs in acrylic-type pressure-sensitive adhesive matrix. II. Influence of interaction. J Control Release 1992; 18:113.
45. Saleem M, Asfour A-FA, De Kee D. Diffusion of organic penetrants through low density polyethylene (LDPE) films: effect of size and shape of the penetrant molecules. J Appl Polym Sci 1989; 37:617.
46. Byrn S, Pfeiffer RR, Ganey M, Hoiberg C, Poochikian G. Pharmaceutical solids: a strategic approach to regulatory considerations. Pharm Res 1995; 12:945.
47. Hancock BC, Zografi G. The relationship between the glass transition temperature and the water content of amorphous pharmaceutical solids. Pharm Res 1994; 11:471.
48. Leuner C, Dressman J. Improving drug solubility for oral delivery using solid dispersions. Eur J Pharm Biopharm 2000; 50:47.

49. Dubernet C. Thermoanalysis of microspheres. Thermochim Acta 1995; 248:259.
50. Ford JL. The use of thermal analysis in the study of solid dispersions. Drug Dev Ind Pharm 1987; 13:1741.
51. Jenquin MR, McGinity JW. Characterization of acrylic resin matrix films and mechanisms of drug–polymer interactions. Int J Pharm 1987; 101:23.
52. Dubernet C, Rouland JC, Benoit JP. Ibuprofen-loaded ethylcellulose microspheres: analysis of the matrix structure by thermal analysis. J Pharm Sci 1991; 80:1029.
53. Wu C, McGinity JW. Non-traditional plasticization of polymeric films. Int J Pharm 1999; 177:15.
54. Jenquin MR, Liebowitz SM, Sarabia RE, McGinity JW. Physical and chemical factors influencing the release of drugs from acrylic resin films. J Pharm Sci 1990; 79:811.
55. Lin S-Y, Chen K-S, Run-Chu L. Organic esters of plasticizers affecting the water absorption, adhesive property, glass transition temperature and plasticizer permanence of Eudragit acrylic films. J Control Release 2000; 68:343.
56. Lähde A, Raula J, Kauppinen EI, Watanabe W, Ahonen PP, Brown DP. Aerosol synthesis of inhalation particles via a droplet-to-particle method. Part Sci Technol 2005; 24:71.
57. Rodríguez-Hornedo N, Murphy D. Significance of controlling crystallization mechanisms and kinetics in pharmaceutical systems. J Pharm Sci 1999; 88:651.
58. Raula J, Kurkela JA, Brown DP, Kauppinen EI. Study of the dispersion behavior of L-leucine containing microparticles synthesized with an aerosol flow reactor method. Powder Technol 2006.
59. Weissbuch I, Frolow F, Addadi L, Lahav M, Leiserowitz L. Oriented crystallization as a tool for detecting ordered aggregates of water-soluble hydrophobic α-amino acids at the air–solution interface. J Am Chem Soc 1990; 112:7718.
60. Matubayasi N, Miyamoto H, Namihira J, Yano K, Tanaka T. Thermodynamic quantities of surface formation of aqueous electrolyte solutions.V. Aqueous solutions of aliphatic amino acids. J Colloid Interface Sci 2002; 250:431.
61. Svec HJ, Clyde DD. Vapour pressures of some amino acids. J Chem Eng Data 1965; 10:151.

9 Supercooled Smectic Nanoparticles

Heike Bunjes and Judith Kuntsche
*Department of Pharmaceutical Technology, Institute of Pharmacy,
Friedrich Schiller University Jena, Jena, Germany*

INTRODUCTION

Among the different types of nanoparticulate drug carrier systems, lipid nanoparticles are particularly promising with regard to physiological compatibility as they can be prepared predominantly or even exclusively on the basis of physiological compounds. Colloidal lipid emulsions and solid lipid nanoparticles are the classical examples of matrix-type lipid nanoparticles, which are mainly under investigation as carriers for poorly water-soluble and lipophilic drugs. These two types of nanodispersions each have their own advantages and disadvantages with regard to their use as drug carrier systems. For example, colloidal lipid emulsions of natural and semisynthetic oils have a solid basis of technological know-how and a well-documented record of physiological compatibility arising from their decade-long use in parenteral nutrition (1). Also their interactions with drugs have been characterized, and some drug-loaded formulations are commercially available (1–3). The drug incorporation capacity of the liquid droplets is comparatively high in comparison with solid lipid nanoparticles and can be modified by variation of the oil compound. On the other hand, the liquid nature of the emulsion droplets may lead to disadvantages. In cases of insufficient stabilization, the droplets may grow by coalescence; incorporated drug molecules have a high mobility and can easily migrate into the surfactant layer or leak into the aqueous phase. Solid lipid nanoparticles with their rigid core were developed to overcome these limitations (4,5). It has, however, turned out that the usually crystalline nature of the solid particle core counteracts incorporation of larger amounts of drugs so that the drug carrier capacity of these particles is frequently rather low (6). Moreover, the physical behavior of the systems is often quite complex (e.g., with regard to crystallization, polymorphic transitions, and interparticle interactions) and certain proposed advantages of solid lipid nanoparticles, such as the ability to provide better control of drug release, still remain to be proven.

In search of an alternative lipid carrier system, which could combine the advantages of lipid emulsions and solid lipid nanoparticles, we were aiming to prepare carrier particles with a less ordered state than solid lipid nanoparticles in order to achieve a higher incorporation capacity for foreign substances. The particles should, however, still reduce the mobility of incorporated drugs and surface active agents as much as possible. We focused our interest on liquid crystalline phases (also called mesophases), which combine a certain mobility on the molecular level with an often rather high macroscopic viscosity. Formation of liquid crystalline phases can be induced by addition of solvents (lyotropic mesophases) or by temperature (thermotropic mesophases). Whereas lyotropic mesomorphism is frequently encountered and also utilized in the area of pharmaceutics (7,8), thermotropic mesophases have not yet received much attention in this field, although thermotropic mesomorphism has been described for some drug substances (9). The solvent-free character of lipophilic thermotropic mesophases makes them similar to the dispersed phase of colloidal lipid emulsions and suspensions, and thus promising to be explored as potential matrix materials in colloidal drug delivery systems.

THERMOTROPIC MESOPHASES

While lyotropic mesophases are formed by amphiphilic molecules in the presence of a suitable solvent, thermotropic mesomorphism is a specific property of certain substances with strongly anisometric molecular shape that does not require any additives and occurs in dependence on temperature (10). Thermotropic mesophases are classified into two main groups: calamitic (formed by molecules with rod-like shape, Fig. 1) and discotic (molecules with disc-like shape) mesophases. Two main calamitic mesophases, the smectic and the nematic phases, can be distinguished. When a substance forms a smectic as well as a nematic phase, the smectic phase always exists at lower temperatures. In the smectic phase, the molecules are aligned side by side forming a layered structure. Different modifications of the smectic phase have been described, for example, the molecules can be arranged perpendicular (smectic A phase) or tilted (smectic C phase) with respect to the smectic layers. Smectic A phases are typical for saturated cholesterol esters such as cholesteryl myristate (CM) and palmitate (CP); for cholesteryl oleate (CO), a smectic C phase is assumed (12). In the nematic phase, the molecules are arranged nearly in parallel but not in specific layers. The cholesteric phase, which is characteristic of cholesterol esters, can be regarded as a twisted nematic phase. Individual nematic molecular layers are twisted against each other in a certain angle forming a helical structure. The distance between the molecular layers with the same orientation (pitch) depends on temperature and is often in the range of the wavelength of visible light leading to characteristic color effects.

Thermotropic mesophases are broadly applied in the technical field, for example, for liquid crystal displays, and, consequently, most known thermotropic mesogens have been developed for technical applications (13). Cholesterol fatty acid esters as a class of physiological substances are, however, also capable of forming thermotropic mesophases (12). As their smectic phase has a high viscosity, it appeared promising to provide the desired characteristics for the development of the novel type of lipid nanoparticles.

CHOLESTERYL MYRISTATE NANOPARTICLES: GENERAL PROPERTIES AND PHASE BEHAVIOR

For first investigations on the preparation of smectic nanoparticles, the physiological ester CM was used as model matrix lipid due to its fully reversible and

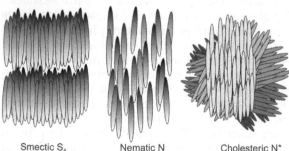

Smectic S_A Nematic N   Cholesteric N*

FIGURE 1 Structures of thermotropic calamitic mesophases. *Source*: Adapted from Ref. 11.

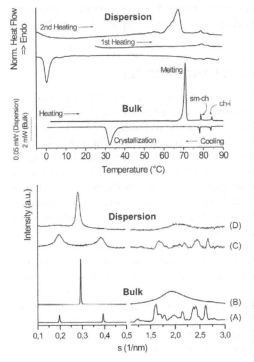

FIGURE 2 *(Top)* Differential scanning calorimetry heating and cooling curves (5°C/min) of CM in bulk and in colloidal dispersion (5% CM, 3.2% S100, 0.8% SGC). The samples were heated to the isotropic melt (curve not shown for the bulk material), cooled down below the crystallization temperature, and heated again (sm-ch: smectic–cholesteric, ch-i: cholesteric–isotropic phase transition). *(Bottom)* Small- and wide-angle X-ray diffraction patterns of CM in bulk and in colloidal dispersion (5% CM, 3.2% S100, 0.8% SGC). Bulk: crystalline powder **(A)** at 20°C and smectic mesophase **(B)** at 60°C (formed upon cooling the isotropic melt). Dispersions: stored at 4°C **(C)** and at 23°C **(D)** measured at 20°C. The graphs of the bulk material and the dispersions are not on the same linear intensity scale ($s = 1/d = 2 \sin \Theta / \lambda$ where 2Θ is the scattering angle and λ is the wavelength, equal to 0.15 nm). *Abbreviations*: CM, cholesteryl myristate; SGC, sodium glycocholate; S100, purified soy bean lecithin Lipoid S100 (Lipoid KG, D-Ludwigshafen).

well-characterized phase behavior (11,14). Crystalline CM melts around 72°C into a smectic phase, transforms into the cholesteric phase around 79°C, and finally melts into an isotropic liquid around 84°C (Fig. 2). Upon cooling the melt, the liquid crystalline phase transitions are observed at about the same temperatures as upon heating. Crystallization occurs between about 40°C and 30°C. Thus, the smectic phase of bulk CM does not exist under pharmaceutically relevant conditions such as body and room temperature. For colloidal particles of CM, the same phase transitions are, in principle, observed as for the bulk material except for the distinctly higher supercooling of the smectic phase upon cooling (Fig. 2). The fact that CM crystallization starts only below 20°C in the colloidal state is the basis for the preparation of smectic nanoparticles. When the hot dispersions are only cooled to room temperature and stored under this condition, their smectic state can be retained for many months (11,14). Upon heating of a stable smectic CM dispersion, only the liquid crystalline phase transitions are observed. These transitions are very small and, for the colloidal dispersions, broad and not well separated, making their quantification difficult. As an additional feature to characterize the smectic state of the nanoparticles, the very sharp small-angle X-ray reflection arising from the layered structure of the smectic phase can be used (Fig. 2). This smectic reflection is broader and less intensive for the nanoparticles, but its position is comparable with that of the bulk material when measured under comparable conditions. As the repeating unit (spacing) of the smectic phase increases with decreasing temperature (15), a larger spacing of the strongly supercooled smectic nanoparticles is measured at 20°C (11). In the wide-angle range, only diffuse X-ray scattering is observed because of the lack of molecular order. For the crystalline material (the nanoparticles can be crystallized by storage at, e.g., 4°C), characteristic wide-angle reflections are visible beside small-angle reflections of first and higher orders. For the crystalline nanoparticles, the reflections are less sharp, but their positions are comparable with those of the bulk lipid.

PREPARATION METHODS FOR SMECTIC NANOPARTICLES

Aqueous dispersions of smectic cholesterol ester nanoparticles can be prepared by high-pressure homogenization of a hot pre-emulsion (obtained, e.g., by ultra-turrax vortexing) at temperatures above the melting point of the respective matrix lipid in the presence of emulsifiers. The process, known as high-pressure melt-homogenization, is also commonly used for the preparation of solid lipid nanoparticles (4,5) and, in principle, similar to the preparation of colloidal fat emulsions (3,16). After homogenization (using a microfluidizer or piston-gap homogenizer), the hot nanoparticle dispersions are usually filtered (0.2 or 5 μm). High-pressure melt-homogenization yields dispersions of smectic nanoparticles with mean particle sizes between 100 and 200 nm, avoiding the use of organic solvents (11,14).

The high temperature during the process of melt-homogenization may lead to a partial degradation of thermally sensitive compounds and drugs. To avoid this problem and for the preparation of dispersions with smaller particles, a modification of the so-called emulsification solvent-evaporation method (17) can be used. The lipid and lipophilic stabilizers are dissolved in an organic solvent, which is not miscible with water, for example, cyclohexane. A crude pre-emulsion with the aqueous phase (containing hydrophilic surfactants) is prepared by ultra-turrax vortexing and the dispersion is high pressure homogenized, for example, using a microfluidizer. The whole process is carried out at room or slightly lower temperature. The organic solvent is removed under reduced pressure and at slightly elevated temperature. The dispersions are filtered and heated above the melting temperature of the matrix lipid for about 10 minutes to ensure the smectic state of the nanoparticles. With this method, dispersions with mean diameters distinctly below 100 nm can be prepared (11). Residual organic solvent in the dispersions may, however, be a disadvantage of this procedure (18,19).

Particle size is a crucial point in the development of dispersions that are stable upon storage with regard to the metastable smectic state of the matrix material, as has been shown for CM dispersions stabilized on the basis of phospholipids. Dispersions of smaller particles are more stable against recrystallization upon storage than dispersions with larger particle sizes (14). Moreover, the storage temperature has to be adjusted to the dispersion properties: If the dispersions are stored too close to the recrystallization temperature of the nanoparticles, the matrix lipid will crystallize during storage.

For administration of nanoparticles via the parenteral or ocular route, sterility of the dispersions is an important issue. First studies indicate that dispersions of supercooled smectic nanoparticles can be sterilized by autoclaving at 121°C without increase in particle size (stabilization with phospholipid/bile salt mixtures) or with only a small increase in particle size [stabilization with poloxamer 188 or poloxamine (Tetronic 908, BASF, D-Ludwigshafen)]. Small-sized dispersions can also be filtered through 0.2-μm filters as outlined above.

INFLUENCE OF THE STABILIZER SYSTEM

Colloidal dispersions are thermodynamically unstable systems because of their high interfacial energy. For the preparation and stabilization of colloidal lipid particles, surface active agents, which accumulate in interfaces and reduce the interfacial energy, are required. Depending on the properties of the surface active agent, stabilization occurs by electrostatic (charged surfactants) or steric (e.g., amphiphilic polymers) stabilization or a combination of both. Stabilizers may also influence the phase behavior of dispersed lipids, like their crystallization and polymorphic behavior (20–22). Furthermore, the stabilizer system determines the surface properties influencing the fate of the nanoparticles in vivo (23,24). For the stabilization of smectic CM nanoparticles, purified phospholipids (soybean and egg-yolk phospholipids) alone or in combination with the bile salt sodium glycocholate, sodium glycocholate alone, sodium oleate, different polymers [poloxamer, poloxamine, partially acetylated polyvinyl alcohol (PVA)], Tween 80, a sucrose ester mainly containing sucrose monolaurate, sodium caseinate, and gelatin polysuccinate have been tested so far. With exception of the sugar ester, all stabilizers led to stable colloidal dispersions after melt-homogenization with respect to macroscopic appearance and particle size upon long-term storage. The smectic state of these nanoparticles could clearly be identified by the characteristic small-angle X-ray reflection without influence of the stabilizer system on the position of the reflection.

The stabilizer system does, however, strongly influence the phase behavior of CM nanoparticles, particularly the crystallization process (25). On the basis of the crystallization pattern and the recrystallization tendency upon storage, two groups of stabilizers can be distinguished:

- Stabilizers inducing a multiple crystallization event depending on the thermal history of the sample and a high recrystallization tendency upon storage (phospholipids, sodium oleate, sucrose monolaurate).
- Stabilizers inducing a monomodal crystallization event mostly independent of the thermal history of the sample and a low recrystallization tendency upon storage (sodium glycocholate, synthetic polymers, gelatin polysuccinate, sodium caseinate).

The common feature of stabilizers resulting in smectic nanoparticles with a multiple crystallization pattern, and a comparatively high recrystallization tendency upon storage is the presence of an acyl chain in the molecule. All corresponding dispersions show a very complex crystallization behavior (Fig. 3), which is probably caused by particles of different shapes (spherical and cylindrical) present in the dispersions as observed in electron microscopy (see below) (14). In contrast, smectic nanoparticles stabilized with polymers and sodium glycocholate alone have a distinctly lower crystallization tendency upon storage despite their relatively high crystallization temperature (Fig. 3). Electron microscopic investigations of these dispersions indicate a more homogeneous particle structure (see below). The dispersion stabilized with Tween 80 (a stabilizer which also contains an acyl chain) cannot be clearly classified into one of the groups mentioned above. Although stored smectic nanoparticles stabilized with Tween 80 display only one crystallization event upon cooling in differential scanning calorimetry (DSC) and the recrystallization tendency of these smectic nanoparticles is low, freshly melted nanoparticles give a bimodal crystallization pattern upon cooling.

INFLUENCE OF THE MATRIX COMPOSITION

CM nanoparticles are excellent model systems for studying the influence of parameters such as particle size and stabilizer system on storage stability and phase behavior. Their comparatively high crystallization temperature, which is observed

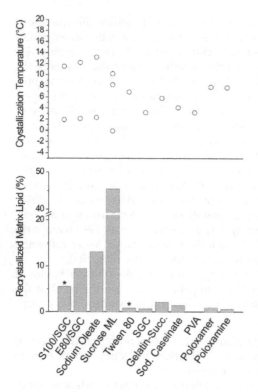

FIGURE 3 Crystallization onset temperatures (differential scanning calorimetry, cooling of thermally untreated samples, 5°C/min) (*top*) and amount of recrystallized matrix lipid after storage (*bottom*) for nine months (eight months for samples marked with an *asterisk*) in dependence on the stabilizer system. All dispersions contain 5% CM and, with exception of SGC (2%), 4% stabilizers. *Abbreviations*: CM, cholesteryl myristate; E80, purified egg yolk lecithin Lipoid E80; PVA, polyvinyl alcohol; S100, purified soybean lecithin Lipoid S100; SGC, sodium glycocholate; sucrose ML, sucrose monolaurate.

even in optimized systems, precludes, however, their development into a robust drug delivery system for practical use. Such a system should display a high stability against recrystallization upon storage, preferably also at temperatures down to about 0°C which can occur during transport and may be required during storage to protect sensitive drugs or excipients, for example, phospholipids, from degradation. Therefore, cholesteryl nonanoate (CN), an ester with nine carbon atoms in the acyl chain, and CO, containing an unsaturated C18 chain, were tested as alternative matrix materials to increase the crystallization stability of smectic nanoparticles (26). Both esters do not crystallize in the colloidal state, neither during cooling to −10°C nor upon storage (even not at refrigerator temperatures). Pure CO is, however, unsuitable as matrix lipid, because its liquid crystalline to isotropic phase transition is very close to body temperature so that CO nanoparticles would lose their smectic state upon administration. The use of CN seems to be very promising from the physicochemical point of view, but its nonphysiological nature requires some safety issues to be resolved prior to its use as drug carrier.

Both esters can also be used as additives to longer-chained cholesterol esters such as CM or CP, which has an even higher crystallization tendency than CM, for the preparation of smectic nanoparticles being more stable against recrystallization. The admixture of already relatively small amounts of these esters to CM (10%, 20%, 40% CN, 20% CO related to the whole matrix lipid) or CP (40%, 50% CN, 50% CO related to the whole matrix lipid) leads to smectic nanoparticles which are stable against recrystallization over at least 18 months at 23°C although the crystallization temperature is only slightly decreased particularly for the CM-based dispersions

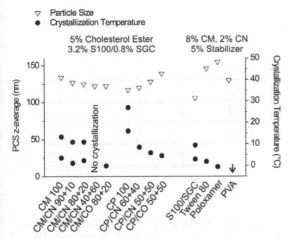

FIGURE 4 Particle size [photon correlation spectroscopy (PCS)] and crystallization onset temperatures of freshly molten samples (differential scanning calorimetry, 5°C/min) in dependence on the matrix composition (*left*) and stabilizer system (*right*). For the dispersion with a CM/CN-matrix stabilized with polyvinyl alcohol, only the very beginning of the crystallization event was recorded so that the onset temperature (<0°C) could not be exactly determined. *Abbreviations*: CM, cholesteryl myristate; CN, cholesteryl nonanoate; CO, cholesteryl oleate; CP, cholesteryl palmitate; PVA, polyvinyl alcohol; SGC, sodium glycocholate; S100, purified soy bean lecithin Lipoid S100.

(Fig. 4). In contrast, the amount of recrystallized matrix lipid was 8% and 94% for the dispersions with a pure CM or CP matrix, respectively. Admixture of higher amounts of CN (60% of the matrix) to CM smectic nanoparticles resulted in dispersions which could be stored at 4°C without nanoparticle recrystallization. The crystallization temperature-suppressing effect of CN admixture can be further increased by the use of polymeric stabilizers such as PVA and poloxamer in dispersions with a mixed cholesterol ester matrix (Fig. 4).

INCORPORATION OF MODEL DRUGS

Ibuprofen, miconazole, etomidate, and progesterone were used as poorly water-soluble model drugs for the preparation of drug-loaded smectic nanoparticles (11). The dispersions containing 5% CM as matrix lipid and a phospholipid/bile salt mixture (3.2/0.8%) as stabilizers were prepared by high-pressure melt-homogenization. The lower melting drugs ibuprofen, miconazole, and etomidate could be incorporated in an amount of 10% relative to the lipid matrix by dissolving the drug in the cholesterol ester melt. Higher drug loads have not been investigated yet but a drug load of 10% is already higher than achieved for solid lipid nanoparticles with miconazole and ibuprofen (27). Progesterone, which melts above 100°C, could be dissolved only at a concentration of 1% in the CM melt within an appropriate time (<30 minutes).

Drug incorporation into the dispersions did not influence the occurrence and position of the small-angle X-ray reflection characteristic of the smectic nanoparticle state. Particularly the liquid crystalline phase transitions were, however, shifted to lower temperatures in DSC, indicating an interaction of the drug molecules with the

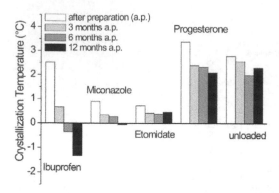

FIGURE 5 Crystallization onset temperatures (differential scanning calorimetry, 5°C/min, freshly molten samples, main crystallization event) of drug-loaded dispersions in comparison to those of a corresponding drug-free dispersion with comparable particle size in dependence on storage time.

smectic phase. The decrease of the liquid crystalline phase transition temperatures was different and least pronounced in the dispersion with 1% progesterone. Except for the dispersion loaded with progesterone, the crystallization temperature was also decreased in the presence of drug (Fig. 5), indicating that drug incorporation may have a beneficial effect on the recrystallization tendency.

The drug-loaded dispersions were stable upon storage for at least 12 months with respect to particle size, macroscopic appearance, and recrystallization of matrix material. Only in the progesterone-loaded dispersion was a small amount of recrystallized matrix lipid (4%) detected after 12 months of storage.

First preliminary studies point to a rapid release of at least a major fraction of ibuprofen and etomidate from the smectic nanoparticles into the aqueous phase. Such behavior would lead to carrier-independent drug distribution after IV administration as is also often observed for lipid emulsions (3). The use of more lipophilic prodrugs (e.g., esters) or ion-pairs is expected to enhance drug retention after administration and might also allow loading with comparatively hydrophilic compounds (28–31).

ULTRASTRUCTURE OF CHOLESTERYL MYRISTATE NANOPARTICLES

Different electron microscopic techniques can be used for the investigation of the ultrastructure of colloidal lipid particles. In cryoelectron microscopy, a thin film of rapidly frozen dispersion is viewed directly, and a good impression of the shape of the projected particles is obtained. In contrast, freeze-fracturing, where the frozen sample is fractured, and the fracture plane shadowed with a thin heavy metal layer leads to images that yield information also about the inner structure of the particles.

Electron microscopic images indicate a mostly nonspherical, nearly cylindrical shape of the CM nanoparticles. The particle shape is strongly influenced by the stabilizer system ranging from nearly exactly cylindrical particles to "paving stone-like" ones (Fig. 6). In dispersions stabilized on the basis of phospholipids and with sodium oleate, an additional particle fraction was observed in cryo-preparations which was very unstable in the electron beam. An onion-like internal structure detected for some particles in freeze-fractured specimen of phospholipid-stabilized dispersions points to a spherical shape of these particles. Consequently, these dispersions seem to contain two different types of smectic nanoparticles—cylindrical and spherical ones. Owing to the layered structure of the smectic phase, a cylindrical particle shape should be energetically more favorable than a spherical one and,

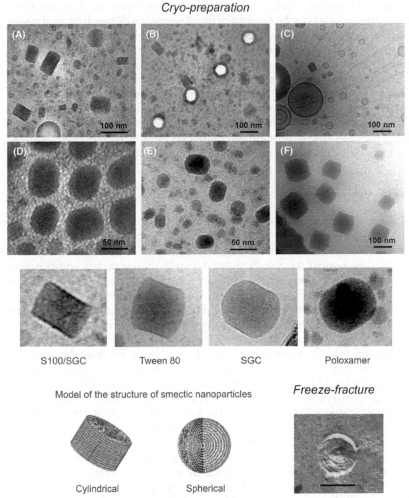

FIGURE 6 Cryoelectron micrographs of selected dispersions containing 5% CM. (**A** and **B**) Dispersion stabilized with the phospholipid/bile salt system (3.2/0.8%). (**B**) The fraction of instable, "bubbling" particles is clearly visible. (**C**) Dispersion stabilized with 4% sodium oleate. (**D**) Dispersion stabilized with 4% polyvinyl alcohol. (**E**) Dispersion stabilized with 4% poloxamer 188. (**F**) Dispersion stabilized with 4% Tween 80. Magnifications illustrate the dependence of the particle shape on the stabilizer system. The freeze-fracture micrograph shows an image of a CM particle with an onion-like inner structure (3.2% S100, bar = 140 nm). A schematic model representation of the structure of cylindrical and spherical CM nanoparticles is also given. *Abbreviations*: CM, cholesteryl myristate; S100, purified soy bean lecithin Lipoid S100; SGC, sodium glycocholate.

therefore, the increased sensitivity of the spherical particles toward the electron beam might be caused by a higher energy level of these particles. A cylindrical shape has also been observed in cryoelectron microscopic investigations of native low-density lipoprotein (LDL) particles (32,33) which contain a core of cholesterol esters that should be in the smectic phase under the conditions used for sample preparation at room temperature (34,35).

Besides smectic nanoparticles, other colloidal structures such as micelles, mixed micelles, and vesicles can be present in the dispersions depending on the self-association characteristics of the stabilizers used. Particularly in the dispersion stabilized with sodium oleate, a variety of different structures was observed in agreement with literature data on cholesterol ester-free samples (36) (Fig. 6). The presence of such other colloidal structures is generally not desirable as they may also solubilize lipophilic drugs and could induce redistribution processes of incorporated drugs upon storage. Moreover, they may lead to additional physiological effects. For example, liposomes formed by an excess of phospholipids used for the stabilization of colloidal fat emulsions for parenteral nutrition (37) influence fat metabolism and can lead to a decreased degradation of the fat emulsion particles (38).

SUMMARY AND CONCLUSION

Supercooled smectic cholesterol ester nanoparticles are a promising new carrier system for the delivery of lipophilic drugs. They can be prepared by different methods, for example, with the established high-pressure melt-homogenization technique. Their stability against recrystallization depends on the matrix composition, emulsifier system, and on the particle size. If properly designed with respect to composition, preparative, and storage parameters, they are stable on storage in liquid dispersion with regard to particle size and liquid crystalline state of the matrix material for pharmaceutically relevant periods of time. The high viscosity of the liquid crystalline matrix is expected to counteract coalescence processes. Lipophilic drugs can be loaded into the nanoparticles as shown above for ibuprofen, etomidate, and miconazole which can be incorporated at considerable concentration. Although basic knowledge has already been collected on the characteristics of this new type of particles, they are still in an early stage of development as drug delivery systems. Future activities will focus on the further optimization of their composition, in particular with respect to stability against recrystallization, drug incorporation, and retention as well as their surface characteristics.

The lipidic nature and small particle size of supercooled smectic nanoparticles offer several interesting possibilities with virtually all ways of administration (e.g., parenteral, ocular, dermal, or peroral). In future, corresponding interactions with biological systems will have to be studied in detail. First cytotoxicity studies have already revealed promising results. Concerning parenteral, in particular intravenous administration, the influence of the new type of matrix structure on the pharmacokinetics and biodistribution requires intensive investigation. As supercooled smectic nanoparticles show similarities in composition and structure with the protein-free core of LDLs (32,33), they may have interesting potential as easily accessible artificial constructs with similar properties, for example, for drug targeting to certain tumors or the brain via the LDL receptor (39–41).

REFERENCES

1. Lyons RT, Carter EG. Lipid emulsions for intravenous nutrition and drug delivery. In: Gunstone FD, Padley FB, eds. Lipid Technologies and Applications. New York: Marcel Dekker, 1997:535–556.
2. Washington C. Stability of lipid emulsions for drug delivery. Adv Drug Deliv Rev 1996; 20:131.

3. Klang S, Benita S. Design and evaluation of submicron emulsions as colloidal drug carriers for intravenous administration. In: Benita S, ed. Submicron Emulsions in Drug Targeting and Delivery. Amsterdam: Harwood Academic Publishers, 1998:119–152.
4. Mehnert W, Mäder K. Solid lipid nanoparticles: production, characterization and applications. Adv Drug Deliv Rev 2001; 47:165.
5. Bunjes H, Siekmann B. Manufacture, characterization and applications of solid lipid nanoparticles as drug delivery systems. In: Benita S, ed. Microencapsulation. 2nd ed. New York: Marcel Dekker, 2006:213–268.
6. Westesen K, Bunjes H, Koch MHJ. Physicochemical characterization of lipid nanoparticles and evaluation of their drug loading capacity and sustained release potential. J Control Release 1997; 48:223.
7. Malmsten M. Liquid crystalline phases. In: Malmsten M, ed. Surfactants and Polymers in Drug Delivery. New York: Marcel Dekker, 2002:51–86.
8. Müller-Goymann CC. Liquid crystals in drug delivery. In: Swarbrick J, Boylan JC, eds. Encyclopedia of Pharmaceutical Technology. New York: Marcel Dekker, 2002:834–853.
9. Bunjes H, Rades T. Thermotropic liquid crystalline drugs. J Pharm Pharmacol 2005; 57:807.
10. Kelker H, Hatz R. Handbook of Liquid Crystals. Weinheim: Verlag Chemie, 1980.
11. Kuntsche J, Westesen K, Drechsler M, Koch MHJ, Bunjes H. Supercooled smectic nanoparticles: a potential novel carrier system for poorly water soluble drugs. Pharm Res 2004; 21:1834.
12. Ginsburg GS, Atkinson D, Small DM. Physical properties of cholesteryl esters. Prog Lipid Res 1984; 23:135.
13. Madhusudana NV. Recent advances in thermotropic liquid crystals. Curr Sci 2001; 80:1018.
14. Kuntsche J, Koch MHJ, Drechsler M, Bunjes H. Crystallization behavior of supercooled smectic cholesteryl myristate nanoparticles containing phospholipids as stabilizers. Colloid Surf B 2005; 44:25.
15. Wendorff JH, Price FP. The structure of mesophases of cholesteryl esters. Mol Cryst Liq Cryst 1973; 24:129.
16. Bock T, Kleinebudde P, Müller BW. Manufacture of emulsions by means of high-pressure homogenization: influence of homogenization parameters, oils and surfactants. In: Müller RH, Benita S, Böhm B, eds. Emulsions and Nanosuspensions for the Formulation of Poorly Soluble Drugs. Stuttgart: Medpharm Scientific Publ., 1998:201–236.
17. Sjöström B, Kronberg B, Carlfors J. A method for the preparation of submicron particles of sparingly water soluble drugs by precipitation in o/w-emulsions. I. Influence of emulsification and surfactant concentration. J Pharm Sci 1993; 82:579.
18. Sjöström B, Westesen K, Bergenståhl B. Preparation of submicron drug particles in lecithin-stabilized o/w emulsions. II. Characterization of cholesteryl acetate particles. Int J Pharm 1993; 94:89.
19. Sjöström B, Kaplun A, Talmon Y, Cabane B. Structures of nanoparticles prepared from oil-in-water emulsions. Pharm Res 1995; 12:39.
20. Garti N, Yano J. The roles of emulsifiers in fat crystallization. In: Garti N, Sato K, eds. Crystallization Processes in Fats and Lipid Systems. New York: Marcel Dekker, 2001:211–250.
21. Ueno S, Hamada Y, Sato K. Controlling polymorphic crystallization of n-alkane crystals in emulsion droplets through interfacial heterogeneous nucleation. Cryst Growth Des 2003; 3:935.
22. Bunjes H, Koch MHJ. Saturated phospholipids promote crystallization but slow down polymorphic transitions in triglyceride nanoparticles. J Control Release 2005; 107:229.
23. Illum L, West P, Washington C, Davis SS. The effect of stabilizing agents on the organ distribution of lipid emulsions. Int J Pharm 1989; 54:41.
24. Liu F, Liu D. Long-circulating emulsions (oil-in-water) as carriers for lipophilic drugs. Pharm Res 1995; 12:1060.
25. Kuntsche J, Westesen K, Bunjes H. Supercooled smectic nanoparticles—influence of the stabilizer system on physicochemical properties. Proc Int Symp Control Release Bioact Mater 2003; 30:199.

26. Kuntsche J, Westesen K, Bunjes H. Supercooled smectic nanoparticles—influence of the matrix composition on the phase behavior. Proc Int Symp Control Release Bioact Mater 2003; 30:182.

27. Bunjes H. Influence of different factors on the structure and properties of nanoparticles from solid triglycerides. Ph.D. Thesis. University of Jena, 1998.

28. Cavalli R, Caputo O, Gasco MR. Solid lipospheres of doxorubicin and idarubicin. Int J Pharm 1993; 89:R9.

29. Murtha JL, Ando HY. Synthesis of the cholesteryl ester prodrugs cholesteryl ibuprofen and cholesteryl flufenamate and their formulation into phospholipid microemulsions. J Pharm Sci 1994; 83:1222.

30. Meyer JD, Manning MC. Hydrophobic ion pairing: altering the solubility properties of biomolecules. Pharm Res 1998; 15:188.

31. Versluis AJ, Rump ET, Rensen PCN, van Berkel TJC, Bijsterbosch MK. Synthesis of a lipophilic daunorubicin derivate and its incorporation into lipidic carriers developed for LDL receptor-mediated tumor therapy. Pharm Res 1998; 15:531.

32. van Antwerpen R, Gilkey JC. Cryo-electron microscopy reveals human low density lipoprotein substructure. J Lipid Res 1994; 35:2223.

33. van Antwerpen R, Chen GC, Pullinger CR, et al. Cryo-electron microscopy of low density lipoprotein and reconstituted discoidal high density lipoprotein: imaging of the apolipo-protein moiety. J Lipid Res 1997; 38:659.

34. Deckelbaum RJ, Shipley GG, Small DM. Structure and interactions of lipids in human plasma low density lipoproteins. J Biol Chem 1977; 252:744.

35. Kroon PA. The order–disorder transition of the core cholesteryl esters of human plasma low density lipoprotein: a proton nuclear magnetic resonance study. J Biol Chem 1981; 256:5332.

36. Edwards K, Silvander M, Karlsson G. Aggregate structure in dilute aqueous dispersions of oleic acid/sodium oleate and oleic acid/sodium oleate/egg phosphatidylcholine. Langmuir 1995; 11:2429.

37. Rotenberg M, Rubin M, Bor A, Meyuhas D, Talmon Y, Lichtenberg D. Physico-chemical characterization of intralipid emulsions. Biochim Biophys Acta 1991; 1086:265.

38. Bach AC, Férézou J, Frey A. Phospholipid-rich particles in commercial parenteral fat emulsions: an overview. Prog Lipid Res 1996; 35:133.

39. Firestone RA. Low-density lipoprotein as a vehicle for targeting antitumor compounds to cancer cells. Bioconjugate Chem 1994; 5:105.

40. Dehouck B, Fenart L, Dehouck MP, Pierce A, Torpier G, Cecchelli R. A new function for the LDL receptor: transcytosis of LDL across the blood–brain barrier. J Cell Biol 1997; 138:877.

41. Kreuter J. Nanoparticulate systems for brain delivery of drugs. Adv Drug Deliv Rev 2001; 47:65.

10 Biological and Engineering Considerations for Developing Tumor-Targeting Metallic Nanoparticle Drug-Delivery Systems

Giulio F. Paciotti and Lawrence Tamarkin
CytImmune Sciences, Inc., Rockville, Maryland, U.S.A.

INTRODUCTION

Currently, first-line treatment of resectable solid tumors most commonly involves surgery followed by a regimen of chemotherapy and/or radiation. Unfortunately, this strategy often fails because of recurrent or metastatic disease. To change this paradigm, new cancer therapies must deliver multifunctional therapeutics capable of destroying the heterogeneous population of tumor cells present within solid tumors.

Targeting cancer therapeutics to solid tumors is facilitated by particle-delivery systems capable of escaping phagocytic clearance by the reticuloendothelial system (RES) (1–3). Under ideal conditions, such delivery systems preferentially extravasate the tumor vasculature and accumulate within the tumor microenvironment (4,5). Additionally, these nanotherapeutics may be engineered to contain tumor-targeting ligands that bind to specific cells within solid tumors to anchor the nanoparticle within the solid tumor. By design, particle-delivery systems capable of sequestering cancer drugs solely within a tumor may also reduce the accumulation of the drugs in healthy organs (1–5). Consequently, these delivery systems may increase the relative efficacy or safety of cancer therapies, and thus serve to increase their therapeutic index.

In recent years, the field of nanoparticle-based drug delivery has been reinvigorated by a convergence of nanotechnology and medicine (6–9). In essence, the blending of these fields is leading to the generation of innovative synthetic vectors with the potential of achieving the long sought after goal of tumor-targeted drug delivery: getting the active agent(s) solely where they are needed, the solid tumor. Furthermore, the versatility of these nanoparticle systems may for the first time lead to the development of multifunctional nanotherapeutics (Fig. 1) that detect and attack the heterogeneous population of tumor cells present in a solid tumor. As shown in Figure 1, these putative vectors may consist of an immune-avoidance moiety (a "stealth" moiety), a tumor-targeting motif, multiple therapeutics, and a diagnostic/sensing component, all of which are delivered on a single nanoparticle no larger than 50 nm.

Over the past 20 years, the field of nanoparticle-based drug delivery focused on two chemically distinct colloidal particles: liposomes and biodegradable polymers (10–14). Both delivery systems encapsulate/entrap the active drug within their structures and release the active agent as the particle lyses, in the case of liposomes, or disintegrates as described for biodegradable polymers. A recent newcomer to this field is the metallic nanoparticle. Like their organic counterparts, the metallic particles have a long history of use in biology; however, only recently have they been formulated into tumor-targeting vectors.

This chapter is divided into three parts. The "Biological Considerations" section focuses on the biological barriers facing metallic-nanoparticle-based, tumor-targeted

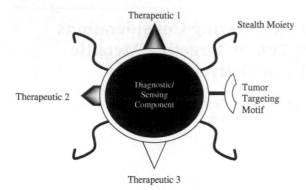

Therapeutic 1

Stealth Moiety

Therapeutic 2

Diagnostic/
Sensing
Component

Tumor
Targeting
Motif

Therapeutic 3

FIGURE 1 Schematic representation of a multifunctional nanoparticle therapeutic.

drug delivery, and will center on the delivery of protein and small-molecule-based therapies. Some of these barriers are naturally present in healthy portions of the body, whereas others are established during tumor growth and progression. The section "Metallic Nanoparticle Drug-Delivery Systems" will describe three examples of metallic-nanoparticle-based, tumor-targeted drug delivery and the specific means used to overcome these barriers. Specifically, an overview of magnetic-iron and colloidal gold-based nanoparticle drug-delivery systems will be discussed. The final section will focus on the design and manufacturing of multifunctional metallic nanoparticles that target the delivery of multiple cancer therapies with a single metallic nanoparticle.

BIOLOGICAL CONSIDERATIONS
Clearance by the Reticuloendothelial System
The painstaking lessons learned from the liposomal- and polymer-based drug-delivery systems must be considered in the formulation of the metallic nanoparticles. There is ample precedent suggesting that immediately after their exposure to the circulation, unprotected metallic nanoparticles will most likely undergo opsinization in the blood and clearance by the RES. Opsinization is the process by which blood-borne proteins, known as opsins, bind to the metallic nanoparticle surface. Opsonic proteins include immunoglobulins, complement proteins C1 and C3, apolipoproteins, von Willebrand factor, thrombospondin, fibronectin, and mannose-binding protein (15–19).

Once bound to the surface of the particles, opsins act as ligands that are recognized, bound, and internalized by a class of macrophages known as Kupffer cells. Kupffer cells are specialized macrophages that reside in the liver and represent the primary cellular component of the scavenging system of the body, known as the RES. Under physiologic conditions, the RES rapidly and very efficiently clears opsinized particulates, such as bacteria and colloidal particles, from the body. For example, in mice intravenously injected with unprotected colloidal gold nanoparticles (i.e., colloidal gold nanoparticles that contain only drug bound to their surface), we observed that 90% to 95% of these gold nanoparticles are cleared from the circulation within 5 to 10 minutes after injection. These observations are consistent with the historical biodistribution data of unprotected liposomes.

Early work in the field of particle-based drug delivery demonstrated that RES clearance was saturable, because pretreating animals with high doses of drug or placebo nanoparticle vectors (i.e., vectors lacking the active product ingredient) exceeded the phagocytic capacity of the RES (20–24). Consequently, nanoparticles not trapped in the liver or spleen were available to deliver drugs to solid tumors. A more practical approach to address RES uptake and clearance is the modification of the nanoparticle surface to include hydrophilic blockers such as polyethylene glycol (PEG) as well as block copolymers of the tetronic and pluronic families of surfactants. Grafting/binding these hydrophilic moieties onto the surface of the colloidal nanoparticles made them "invisible" to the RES. Typically, such sterically stabilized nanoparticles exhibit prolonged circulatory half-life and as discussed below such nanoparticle formulations may passively accumulate in solid tumors through extravasation of the leaky vasculature that feed them (25–28).

The nature and conformation of potential stealth molecules influence the ability of the immune system to detect and clear nanoparticles. As an example, Moghimi (29) demonstrated that the concentration and conformation of one such polymer, poloxamer 407, significantly altered the biodistribution of polystyrene nanoparticles after subcutaneous injection. When the ethylene oxide (ETOX) tails of the poloxamer polymer were grafted at relatively low concentrations, the molecule assumed a flat or mushroom-like configuration on the surface of the particles, whereas at higher polymer concentrations the closely packed ETOX tails assumed a brush-like conformation on the surface of the particles. The particles with the mushroom-like configuration were readily picked up by the macrophages present in the primary or secondary lymph nodes, whereas those carrying the brush-like configuration evaded the lymph nodes, traveled through the lymphatic system and reentered the circulation.

In our laboratory, we also observed that the manner by which a stealth molecule binds to drug-coated colloidal gold nanoparticles influences their biodistribution (30). As described above, 95% of various formulations of drug-stabilized, monodispersed colloidal gold nanoparticles [nanoparticles bound with a saturating amount of the protein therapeutic, tumor necrosis factor (TNF) alpha], were cleared by the RES within 5 to 10 minutes of intravenous injection. The fate of these monodispersed nanoparticles was evident upon animal necropsy as both the livers and spleens were black with aggregated colloidal gold precipitates. Several block copolymers including pluronic, tetronic, carbowax, and monothiolated forms of PEG (PEG-THIOL) were tested for their ability to block RES uptake and clearance. Although all four classes of polymers bound and stabilized the colloidal gold nanoparticles in a test tube, only PEG-THIOL prevented RES uptake and clearance when injected intravenously. Unlike the poloxamer-stabilized nanoparticles, we believe that the pluronic-, tetronic-, and carbowax-based polymers were unable to bind to the surface of the colloidal gold nanoparticle. However, the presence of the single sulfhydryl group on the PEG molecule (PEG-THIOL) allowed it to bind directly to the surface of the particle, interspersed between the protein therapeutic. In this case, we believe that the molecules of PEG-THIOL assumed a brush-like configuration on the surface of the nanoparticles, and the biological response (i.e., avoiding immune recognition) was similar to that seen in the example above.

Surface characteristics including size, surface contour/facets, and charge may also regulate which opsins bind and the extent to which they adhere to the surface of the particles. Particle size can affect particle clearance by two mechanisms (31–34). First, larger particles more efficiently activate the complement pathway for clearance by the RES. Second, in the red pulp of the spleen, the interendothelial slits present on the endothelial cells of the venous sinusoids may filter particles, merely based on size (larger than 200 nm). The latter effect seems more problematic for the earlier formulations of liposomes rather than metallic nanoparticles as metal-based nanoparticles range in size from 5 to 40 nm. Also, as described below, particle size may influence the ability of nanoparticles to effectively deliver drugs to the tumor interstitium.

Surface charge must also be considered in formulating metallic nanoparticles because the overall surface charge may determine the degree to which particles are cleared by the RES, as well as their ability to interact with endothelial cells that form the tumor neovasculature. For example, the RES readily clears anionic lipid particles, whereas neutral lipid particles are not readily cleared (18,33–35). Cationic liposomes containing an RES-avoidance system (i.e., PEG) preferentially bind to the surface of tumor endothelia (36,37).

The process of particle opsinization and RES clearance is an active process by which particle-bound opsins are recognized, bound, and internalized by the macrophages present in the liver and spleen. Overcoming this biological barrier is just the first step in tumor-targeted drug delivery. So, even when RES clearance is adequately addressed, the physical barriers established during solid tumor formation and progression must next be addressed for the development of a successful tumor-targeted metallic drug delivery vector.

Tumor Angiogenesis and Vascularization

In 1971, Folkman (38) laid out his hypothesis describing the angiogenic model of tumor growth and metastases. A central component of this hypothesis is that solid tumors, in response to physiologic stresses such as hypoxia, secrete factors that cause new blood vessels to sprout and grow from existing blood vessels toward the tumor. Eventually these angiogenic blood vessels become inexorably entwined in the solid tumor mass. Such angiogenesis is required to ensure continued tumor growth and progression, and this process is currently the focus of many novel cancer therapies.

Angiogenesis, the process by which new blood vessels sprout from existing normal blood vessels, occurs in a variety of disease states including cancer and inflammation as well as during normal physiological events such as the thickening of the uterine wall, follicle development, and wound healing. During wound healing, for example, angiogenesis and clot formation are highly interconnected processes that are regulated by platelets and soluble blood proteins (39).

Upon injury, tissue factor is released and induces clot formation through the well-characterized cascade of clotting factors that ultimately lead to the formation of a clot by the thrombin-mediated conversion of fibrinogen to fibrin. Thrombin also activates platelets to release a variety of potent pro-angiogenic factors including various forms of vascular endothelial growth factors A, B, and C (VEGF A, B, and C, respectively), fibroblast growth factor-2, and angiopoietin-2. Finally, thrombin stimulates endothelial cells to secrete a variety of enzymes responsible for the degradation of the basement membrane causing the release of VEGF from these compartments (39,40).

Platelets may also be recruited and activated to secrete these pro-angiogenic factors by interaction with collagen or indirectly through interaction with von Willebrand factor. These pro-angiogenic factors signal the surrounding vascular endothelial cells to grow and migrate through the fibrin clot (41). To keep the angiogenic process in check, platelets also secrete antiangiogenic factors such as thrombospondin-1, plasminogen, and TGFβ-1, which serve to block angiogenesis, and induce the expression of enzymes that help break down the clot. Tight control between the pro- and antiangiogenic signals ensures that as the process of tissue repair and remodeling is completed, angiogenesis is terminated.

Within solid tumors, however, the homeostatic mechanism for controlling new blood vessel formation is aberrant, often favoring angiogenesis and continued tumor growth and metastasis. For example, the constitutive expression of tissue factor by tumor and supporting stromal cells may induce the clotting mechanism by circulating coagulating factors, such as factor VIIa, to ultimately cause platelet-mediated coagulation and release of VEGF (42,43). Indeed there is a reasonable precedent in the literature showing a potential link between the state of coagulation and tumor progression (44,45). Gasic et al. (46) demonstrated this potential link by showing that antibodies which blocked platelet function inhibited the formation of pulmonary metastases. More recently, Cramerer et al. (47) highlighted a model in which circulating tumor cells use secreted tissue factor as a means of inducing the clotting mechanism to arrest their migration from the normal vasculature, to traverse the endothelial cell barrier, and ultimately to form secondary metastases.

A newly identified and more problematic cell type may provide solid tumors with not only angiogenic support, but also with strong protection against the ability of the immune system to induce an antitumor response. Tumor-associated macrophages (TAMs) are monocyte-derived macrophages that migrate from the vasculature to regions of hypoxia in solid tumors. Unlike wild-type macrophages that are present in normal tissues and in well-oxygenated areas of tumors, TAMs exhibit altered phenotypes. For example, TAMs secrete immunosuppressive cytokines, such as IL-10, TGFβ, and prostaglandins (48–50). Finally, TAMs residing in the hypoxic centers of tumors are not effective at antigen presentation (51). Thus, TAMs may indirectly support tumor growth by blunting the ability of the immune system to mount an effective antitumor response.

In fact, once trapped in the hypoxic regions of tumors, TAMs may actually begin to support tumor growth. In response to the low oxygen tension present in the hypoxic regions of solid tumors, TAMs upregulate the expression of hypoxia-inducible factors one and two (HIF-1 and HIF-2, respectively) (52–54). Tumor cells also express these factors in response to hypoxia (55). The HIF family of proteins are transcription factors that translocate to the nucleus, bind specific DNA regions known as hypoxia-response elements to stimulate gene expression, and ultimately lead to VEGF secretion by the macrophages and tumor cells (52,55,56).

Vascular Endothelial Growth Factor

VEGF was identified in the late 1970s for its ability to induce vascular permeability of venules and small veins present in the postcapillary plexus. VEGF-induced permeability is mediated by the formation of vesicular vacuolar organelles (VVOs) (57–59). VVOs are a series of interconnected vesicles and vacuoles that span the entire distance of endothelial cells from the lumenal to the abluminal side of the endothelial cells. In the absence of VEGF, access of macromolecules to the VVOs is limited by the presence of a membrane-covered stomata which is connected to the plasma membrane of the endothelial cell. In response to VEGF stimulation, the stomata open to allow passage of tracer elements, plasma, and plasma proteins from the lumenal side of the endothelial cell, through the VVOs, to the extravascular space of tissues.

Additional structures such as intercellular openings and intracellular holes may also increase the permeability of tumor blood vessels. For example, Hashizume et al. (60) described round or oval openings between the endothelial blood vessel cells supporting the growth of MCa-IV tumors. These openings are much larger than the fenestrations (50–80 nm) (60) reported for tumor blood vessel endothelium and ranged from 0.3 to 4.7 μm with an average of 1.7 μm. In addition, transcellular holes ranging from 0.2 to 0.9 μm were also reported. Although additional study is needed, the presence of such extra-fenestral openings suggests a potential mechanism by which nanoparticle-delivery systems passively accumulate in solid tumors rather than other healthy filtering organs such as the liver, an organ in which fenestrae ranging from 50 to 300 nm have been described.

The increase in vascular permeability and the deposition of a fibrin clot are among the responses attributed to VEGF-mediated angiogenesis. Within the fibrin clot, VEGF-mediated angiogenesis starts with the generation of a mother vessel, a vessel characterized by poor coverage with both a basement membrane and pericytes. Subsequently, the formation of new blood vessels may occur by one of three mechanisms. First, the mother vessel may undergo sprouting, endothelial cell migration, and proliferation. Second, the mother vessel may undergo bridging in which translumenal bridges, formed between the endothelial cells, serve to divide the lumen of the mother vessels into smaller channels. Ultimately, these multichannel vessels give rise to new daughter vessels. Finally, during intussusceptive vessel formation, the mother vessel invaginates to give rise to two vessels.

Characterization of the Angiogenic Tumor Blood Vessels

During normal physiologic conditions, the neonatal vasculature is under the tight control of two processes: vasculogenesis and angiogenesis. Vasculogenesis, the de novo generation of blood vessels, is initiated from a precursor stem cell or angioblast, whereas during angiogenesis these newly formed vessels are instructed to undergo branching and sprouting by signals including VEGF. These fragile, newly formed blood vessels are reinforced by a cast of supporting cellular (mural cells) and structural elements including pericytes, smooth muscle cells, and the extracellular matrix, a process which is regulated and coordinated by extracellular signals including PDGF, EDG1, and S1P1 (61). Finally, during embryonic development, the vasculature is tailored and remodeled to fit the needs of the organ it supplies by the localized expression of chemoattractants and repellents such as ephrins and neuropilins (62–64). Overall, the process results in the formation of highly ordered vascular beds comprised of arteries, arterioles, capillaries, venules, and veins.

In tumors, however, the organization of angiogenic blood vessels resembles haphazard arrays of sprouting blood vessels, tumor cells, and pericyte-like cells which collectively form a vessel that oftentimes lacks an organized extracellular matrix. The hyperpermeability of these blood vessels, a process which is in part mediated by VEGF, allows the extravasation of colloidal particles such as colloidal carbon and colloidal gold, as well as tracer molecules including radioisotopes, fluorescently labeled dextrans, and albumin (58,65–67). In certain instances, erythrocytes cross the vascular bed and pool to form vascular lakes of blood cells (60).

Recently, the tumor cells themselves were reported to form the so-called "tumor blood vessels." Chang et al. (68) described the presence of "mosaic" blood vessels in a murine colon tumor model. These mosaic blood vessels consisted of both tumor and endothelial cells which were distinguished by fluorescence. In these studies, Chang implanted LS174T murine colon carcinoma tumor cells, which were stably transfected to express green fluorescence protein (GFP), into SCID mice.

With tumor formation, the intracellular expression of GFP was used to identify the tumor cells, whereas Cy5 and rhodamine-conjugated anti-CD31/105 systems were used to identify the endothelial cells. They report that nearly 15% of the vessels examined did not show any endothelial cell staining, but did show the green fluorescence of the implanted tumor cell line, creating the lumen of the "tumor blood vessel." In contrast to the data reported by Monsky et al. (69) (see later), who reported that the permeability of angiogenic blood vessels was influenced by the location of tumor cell implantation, the location of tumor cell implantation in the studies conducted by Chang et al. did not affect the presence or percentage of the mosaic cells. These mosaic blood vessels are thought to represent one mechanism by which shedding tumor cells enter the circulation in formation of metastases. Furthermore, given that mosaic cells, similar to those described above, were also identified in biopsies of colon cancer patients (68) has significant implications for angiogenic-targeted cancer therapies, because the main target for these therapies, the newly formed blood vessels, may not be present in all cases.

Tumor Angiogenesis and Interstitial Fluid Pressure
For some time now the inherent leakiness of the tumor vasculature has been a target for developing nanoparticle-based, tumor-targeted delivery vectors. Because of their size, these particle-based therapeutics may passively extravasate the leaky tumor vasculature to accumulate within solid tumors. Tumor–host interactions are also shown to control the degree of endothelial cell leakiness. Monsky et al. (69) demonstrated that the degree of tumor blood vessel porosity is dependent not only on the tumor type, but also on its location. For example, the inherent vascular permeability of human breast cancer tumors was dependent on the site of implantation. Although tumors implanted in the cranial wall were highly angiogenic, when compared with the same tumors implanted in mammary fat pad, they were also less permeable to fluorescently labeled indicators.

Nevertheless, the formation of an intratumor clot, in the presence of continued angiogenesis, and a late-forming lymphatic system combine to increase the interstitial fluid pressure (IFP) of solid tumors. This hypertensive state represents a major obstacle for the penetration of macromolecular- or nanoparticle-based therapies to solid tumors. To effectively overcome this barrier, nanoparticle-based delivery systems must contain elements that break down this interstitial pressure gradient. Described below are two classes of therapeutic compounds shown to disrupt the IFP gradient.

Antiangiogenic Therapies
One clear choice for reducing the IFP in solid tumors is to block VEGF signaling. Preclinical and clinical studies with monoclonal antibodies designed to block the interaction of VEGF with its receptor show that the antibody not only inhibits the formation of new blood vessels, but also causes the regression of already established vessels, an observation which is consistent with the role that VEGF serves as a survival factor for newly formed blood vessels (70,71).

More interestingly, treatments with such monoclonal antibodies cause an apparent reorganization and restructuring of the blood vessels within solid tumors. This process, termed normalization (70,72), involves a pruning of existing blood vessels, improved covering of the normalizing blood vessels with pericytes, and reestablishment of basement membrane. Overall, normalization results in improved blood flow in solid tumors, decreases the IFP of tumors (an observation which has also been demonstrated in colon cancer patients), and establishes a hydrostatic pressure gradient across the vascular wall. The combination of these events improves the accumulation and efficacy of secondary therapies, such as chemotherapy.

There is, however, one caveat associated with the anti-VEGF-induced normalization of the tumor vasculature and its proposed synergy with chemotherapy. Apparently, there is a period of time, known as the "normalization window" (71), in which synergy of anti-VEGF therapy with radiation or chemical therapies is optimal. This period of time is temporally flanked (i.e., prior to and immediately following the normalization window) by two time periods in which the combination is less effective. Not surprisingly, prior to normalization, when solid tumors are supported by their torturous/leaky circulation vasculature, the synergy of anti-VEGF treatment and chemotherapy proves ineffective. During normalization, the drop in IFP coupled with the reestablishment of a vascular pressure gradient improves the efficacy of secondary therapies. Finally, as the anti-VEGF therapy causes the death of the tumor neovasculature, the efficacy of anti-VEGF and radio or chemotherapies once again decreases. These data, however, suggest that in order to maximize the synergy between anti-VEGF and chemotherapy, the normalization window in cancer patients must be clearly identified to ensure maximal synergy between the two therapies.

Cytokine-Mediated Reduction of Interstitial Fluid Pressure

TNF was initially described as a serum factor isolated from the blood of endotoxin-treated mice, which was capable of inducing hemorrhagic necrosis of solid tumors. Nevertheless, in the 1980s hopes of using TNF as a cancer therapy were nearly dashed by the life-threatening toxicities it induced (72), a fate shared by many cytokines showing promise in preclinical tumor models. The major toxicity observed during the systemic administration of TNF is severe hypotension.

Yet the pioneering works of Lienard and Lejuene (73,74) demonstrated vast improvements in the therapeutic index of TNF by limiting its delivery to solid tumors. For TNF, the isolated limb protocol (ILP) demonstrated that the combination of surgically localized delivery of the cytokine with regionally administered chemotherapies induced sustainable antitumor responses in patients failing traditional standards of care (72–74). By localizing the delivery of TNF to solid tumors, Lienard and Lejuene harnessed TNF to induce at least one of the possible mechanisms by which the cytokine induces an antitumor response. For example, TNF may directly cause apoptosis of various tumor cell types (75,76), activate and drive immune-based antitumor responses (77), and induce vascular leak in tumor blood vessels (78,79), leading to a destruction of the IFP gradient in solid tumors (80,81).

The clinical observations made on the timing/order of TNF and chemotherapy treatment is consistent with a reduction in the IFP. In order to achieve maximal antitumor responses, TNF treatment either preceded or was given simultaneously with chemotherapy. Reversing the order, that is, giving the chemotherapy first followed by TNF treatment, produced less than optimal results. In effect, ILP with TNF served to sensitize the tumors to chemotherapy, and in preclinical models, this observation correlated with improved uptake of chemotherapeutic agents by the solid tumors (82). In the following section, we will describe our recent efforts to simulate the ILP using colloidal gold-based nanotherapeutics that sequester not only TNF, but also a chemotherapeutic (i.e., paclitaxel) in murine tumors.

Barriers Within the Tumor Interstitium: Intratumor Barriers

In order to achieve effective delivery of antineoplastic agents to solid tumors, nanoparticle delivery systems must effectively evade immune detection by the RES, find and extravasate the leaky tumor vasculature, and simultaneously possess methods for reducing the IFP. Yet, even when these prerequisites are met, the intra-tumor microenvironment presents one additional obstacle that may thwart effective drug delivery to the tumor interstitium. These nanotherapeutics must overcome the spatial barrier established by the extracellular matrix of solid tumors. This viscous matrix consists of a fibrous mesh of proteoglycan-assembled collagen fibers in which stromal and tumor cells are suspended.

The orientation of collagen type I fibers present in the extracellular matrix may retard the trafficking and penetration of large macromolecules such as IgG, IgM, and high-molecular-weight dextran and nanoparticle-delivery systems through the tumor interstitium. The main obstacle posed by collagen is the spatial orientation of the individual collagen fibrils and collagen bundles. Depending on the tumor model, the small space between individual collagen fibers may hinder the move-ment of particles larger than 40 nm, whereas the collagen bundles may retard the trafficking of particles that are 75 to 130 nm in diameter. Interestingly, in murine tumor models, the relative contribution of the collagen mesh appears to be con-trolled by tumor–host interactions because the density of collagen and the complex-ity of the mesh are dependent on the site of tumor implantation (83).

Active vs. Passive Tumor Targeting

Passive extravasation through the leaky tumor vasculature is the primary mecha-nism by which nanoparticle vectors gain access to the tumor interstitium. Upon extravasation, these nanotherapeutics rely on diffusion, rather than convection, as the primary mechanism for delivering drugs to cancer cells. In effect, the passive accumulation of the nanotherapeutics is designed to limit the biodistribution of the therapeutics.

To further improve the delivery of the therapeutic payload, the nanoparticles may be engineered to contain tumor-targeting ligands that guide the delivery of these vectors to tumor, endothelial, and potentially stromal cells. Such targeting ligands also assist in the uptake of the nanotherapeutics by tumor cells by receptor-mediated mechanisms including receptor-mediated endocytosis and potolysis. Examples of tumor-targeting ligands include oligosaccharides, folic acid, EGF, and TNF, as well as antibody-directed cell surface receptors (84–89).

Tumor Models

One final challenge in developing nanoparticle therapeutics lies in the extrapolation of preclinical findings, often conducted in rodent tumor models, to the clinical set-ting. Typically, after showing promise in such preclinical studies, candidate drug therapies are tested in FDA-guided GLP toxicology studies, and indeed these stud-ies are requisite to ensure patient safety. Yet, testing such therapeutics in patients with naturally occurring cancer is the critical test. In advance of formal clinical trials, treating companion animals (i.e., pets) with inoperable/unresponsive tumors on a compassionate use basis may provide additional insight to data obtained from animal tumor models. It is estimated that in the U.S.A. alone there are 130 million cats and dogs, of which 10% to 25% present with a variety of naturally occurring solid tumors (90). We believe that such terminally ill animals may serve as sentinels for the human condition and may provide valuable information regarding drug performance in human cancer patients.

METALLIC NANOPARTICLE DRUG-DELIVERY SYSTEMS

Although metallic nanoparticles have a long history of use in biology, their application to tumor-targeted drug delivery has only recently been described. For example, colloidal gold nanoparticles have been used as diagnostic indicators and therapeutics since the early 1950s. Similarly, although the magnetic properties of iron nanoparticles have made them a valuable tool for magnetic resonance imaging (MRI), their use in magnetic-targeted drug delivery to solid tumors has only recently been described. In the following sections, we describe the characterization of these nanoparticulates, toxicologic considerations, and formulation into tumor-targeted drug-delivery vectors.

Primer on the Use of Colloidal Gold and Iron Nanoparticles in Biotechnology
Gold Nanoparticles
In 1857, Michael Faraday (91) when generating multicolored solutions by reacting gold chloride with sodium citrate, he could not have appreciated the fact that he was laying the foundation for the field of nanotechnology. Unbeknownst to him what he actually described was the synthesis of colloidal gold nanoparticles that ranged from 12 to 100 nm in diameter. Since that time gold nanoparticles have been used to meet a variety of needs in science and medicine. In the 1950s, the discovery that the particles bound protein biologics without altering their activity paved the way for their use in hand-held immunodiagnostics and in histopathology (92). Of particular importance to the current discussion was the long-standing use of colloidal gold in the treatment of rheumatoid arthritis as well as the use of radioactive gold nanoparticles to treat liver cancer (see later). More recently, gold nanoparticles have been assembled into scaffolds for use in DNA diagnostics and biosensors (93).

Iron Nanoparticles
Iron nanoparticles have been used in both diagnostics and therapeutics agents, with specific applications as contrasting agents for MRI and magnetically targeted drug delivery. Two types of iron oxide nanoparticles have been used as imaging agents: superparamagnetic iron oxide (SPIO) and ultra-small superparamagnetic iron oxide (USPIO) nanoparticles (94). Typically, these nanoparticles are coated with a variety of stabilizing agents including dextran, albumin, starch, or silicones. The major difference between SIPOs and USPIOs relates to their size and circulatory half-life. Both particles may be used as contrasting agents to image the gastrointestinal tract, liver, spleen, and lymph nodes, although the USPIOs may be used to demonstrate blood pooling in diseases such as brain and myocardial ischemia.

Safety of Metallic Nanoparticle Administration in Man
Unlike biodegradable particles such as liposomes and polymeric-based nanoparticles, metallic nanoparticles are relative newcomers to the field and thus the available toxicology data for each nanoparticle system are limited. From a historical perspective, the question of colloidal gold toxicity may be gleaned from the use of radioactive colloidal gold nanoparticles as a cancer therapy in the late 1950s.

Specifically, radioactive colloidal gold nanoparticles were made from Au^{198} and used for the treatment of liver cancer and sarcoma (95,96). Safety data revealed that the observed toxicities of these intravenously administered radioactive nanoparticles were due to radiation exposure. No demonstrable toxicities were noted from the particles themselves. In other reports, gold was also reported to be inert and biologically compatible (97). Data from our GLP toxicology study on the safety of drug stabilized colloidal gold nanoparticles agree with the historical data (Paciotti et al., unpublished observations). Like gold, iron-based nanoparticles are also biologically inert drug carriers Alexiou (98) and Lubhe (99) showed that dextran-coated magnetite particles exhibit no discernable toxicity (i.e., LD_{50}) in mice and rats (98,99). Furthermore, clinical studies on the use of epirubicin demonstrated that ferrofluids were well tolerated, with toxicity being limited to the active agent, rather than the iron nanoparticles themselves (99,100).

Metallic Nanoparticle-Binding Chemistry
Inherent in the development of metallic nanoparticle drug vectors is an understanding of the binding mechanisms involved in adsorbing proteins and other drugs to the surface of metallic nanoparticles. For colloidal gold, proteins and other drugs bind to the surface of the colloidal gold particle by one of three mechanisms. Two of these mechanisms, ionic and hydrophobic binding, are relatively weak interactions that often result in the generation of poor-quality vectors. The third method involves the formation of a dative/coordinate covalent bond between free sulfhydryl/thiols of the biomolecule and the gold atoms present on the surface of the particles. Dative bonds are very stable, possessing the energy equivalence of a covalent bond, and are only disrupted by strong reducing agents such as dithiothreitol or mercaptoethanol (30,101). Additionally, we recently generated functionalized colloidal gold nanoparticles containing various surface groups that are useful for covalent drug immobilization. These functional groups, which include NH_2, COOH, SH, and OH, may be used to link drugs through well-described cross-linking chemistries such as NHS-based ester formation and EDC-based coupling (Silin et al., unpublished observations).

For iron-based particles, drug binding primarily occurs through indirect coupling of the drug to the polymer coat surrounding the particle. For example, Allport and Weissleder (102) attached the HIV tat peptide to the surface of dextran-coated iron nanoparticles. Alternatively, Jain et al. (103) used a double coating of oleic acid and pluronic F127 around the central iron nanoparticle to allow doxorubicin to partition in this hydrophobic layer while relying upon the pluronic coating to increase the hydrophilic nature of the particle (see earlier). One unique aspect of magnetic particles is that the particles themselves represent a novel therapeutic. For example, through magnetic excitation, the particles become heated and have been shown to be useful in thermal ablation of cancer cells (see later).

Preclinical and Clinical Studies on Gold and Iron Nanoparticle Drug Delivery
Gold Nanoparticles
CYT-6091 is a multivalent drug that is assembled on 26-nm particles of colloidal gold and designed to actively sequester recombinant human TNF alpha within solid tumors (30). The drug is manufactured by covalently linking molecules of TNF and thiol-derivatized polyethylene glycol (PEG-THIOL) onto the surface of the colloidal

gold nanoparticles (30). Following intravenous administration, CYT-6091 rapidly accumulates in MC-38 colon carcinoma tumors and shows little to no accumulation in the livers, spleens (i.e., the RES), or other healthy organs of the animals. The tumor accumulation was evidenced by a marked change in the color of the tumor as it acquired the bright red/purple color of the colloidal gold nanoparticles, and was coincident with the active and tumor-specific sequestration of TNF. Finally, CYT-6091 was less toxic and more effective in reducing tumor burden than native TNF because maximal antitumor responses were achieved at lower doses of the drug. Our experimental data suggest that the inherent leakiness of the tumor neovasculature facilitates the passive extravasation of CYT-6091 into the solid tumor, limiting the biodistribution of TNF and avoiding healthy organs and tissues. Once inside the tumor, each molecule of TNF bound to the surface of PEGylated colloidal gold nanoparticles may serve one of the two functions. First, as expected from TNF's known biological action, CYT-6091 serves as the anticancer therapeutic; second and more importantly, TNF serves as a tumor-targeting ligand. The above studies were conducted in the TNF-sensitive colon carcinoma model, MC-38, and thus the observed antitumor effect may have been due to a direct action/binding of TNF on these tumor cells. However, in human TNF-insensitive B16/F10 melanoma tumors, CYT-6091 exhibited differential pharmacodynamics. Although CYT-6091 caused similar accumulation of TNF in B16/F10 tumors, only transient inhibition of tumor growth was observed. These data combined with the known cellular heterogeneity of solid tumors support the development of multifunctional metallic nanotherapeutics that attack solid tumors on multiple levels. An example of such a vector is presented below.

Iron Nanoparticles
The delivery of the epirubicin-conjugated iron particles was done by intravenous injection of the nanoparticles into a vein, which was located contralateral to the tumor. At the same time, a magnetic field, ranging from 0.5 to 0.8 T, was established and maintained for 45 minutes around the site of the tumor. Preclinical data in rodent models demonstrated that not only could this strategy concentrate the nanoparticle drug vectors within the solid tumor, but also significantly improve the antitumor efficacy of epirubicin treatment. In clinical trials, these studies show similar findings: the magnetic particles were detected in 50% of the patients treated, which correlated with the tumor areas showing the coloring of the iron nanoparticles. These data were further confirmed by histological examination of tumor tissue. Data from preclinical studies revealed that the particles were cleared by the RES after removal of the magnetic field. Other healthy filtering organs such as the lung and the kidney did not show the presence of the nanoparticles (98–101).

Metallic Nanoparticle for the Thermal Ablation of Tumors
In 1957, Gilchrist et al. (104) proposed the use of thermal therapy as a treatment for solid tumors. Data supporting such an approach was later provided by Jordan et al. (105) and Neilsen et al. (106), showing that tumor cells were sensitive to temperatures above 41°C. The means of treating solid tumors with heat has advanced from the use of ultrasonic and microwaves to the use of magnetic nanoparticles that heat in response to alternating magnetic fields. The degree of heating and in turn the strength of treatment is determined by the intensity of the magnetic field and the size of the object being magnetized. Babincova et al. (107) demonstrated that the use of this approach favored the destruction of neoplastic cells over healthy cells.

Two approaches have been tried to improve the efficacy of thermal ablation therapy. The first modification involves coupling of the thermal therapy with more conventional therapies such as chemo- or radiotherapy. The second method increases the maximal treatment temperature from 45 to 47 to 55°C. Nevertheless, at these high temperatures normal cells are affected, a side effect which may be overcome by direct intratumor injection of the particles (see Ref. 93 for review).

Hirsch et al. (108) recently described a second nanoparticle approach for the thermal therapy of solid tumors. They describe the synthesis of a gold/silica nanoshell comprised of an aminated silica core particle which was studded with ultra-small (1–3 nm) gold particles. These small gold nanoparticles are bound to the surface of the silica core through their interaction with the amine group. The ultra-small gold particles were subsequently used as nucleation sites upon which additional gold was reduced to form the encased gold nanoshell. This process allowed for the synthesis of gold-covered particles with a tunable plasmon band in the near-infrared region. Exposing these particles to a light source (i.e., diode laser) with a wavelength of 820 nm causes the electrons present on the gold surface (i.e., plasmons) to become excited, resulting in particle heating. Interstitial injection of these particles near the tumor followed by laser light excitation caused a significant reduction of transmissible venerea tumors (TVT) tumors growing in SCID mice.

Multifunctional Nanotherapeutics

Our previous discussion has centered on the use of metallic nanoparticles to target delivery of singular therapies, whether chemical, biological, or physical (e.g., heat), to solid tumors. Nevertheless, in recent years, it has become increasingly clear that solid tumors may be viewed as unique organs that are constantly adapting to their changing environment by altering their phenotype. As previously discussed, solid tumors represent a collage of cells, which for the most part work in concert to ensure continued tumor growth and metastasis. It seems unlikely that any given single agent, regardless of its ability to perform in experimental tumor models, will yield the exacting results in cancer patients.

Thus, one of the final challenges that metallic nanoparticle drug-delivery systems face is to attack the heterogeneous population of tumor cells present within a solid tumor by delivering multiple therapeutics on a single nanoparticle. Combinational cancer treatments have been a hallmark of recent clinical strategies to treat cancer. One example, previously discussed, the isolated limb perfusion, demonstrates dramatic efficacy of the combination of TNF and chemotherapy to treat refractory cancer patients (72–74). More recently, a similar combination, Avastin and 5-FU, has demonstrated significant benefit in colorectal cancer patients (70,71). Our own experience with CYT-6091 also supports the development of multifunctional metallic nanotherapies. We observed that although CYT-6091 sequestered TNF within B16/F10 tumors, it produced only marginal antitumor effects in this model.

Metallic nanoparticles may deliver these combination therapies either spatially, on the same particle, or temporally, over the course of the disease. Our initial efforts to develop such a therapeutic centered on developing a colloidal gold nanoparticle vector that simulates the ILP on a single nanoparticle. Recall that ILP involves the surgical isolation of the blood supply of a solid tumor to allow for the regional delivery of TNF and a chemotherapeutic, avoiding systemic toxicities.

To accomplish this goal required the binding of a tumor-targeting ligand, a chemotherapeutic, and an RES-avoiding molecule onto the same 25-nm particle of colloidal gold. Specifically, this nanoparticle, termed CYT-21001, uses TNF as the tumor-targeting ligand, a thiolated paclitaxel analog as the therapeutic, and PEG-THIOL as an RES-avoidance molecule. To date, we have observed that CYT-21001 delivers significantly more TNF and paclitaxel to solid tumors growing in mice, when compared to native TNF/paclitaxel. Furthermore, we observed that unlike CYT-6091, which only caused transient tumor inhibition, CYT-21001 induced significant antitumor responses in this TNF-insensitive tumor model (Paciotti et al., unpublished observations).

SUMMARY

Depicted in Figure 1 is a simplified blueprint for developing multifunctional metallic nanotherapeutics. On the basis of the current knowledge of the biology of tumor neovascularization as briefly summarized above, there is a rational strategy for using metallic particles to both target the tumor and to deliver well-known, potent, but potentially toxic cancer therapies to a broad spectrum of solid tumors. Additionally, as new therapies are discovered, the versatility of the metallic nanoparticle surface may allow for the rapid development and evaluation of new vectors in both preclinical and clinical settings. With the development of the first generation of metallic nanoparticle cancer therapies almost ready for clinical trials, the potential promise of these new cancer therapeutics may be realized in years not decades.

REFERENCES

1. Papisov MI. Theoretical considerations of RES-avoiding liposomes: molecular mechanisms and chemistry of liposome interactions. Adv Drug Deliv Rev 1998; 32:119–138.
2. Moghimi SM, Patel HM. Serum-mediated recognition of liposomes by phagocytic cells of the reticuloendothelial system—the concept of tissue specificity. Adv Drug Deliv Rev 1998; 32:45–60.
3. Woodle MC. Controlling liposome blood clearance by surface grafted polymers. Adv Drug Deliv Rev 1998; 32:139–152.
4. Nafayasu A, Uchiyama K, Kiwada H. The size of liposomes: a factor, which affects their targeting efficiency to tumors and therapeutic activity of liposomal antitumor drugs. Adv Drug Deliv Rev 1999; 40:75–87.
5. Maruyama K, Ishida O, Takizawa T, Moribe K. Possibility of active targeting to tumor tissues with liposomes. Adv Drug Deliv Rev 1999; 40:89–102.
6. Salata OV. Applications of nanoparticles in biology and medicine. J. Nanotechnol 2004; 2:3–8.
7. Moghimi SM, Hunter AC, Murray JC. Nanomedicine: current status and future prospects. FASEB J 2005; 19:311–330.
8. Moghimi SM, Hunter AC, Murray JC. Long-circulating and target-specific nanoparticles: theory to practice. Pharmacol Rev 2001; 53:283–318.
9. Ferrari M. Cancer nanotechnology: opportunities and challenges. Nat Rev Cancer 2005; 5:161–171.
10. Müller RH, Mäder K, Gohla S. Solid–lipid nanoparticles (SLN) for controlled drug delivery—a review of the state of the art. Eur J Pharm Biopharm 2000; 50:161–177.
11. Jain R, Shah NH, Malick AW, Rhodes CT. Controlled drug delivery by biodegradable poly(ester) devices: different preparative approaches. Drug Dev Indust Pharm 1998; 24:703–727.
12. Rafferty DE, Elfaki MG, Montgomery PC. Preparation and characterization of a biodegradable microparticle antigen/cytokine delivery system. Vaccine 1996; 14:532–538.
13. Ogawa Y. Injectable microcapsules prepared with biodegradable poly(a-hydroxy) acids for prolonged release of drugs. J Biomater Sci Polym Ed 1997; 8:391–409.
14. Maruyama K, Takizawa T, Takahashi N, et al. Targeting efficiency of PEG-immuniliposome-conjugated antibodies at PEG terminals. Adv Drug Deliv Rev 1998; 24:235–242.

15. Absolom D. Opsonins and dysopsonins: an overview. Methods Enzymol 1986; 132:281–318.
16. Patel HM. Serum opsins and liposomes: their interaction and opsonophagocytosis. Crit Rev Ther Drug Carrier Syst 1992; 9:39–90.
17. Serra MV, Mannu F, Mater A, Turrini F, Arese P. Enhanced IgG and complement-independent phagocytosis of sulfatide-enriched human erythrocytes by human monocytes. FEBS Lett 1992; 311:67–70.
18. Chonn A, Cullis PR, Devine DV. The role of surface charge in the activation of the classic and alternative pathways of complement activation by liposomes. J Immunol 1991; 146:4234–4241.
19. Moghimi SM, Patel HM. Altered tissue specific opsonic activities and opsonophagocytosis of liposomes in tumor bearing rats. Biochem Biophys Acta 1996; 1179:157–165.
20. Abra RM, Bosworth ME, Hunt CA. Liposome disposition in vivo: effect of pre-dosing with liposomes. Res Commun Chem Pathol Pharmacol 1980; 29:349–360.
21. Souhami RL, Patel HM, Ryman BE. The effect of reticuloendothelial blockade on the blood clearance and tissue distribution of liposomes. Biochem Biophys Acta 1981; 674:354–371.
22. Moghimi SM, Davis SS. Innovations in avoiding particle clearance from the blood by Kupffer cells: cause for reflection. Crit Rev Ther Drug Carrier Syst 1994; 11:31–59.
23. Bergqvist L, Sundberg R, Ryden S, Strand SE. The "critical colloid dose" in studies of reticuloendothelial function. J Nucl Med 1987; 28:1424–1429.
24. Bradfield JW. A new look at reticuloendothelial blockade. Br J Exp Pathol 1980; 61:617–623.
25. Baban DF, Seymour LW. Control of tumour vascular permeability. Adv Drug Deliv Rev 1998; 34:109–119.
26. Cleland JL. Protein delivery from biodegradable microspheres. In: Sanders, Hendren, eds. Protein Delivery: Physical Systems. New York: Plenum Press, 1997:1–43.
27. Illum L, Davis SS, Muller RH, Mak E, West P. The organ distribution and circulation time of intravenously injected colloidal carriers sterically stabilized with a block copolymer— poloxamine 908. Life Sci 1987; 40:367–374.
28. Redhead HM, Davis SS, Illum L. Drug delivery in poly(lactide-co-glycolide) nanoparticles surface modified with poloxamer 407 and poloxamine 908: in vitro characterisation and in vivo evaluation. J Control Release 2001; 70:353–363.
29. Moghimi SM. Modulation of lymphatic distribution of subcutaneously injected poloxamer 407-coated nanospheres: the effect of ethylene oxide chain configuration. FEBS Lett 2003; 241–244.
30. Paciotti GF, Myer L, Weinreich D, et al. Colloidal gold: a novel nanoparticle vector for tumor directed drug delivery. Drug Deliv 2004; 11:169–183.
31. Chen LT, Weiss L. The role of the sinus wall in the passage of erythrocytes through the spleen. Blood 1973; 41:529–573.
32. Moghimi SM, Porter CJH, Muir IS, Illum L, Davis SS. Non-phagocytic uptake of intravenously injected microspheres in the rat spleen: influence of particle size and hydrophilic coating. Biochem Biophys Res Commun 1991; 177:861–866.
33. Senior J, Gregoriadis G. Is half-life of circulating small unilamellar liposomes determined by changes in their permeability. FEBS Lett 1982; 145:109–114.
34. Volakanis JE, Wirtz K. Interaction of C-reactive protein with artificial phosphatidylcholine bilayer. Nature (Lond) 1979; 281:115–157.
35. Devine DV, Bradley AJ. The complement system in liposome clearance: can complement deposition be inhibited? Adv Drug Deliv Rev 1998; 32:19–39.
36. Thurston G, McLean JW, Rizen M, et al. Cationic liposomes target angiogenic endothelial cells in tumors and chronic inflammation in mice. J Clin Invest 1998; 101:1401–1413.
37. Campbell RB, Fukuruma D, Brown EB, Mazzola LM, Izumi Y, Jain RK. Cationic charge determines the distribution of liposomes between the vascular and extravascular compartment. Can Res 2002; 61:6831–6836.
38. Folkman J. Tumor angiogenesis: therapeutic implications. N Engl J Med 1971; 285:1182–1186.
39. Daly ME, Markis A, Reed M, Lewis CE. Homeostatic regulators of tumor angiogenesis: a source of antiangiogenic agents for cancer treatment? J Natl Cancer Inst 2003; 95:1660–1673.

40. Heemskerk JW, Bevers EM, Lindhout T. Platelet activation and blood coagulation. Thromb Haemost 2002; 88:186–193.
41. Carmeliet P. Mechanisms of angiogenesis and arteriogenesis. Natl Med 2000; 6:389–395.
42. Pinedo HM, Verheul HM, D'Amato RJ, Folkman J. Involvement of platelets in tumor angiogenesis? Lancet 1998; 352:1775–1777.
43. Chen J, Bierhaus A, Schiekofer S, et al. Tissue factor—a receptor involved in the control of cellular properties, including angiogenesis. Thromb Haemost 2001; 86:334–345.
44. Kakkar AK, Lemoine NR, Scully MF, Tebbutt S, Williamson RC. Tissue factor expression correlates with histological grade in human pancreatic cancer. Br J Surg 1995; 82:1101–1104.
45. Hamada K, Kuratsu J, Saitah Y, Takeshima H, Nishi T, Ushio Y. Expression of tissue factor correlates with grade of malignancy in human glioma. Cancer 1996; 77:1877–1883.
46. Gasic GJ, Gasic TB, Stewart CC. Anti-metastatic effects associated with platelet reduction. PNAS (USA) 1968; 61:46–52.
47. Cramerer E, Qazi AA, Duong D, Cornelissen I, Advincula R, Coughlin SR. Platelets, protease-activated receptors, and fibrinogen in hematogenous metastasis. Blood 2004; 104:397–401.
48. Mantovani A, Sozzani S, Locati M, Allavena P, Sica. Macrophage polarization: tumor-associated macrophages as a paradigm for polarized M2 mononulcear phagocytes. Trends Immunol 2002; 23:549–555.
49. Elgert KD, Alleva DG, Mullins DW. Tumor induced immune dysfunction: the macrophage connection. J Leukoc Biol 1998; 64:2765–290.
50. Watson GA, Fu YX, Lopez DM. Splenic macrophages from tumor-bearing mice co-expressing MAC-1 and MAC-2 antigens exert immunoregulatory functions via two distinct pathways. J Leukoc Biol 1991; 49:126–138.
51. Watson GA, Lopez DM. Aberrant antigen presentation by macrophages from tumor-bearing mice is involved in the downregulation of their T-cell responses. J Immunol 1995; 155:124–134.
52. Burke B, Tang N, Corke KP, et al. Expression of HIF-1a by human macrophages: implications for the use of hypoxia-regulated cancer therapy. J Pathol 2002; 196:204–212.
53. Murdoch C, Giannoudis A, Lewis CE. Mechanism of regulating the recruitment of macrophages into hypoxic areas of tumors and other ischemic tissues. Blood 2004; 104:2224–2234.
54. Burke B, Giannoudis A, Corke KP, et al. Hypoxia-induced gene expression in human macrophages: implications for ischemic tissues and hypoxia regulated gene therapy. Am J Pathol 2003; 163:1233–1243.
55. Koshikawa N, Iyozumi A, Gassmann M, Takenaga K. Constitutive upregulation of hypoxia-inducible factor-1 alpha mRNA occurring in highly metastatic carcinoma cells leads to vascular endothelial growth factor overexpression under hypoxic exposure. Oncogene 2003; 22:6717–6724.
56. Kuwai T, Tanaka KY, Tanaka S, et al. Expression of hypoxia-inducible factor-1 alpha is associated with tumor vascularization in human colorectal carcinoma. Int J Cancer 2003; 105:176–181.
57. Kohn S, Nagy JA, Dvorak HF, et al. Pathways of macromolecular tracer transport across venules and small veins: structural basis for the hyperpermeability of tumor blood vessels. Lab Invest 1992; 67:596–607.
58. Dvorak AM, Kohn S, Morgan ES, et al. The vesiculo-vacuolar organelle (VVO): a distinct endothelial cell structure that provides a transcellular pathway for macromolecular extravasation. J Leukoc Biol 1996; 59:100–115.
59. Feng D, Nagy J, Hipp J, et al. Vesiculo-vacuolar organelles and the regulation of venule permeability to macromolecules by vascular permeability factor, histamine, and serotonin. J Exp Med 1996; 183:1981–1986.
60. Hashizume H, Baluk P, Morikawa S, et al. Openings between defective endothelial cells explain tumor vessel leakiness. Am J Pathol 2000; 156:1363–1380.
61. Jain RK. Molecular regulation of vessel maturation. Nat Med 2003; 9:685–693.
62. Mukouyama YS, Shin D, Britsch S, Tabiguchi M, Anderson DJ. Sensory nerves determine the pattern of arterial differentiation and blood vessel branching in the skin. Cell 2002; 109:693–705.

63. Neufeld G, Cohen T, Shraga N, Lange T, Kessler O, Herzog Y. The neuropilins: multi-functional semaphorin and VEGF receptors that modulate axon guidance and angiogenesis. Trends Cardiovasc Med 2002; 12:13–19.
64. Eichmann A, Le Noble F, Autiero M, Carmeliet P. Guidance of vascular and neural network formation. Curr Opin Neurobiol 2005; 15:108–115.
65. Nagy JA, Masse EM, Herzberg KT, et al. Pathogenesis of ascites tumor growth: vascular permeability factor, vascular hyperpermeability, and ascites fluid accumulation. Cancer Res 1995; 55:360–368.
66. Lichtenbeld HC, Yuan F, Michel CC, Jain RK. Perfusion of single tumor microvessels: application to vascular permeability measurement. Microcirculation 1996; 3:349–357.
67. Dvorak HF, Nagy JA, Feng D, Brown LF, Dvorak AM. Vascular permeability factor vascular endothelial growth factor and the significance of microvascular hyperpermeability in angiogenesis. Curr Top Microbiol Immunol 1999; 237:97–132.
68. Chang YS, diTomaso E, McDonald DM, Jones R, Jain RK. Mosaic blood vessels in tumors: frequency of cancer cells in contact with flowing blood. PNAS 2000; 97:14608–14613.
69. Monsky WL, Carreira CM, Tsuzuki Y, Gohongi T, Fukumara Y, Jain RK. Role of host microenvironment in angiogenesis and microvascular functions in human breast cancer xenografts: mammary fat pad versus cranial tumors. Clin Cancer Res 2002; 8:1008–1013.
70. Tong RT, Yves Boucher Y, Sergey V, et al. Vascular normalization by vascular endothelial growth factor receptor 2 blockade induces a pressure gradient across the vasculature and improves drug penetration in tumors. Cancer Res 2004; 64:3731–3736.
71. Jain RK. Normalization of tumor vasculature: an emerging concept in antiangiogenic therapy. Science 2005; 307:58–62.
72. Alexander HR, Bartlett DL, Libutti SK, Fraker DL, Moser T, Rosenberg SA. Isolated hepatic perfusion with tumor necrosis factor and melphalan for unresectable cancers confined to the liver. J Clin Oncol 1998; 16:1479–1489.
73. Lejeune FJ. High dose recombinant tumour necrosis factor (rTNFa) administered by isolation perfusion for advanced tumors of the limbs: a model for biochemotherapy of cancer. Eur J Cancer 1995; 31:1009.
74. Lienard D, Lejeune F, Ewalenko I. In transit metastases of malignant melanoma treated by high dose rTNF alpha in combination with interferon-gamma and melphalan in isolation perfusion. World J Surg 1992; 16:234.
75. Carswell EA, Old LJ, Kassel RL, Green S, Fiore N, Williamson B. An endotoxin induced serum factor that causes necrosis of tumors. Proc Natl Acad Sci USA 1975; 72:3666.
76. Helson L, Green S, Carswell EA, Old LJ. Effect of tumor necrosis factor on cultured human melanoma cells. Nature 1975; 258:731.
77. Asami T, Iami M, Tanaka Y. In vivo anti-tumor mechanism of natural human tumor necrosis factor involving a T-cell mediated immunologic route. Jpn J Cancer Res 1989; 80:1161.
78. Nawroth PP, Stern DM. Modulation of endothelial cell homeostatic properties by tumor necrosis factor. J Exp Med 1986; 163:740.
79. Brett J, Gerlach H, Nawroth P, Steinberg S, Godman G, Stern D. Tumor necrosis factor/cachectin increases permeability of endothelial cell monolayers by a mechanism involving regulatory G proteins. J Exp Med 1989; 168:637.
80. Kristensen CA, Nozue M, Boucher Y, Jain RK. Reduction of interstitial fluid pressure after TNF-alpha treatment of three human melanoma xenografts. Br J Cancer 1996; 74:533.
81. Nedrebo T, Berg A, Reed RK. Effect of tumor necrosis factor-α, IL-1β, and IL-6 on interstitial fluid pressure in rat skin. Heart Circ Physiol 1999; 46:H1857.
82. van der Veen AH, deWilt JHW, Eggermont AMM, van Tiel ST, Seynhaeve ALB, ten Hagen TLM. TNF-α augments intratumoral concentrations of doxorubicin in TNF-α based isolated limb perfusion in rat sarcoma models, and enhances anti-tumor effects. Br J Cancer 2000; 82:973–980.
83. Pluen A, Boucher Y, Ramanujan S, et al. Role of tumor–host interactions in interstitial diffusion of macromolecules: cranial vs. subcutaneous tumors. PNAS 2001; 98:4628–4633.
84. Cristiano RJ, Roth JA. Epidermal growth-factor mediated DNA delivery into lung-cancer cells via the epidermal growth factor receptor. Cancer Gene Ther 1996; 3:4–10.

85. Gottschalk S, Cristiano RJ, Smith LC, Woo SLC. Folate-mediated receptor mediated DNA delivery into tumor cells—postsomal disruption results in enhanced gene-expression. Gene Ther 1994; 1:185–191.
86. Singh M. Transferrin as a targeting ligand for liposomes and anticancer drugs. Curr Pharm Des 1999; 5:443–451.
87. Curnis F, Sacchi A, Corti A. Improving chemotherapeutic drug penetration in tumors by vascular targeting and barrier alteration. J Clin Invest 2002; 110:475–482.
88. Tuffin G, Waelti E, Huwyler J, Hammer C, Marti HP. Immunoliposomes targeting mesangial cells: a promising strategy for specific drug delivery to the kidney. J Am Soc Nephrol 2005; 16:3395–3305.
89. Sachdeva MS. Drug targeting systems for cancer chemotherapy. Expert Opin Invest Drug 1998; 7:1849–1864.
90. Marketing survey. Robert H. Smith School of Business, University of Maryland College Park, April 2004.
91. Faraday M. Experimental relations of gold (and other metals) to light. Philos Trans R Soc London 1857; 14:145.
92. Chandler J, Robinson N, Whiting K. Handling false signals in gold-based tests. IVD Technol 2001; 7:34.
93. Mirkin CA, Letsinger RL, Mucic RC, Storhoff JJ. A DNA based method for rationally assembling nanoparticles into macroscopic materials. Nature 1996; 382:607.
94. Berry CC, Curtis ASG. Functionalisation of magnetic nanoparticles for applications in biomedicine. J Phys Appl Phys 2003; 36:R198–R206.
95. Rubin P, Levitt SH. The response of disseminated reticulum cell sarcoma to the intravenous injection of colloidal radioactive gold. J Nucl Med 1964; 5:581.
96. Root SW, Andrews GA, Knieseley RM, Tyor MP. The distribution and radiation effects of intravenously administered colloidal Au 198 in man. Cancer 1954; 7:856.
97. Tang L, Liu L, Elwing HB. Complement activation and inflammation triggered by model biomaterial surfaces. J Biomed Mater Res 1998; 41:333–340.
98. Alexiou C, Arnold W, Klein RJ, et al. Locoregional cancer treatment with magnetic targeting. Can Res 2001; 60:6641–6648.
99. Lubbe AS, Alexiou C, Bergemann C. Clinical applications of magnetic drug targeting. J Surg Res 2001; 95:200–206.
100. Lubbe AS, Alexiou C, Reiss H, et al. Clinical experiences with magnetic drug targeting: a phase I study with 4′-epidoxorubidin in 14 patients with advanced solid tumors. Cancer Res 1996; 56:4686–4693.
101. Hermanson GT. Bioconjugate Techniques. Academic Press, 1996:594–597.
102. Allport JR, Weissleder. In vivo imaging of gene and cell therapies. Exp Hematol 2001; 29:1237–1246.
103. Jain TK, Morales MA, Sahoo SK, Leslie-Pelecky DL, Labhasetwar. Iron oxide nanoparticles for sustained delivery of anticancer agents. Mol Pharm 2005; 2:194–205.
104. Gilchrist RK, Medal R, Shorey WD, Hanselman RC, Parrot JC, Taylor CB. Selective inductive heating of lymph nodes. Ann Surg 1957; 146:596–606.
105. Jordan A, Wust P, Scholz R, et al. Cellular uptake of magnetic fluids particles and their effects on human adenocarcinoma cells exposed to AC magnetic fields in vitro. Int J Hyperthermia 1996; 12:705–722.
106. Neilsen OS, Horsman M, Overgaard J. A future for hyperthermia in cancer treatment? Eur J Cancer 2001; 37:1587–1589.
107. Babincova M, Sourivong P, Leszczynska D, Babinec P. Blood-specific whole-body electromagnetic hyperthermia. Med Hypotheses 2000; 55:459–460.
108. Hirsch LR, Stafford RJ, Bankson JA, et al. Nanoshell-mediated near infra-red thermal therapy of tumors under magnetic resonance guide. PNAS 2003; 100:13549–13554.

Biological Requirements for Nanotherapeutic Applications

Joseph F. Chiang
Department of Chemistry and Biochemistry, State University of New York at Oneonta, Oneonta, New York, U.S.A., and Department of Chemistry, Tsinghua University, Beijing, China

INTRODUCTION

In order to discuss the biological requirements for nanotherapeutic application, a brief discussion of cellular and tissue structure is necessary to provide some basic background for readers. Understanding the structure and the function of living cells and their interactions with their environments is essential to understand the "biological requirement" and the interactions of nanotherapeutic devices with living systems. Cells are alive and are the smallest units that exhibit the property of life. They can be cultured in vitro and could die by themselves. The structure of cells is a very complex and well-organized system. Cells perform many functions in living things. The following are functions of cells:

1. self-replications and regulations,
2. taking energy from the metabolites,
3. carrying out mechanical and translocation works, and
4. producing metabolic functions and chemical reactions using enzymes.

There are two classes of cells: prokaryotic and eukaryotic. They have different sizes and different internal structures. The former, such as bacteria, is simpler, and the latter, such as fungi, plants, and animals, is more complex in structure. The contents of a cell are called "protoplasm." They can be further divided into *cytoplasm* (all the protoplasm except the contents of the nucleus) and *nucleoplasm* (all of the materials, plasma and DNA, etc. within the nucleus).

STRUCTURE OF CELLS

Every cell has three major components: plasma (cell) membrane, cytoplasm, and nucleus (Fig. 1).

Plasma (Cell) Membrane

Plasma membrane is a semipermeable outer boundary of cells. It is a bilayer chain of molecules (phospholipids). The membrane has a hydrophobic tail pointing inward, and a hydrophilic head which is in contact with the surrounding environments. Cholesterol is also a component of the membrane in the hydrophobic part of the membrane. Plasma membrane controls the transport of nutrients, water, and ions, such as Na^+, K^+, $Ca2^+$, $Mg2^+$, and so on.

Cytoplasm

All parts are within the cell membrane. The fluids contain salts, sugars, lipids, vitamins, nucleotides, amino acids, RNA, and proteins. Cell metabolism, replication,

Cell Structure

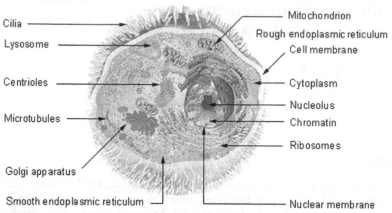

Cilia

Lysosome

Centrioles

Microtubules

Golgi apparatus

Smooth endoplasmic reticulum

Mitochondrion

Rough endoplasmic reticulum

Cell membrane

Cytoplasm

Nucleolus

Chromatin

Ribosomes

Nuclear membrane

FIGURE 1 (*See color insert.*) Structure of a typical cell.

and growth all occur within the cytoplasm. Cytosol is a part of cytoplasm, which refers to a protein-rich environment. Cytoskeleton is the network fibers of proteins, which maintain the shape of the cell. Ribosomes are the sites for protein synthesis and consist of ribosomal RNA (rRNA) and structural proteins. Mitochondria, lysosomes, peroxisomes, and chloroplast (in plants only) are also located in the cytoplasm. Peroxisomes are membrane-bound vesicles containing enzymes to regulate hydrogen peroxide in the cells. Endoplasmic reticulum is the interconnected membrane function for protein synthesis and transport. Rough endoplasmic reticulum (Rough ER) is connected to the nuclear envelop. The smooth ER is involved in transport and other cell functions. The Golgi body functions as an intracellular tool for sorting new proteins made from Rough ER. Lysosomes are used in phagocytosis in which foreign materials are brought into the cell for breakdown of the materials. Mitochondria, (organelles in globular shape) have two membranes. They serve as sites of energy release and adenosine triphosphate (ATP) formation. Organisms in storage areas use vacuoles, single-membrane organelles.

Nucleus

The nucleus contains chromatin, DNA–chromosomes, nucleoli, and nuclear proteins. The nucleolus is the site for rRNA gene transcriptions. The nuclear envelope is used to separate cytoplasm and nucleus. It is a structural frame for the nucleus. The nuclear membrane acts as a barrier and prevents free passage of molecules between nucleus and cytoplasm. Nuclear pore complexes regulate the exchange of molecules between nucleus and cytoplasm. Nuclear membranes are associated with Rough ER. Ribosomes are bounded to Rough ER.

THE CHEMICAL COMPOSITIONS OF CELLS

Cells are made of water, organic and inorganic ions, and organic molecules. Water plays an important role in cells. It is a polar molecule with a dipole moment of 1.94 Da. Water has the capability to form hydrogen bonding due to the polarity property, and also interacts with cations and anions. Many organic molecules are nonpolar and are water-insoluble in an aqueous environment. The former is called "hydrophilic," whereas the latter is called "hydrophobic." Inorganic ions in cells containing sodium ion (Na^+), potassium ion (K^+), calcium ion (Ca^{2+}), magnesium ion (Mg^{2+}), monohydrophosphate ion (HPO_4^2), chloride ion (Cl^-), and bicarbonate ion (HCO_3) play critical roles in cell functions. The organic molecules in cells can be classified as small organic molecules and macromolecules. Lipids belong to the small organic molecules category, whereas carbohydrates (the polysaccharides), proteins, and nucleic acids belong to the macromolecules category.

Small Organic Molecules
Lipids
Lipids include triacylglycerol, phosphoglyceride, glycolipid, steroid, wax, terpene, and prostaglandin and are nonpolar molecules which are soluble in organic solvents. The simplest lipids are fatty acids consisting of long hydrocarbon chains of 16 to 18 carbons with a carboxylic group (–COO). The other end contains nonpolar C—H bonds which will not interact with water. There are two types of fatty acids: saturated and unsaturated. Unsaturated fatty acids have one or more double C=C bonds. Phospholipids are the principal components of cell membranes. Two fatty acids and a phosphate are combined with glycerol to form phosphoglycerides. Triacylglycerols, or fats, have three fatty acids bound to a glycerol molecule. Energy sources are stored in fats. Phospholipids are amphipathic molecules, one end is water-soluble and the other end is water-insoluble. Another type of phospholipids is sphingomelin, which is the only nonglycerol phospholipid in the cell membrane.

Macromolecules
Carbohydrates
Simple sugars and polysaccharides are carbohydrates. Simple sugars, such as glucose, serve as major nutrients for cells. The chemical reactions of carbohydrates will provide energy for cells and also provide sources for the synthesis of other cellular products. Polysaccharides are also used for protein transport to and association with other parts of the cellular system. Simple sugar or monosaccharide has the experimental formula $(CH_2O)_n$. Glucose, one of the simple sugars in which with $n = 6$, is the simplest sugar, $(CH_2O)6$, or $C_6H_{12}O_6$. Oligosaccharides are formed by condensation of several simple sugars, whereas polysaccharides are formed with a large numbers of simple sugars. Glycogen is a polysaccharide in animals. Oligosaccharides and polysaccharides are also used for chemical interaction between cells.

Nucleic Acids
Nucleic acids are genetic information materials in cells. DNA (deoxyribonucleic acid) is the genetic material in the nucleus. RNA (ribonucleic acid) is responsible for cellular activities in the cell. There are several types of RNAs. Messenger RNA (mRNA) serves as a template for protein synthesis. It carries genetic information to ribosomes from DNA.

Transfer RNA (tRNA) and ribosomal RNA are also used in protein synthesis. Polymerization of nucleotides, a nucleic acid base attached to a sugar, and phosphate forms DNA and RNA. ATP, a type of nucleotide, is a chemical energy source in cells. A detailed description of DNA, RNA, and related subjects can be found in any cell and molecular biology text. Nucleic acids act in many cellular processes. They can produce their replications, direct protein synthesis, and carry out informational transfer.

Proteins

Proteins are biopolymers consisting of many different amino acids. Amino acids have a general structural formulas of $R\text{-}C(H)(NH_3)^+(COO)$. Condensation of two amino acids between the carboxyl group of one and the amino group of the other forms a peptide bond. The side chains are either straight carbon chains or carbon rings. There are approximately 20 such amino acids. The characteristics of proteins are based on the properties of the amino acids. Some amino acids have nonpolar side chains, such as glycine, alanine, valine, leucine, isoleucine, proline, cysteine, methionine, phenylalanine, and tryptophan. Thus, the side chain of these amino acids will not interact with water or polar molecules. Amino acids serine, threonine, tyrosine, asparagine, and glutamine have polar side chains of either OH group, or amide group ($O{=}C\text{-}NH2$). They are hydrophilic and will form hydrogen bonding with water. Lysine and arginine, with charged groups in the side chain, are hydrophilic and will interact with water. Histidine, acting as a positive charged or neutral amino acid based on the pH value, has the ability to produce H^+ for enzymatic catalysis. Both aspartic acid and glutamic acid have a carboxyl group at the end of the side chain. They are very hydrophilic. In forming proteins, this end is located on the protein surface. Amino acid linked by peptide bonds is called protein. The properties of proteins are based on the sequence of amino acids. The properties of proteins also depend on the conformation of the proteins. Many proteins perform enzyme catalytic reactions within the cells. A catalyst can either increase or slow down the reaction rate without consuming the catalyst. Such a catalyst is called an "enzyme" in biological reaction systems. The catalytic action of enzymes usually increases the rate of reaction. A basic knowledge of chemical kinetics is essential to understanding any enzymatic process.

DEVELOPMENT OF NANOTECHNOLOGY

Nanotechnology had a fast pace of development for the past decade. It has been used to rearrange molecules so that every atom can be placed in the most efficient way. Another term for such arrangement is "molecular nanotechnology" or molecular manufacturing. Thus, it can be used to construct shapes, machines, and products at the atomic level. Nanotechnology can also be defined as the application of science that deals with materials in 100-nm size, but it is not a miniaturization. At this range, materials produced will exhibit new properties we are looking for. In this range, the surface area increases drastically, which will exhibit new chemical and physical properties. Nanotechnology also provides applications in energy storage, energy production, agriculture, air pollution, nanoelectronics, and healthcare. In the healthcare application, use of nanotechnology as tools to manipulate biomolecules to regulate life and death, illness, and health will be the main goal to achieve. One of the examples is the use of molecular diagnostics, which will enable selection of the most efficient treatment for each individual. Nanoparticles are thought to have potential as novel intravascular probes for diagnostics (e.g., imaging) and therapeutic purposes (e.g., drug delivery). The critical requirement is the ability to target specific tissues and cell types and escape from biological particulate filters. This is the so-called "reticuloendothelial system." The advantage of nano-technology over microsystems is that nanotherapeutics has higher intracellular uptakes, allowing drug release in different cellular compartments such as cytoplasm and nucleus. It can also be conjugated with a ligand to favor a targeted therapeutic approach. Practically, drug load is a science based on size and structure of device. Examples are the use of nanoparticles as controlled drug delivery for cancer treatment. A combination of micro- and nanoparticles can also be used for drug-delivery systems, such as micro/nanospheres, micro/nanocapsules, and liposomes. Such combinations will differ in structure and biopharmaceutical properties for different therapeutic uses. Liposomes discovered by Baughman (1) are the smallest artificial vesicles of spherical shape that can be produced from natural untoxic phospholipids and cholesterols. Liposomes can be used as drug carriers and loaded with a variety of molecules, such as small drug molecules, proteins, nucleotides, plasmids, and carriers for lipophilic-antitumor drug N-octadecyl-1-β-arabinofuranosyl cystine (2), azidothymidine, and dideoxycytidine. There are other drug-delivery system approaches in addition to liposomes, such as polymer microcapsules, microspheres, polymer conjugates, and nanoparticles as mentioned previously. The most fundamental requirement for nanotherapeutic devices is to deliver any drug at the right time and in the target where it is needed and at the level that is required. Development of drug-delivery systems is also aiming at the therapeutic and toxicological properties of existing chemotherapies. Nanoporous membranes with 7 to 9 nm pores offer size-based exclusion and controlled diffusion of molecule drugs. Common technology for drug administration and devices include: subcutaneous, implants, surgical, oral, intravenous, and possible pulmonary inhalation, whereas the characteristics of common routes of drug administration are shown in Table 1.

Research and technology development at nanoscale provides a fundamental understanding of materials at nanoscale in order to create devices and systems in medicine–nanomedicine. Recently, a professional organization "American Academy of Nanomedicine (AANM)" was established in Baltimore, Maryland, on August 15, 2005. AANM is devoted to the study of nanomedicine and nanotherapeutic devices.

FABRICATION OF NANODEVICES

It is worthy to review and introduce the two approaches in fabrication of nanodevices and any nanoparticles at this point. The first one is the top-down approach and the second one is called bottom-up. The top-down approach involves the reduction of materials from bulk size to micro- and to nanoscale. For a three-dimensional case, if two dimensions are kept in macroscale, but the third one is reduced to nanoscale, the structure is known as quantum well. If one dimension is kept in macroscale and the other two are reduced to nanoscale, this is called nanowire. If all three dimensions are reduced to nanoscale, it is referred to as quantum dot. The top-down approach begins with a reduction of macroscale substance to nanoscale product. Lithographic technique as used in microchip fabrication is an example. The standard process is listed below. An n-type silicon wafer doped with p-type impurities can be used to create the drain and source of a transistor. A stepwise illustration is shown as follows (Fig. 2).

TABLE 1 Characteristics of Common Routes of Drug Administration

Route	Absorption pattern	Special utility	Limitations and precautions
Intravenous	Absorption circumvented	Valuable for emergency use	Increased risk of adverse effects
	Potentially immediate effects	Permits titration of dosage	Must inject solutions *slowly*, as a rule
		Suitable for large volumes and for irritating substances, if diluted	Not suitable for oily solutions or insoluble substances
Subcutaneous	Prompt, from aqueous solution	Suitable for some insoluble suspensions and for implantation of solid pellets	Not suitable for large volumes
	Slow and sustained, from repository preparations		Possible slough from irritating substances
Intramuscular	Prompt, from aqueous solution	Suitable for moderate volumes oily vehicles, and some irritating substances	Precluded during anticoagulant medication
	Slow and sustained, from repository preparations		May interfere with interpretation of certain diagnostic tests (e.g., creatine phosphokinase)
Oral ingestion	Variable; depends upon many factors	Most convenient, safe, and economical	Requires patient cooperation. Absorption potentially erratic and incomplete for drugs that are poorly soluble and absorbed slowly

1. A silicon wafer is cut from monocrystal silicon (1 1 1) direction.
2. A layer of silicon oxide is deposited on n-silicon.
3. A photosensitive emulsion is doped on SiO_2. The etched area is removed by chemical process.
4. A layer of SiO_2 is formed by oxidation process on top of the silicon. A p-type of impurities is used to cover the area to be metalized.
5. Oxidation is processed again.
6. Removal of the second oxide is performed.
7. Oxidation again on the newly grown areas.
8. Removal of the third layer again.
9. The final metallization will produce the final transistor.

There are many bottom-up processes in use for fabrication of nanomaterials. The following are just a few and include sol–gel process, chemical vapor deposition (CVD), laser pyrolysis, molecular condensation, hydrothermal process, and many other newly developing techniques. A particular method developed by Xu (3) used water-in-oil microemulsion and hydrothermal microemulsion to prepare CdS nanocrystal. The group also prepared NiO nanoring and monodispersed monoclinic zirconia (m-ZrO_2) via hydrothermal method in ethanol–water system (4). A new tool: "Dip-pen nanolithography" was developed by Mirkin and coworkers (5). This new method can be used for direct-write scanning probe-based lithography

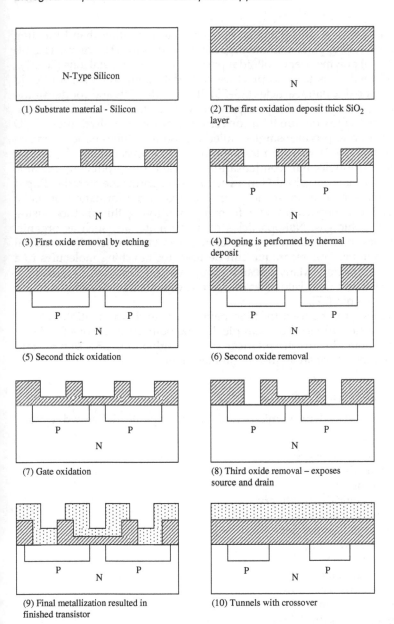

FIGURE 2 Standard method for fabrication of p-channel metal oxide semiconductor field effect transistor (MOSFET).

which uses an atomic force microscopy (AFM) tip to deliver chemical reagents on a target substrate.

AFM is a scanning technique to produce high resolution 3-D image of less than 1 nN sample surface. It can be used to measure the force between an AFM tip and the sample surface (conductor or insulator). The small forces are measured by measuring the motion of a very flexible cantilever beam having an extra small mass.

In AFM, the forces between the tip and sample are detected rather than tunneling current. It is a good tool to pattern many organic molecules (6–11), organic (12–14) and biological (15,16) polymers, and colloidal particles (17–19) to metal ions (20–22).

The sol–gel method is used to produce colloidal nanoparticles from liquid phase, especially for oxide nanoparticles (23–25). It is a hydrolysis and condensation of metal alkoxides process. In hydrolysis, precipitation from solution forms insoluble hydroxides. The hydroxides are then converted to oxides by dehydration. CVD method has been used to produce single-walled carbon nanotubes either at raised temperature (thermal CVD), or with plasma-enhanced chemical vapor deposition (PECVD). Atomic or molecular condensation is used for producing metallic nanoparticles. A raw material is heated in a vacuum to vaporize the material. Rapid coating of the vapor-phase metal in noble gas results in the formation of metal nanoparticles. Oxide nanoparticles will form by modifying this method using oxygen instead of noble gas. Nanoparticles of many materials, such as organic, biological molecules, metals, and inorganic oxides, can be produced by chemical self-assembly technique. This technique can be used for attaching molecules to a specific surface of a substrate. Many research groups use self-assembly as a method. One of them is to fabricate alkylsiloxanes on silicone dioxide (26). Another example is alkanethiolates on gold (27).

Nanotechnology can be used for therapeutics due to the compatible sizes of proteins and nanoscale particles. For example, hemoglobin has a size of 4.5×7 nm^2 dimension; lipoprotein, 20 nm^2 in spherical shape; α-globulin, 4.3×26 nm^2; and fibrinogen, 4×76 nm^2. These are in the nanometer range.

NANOTHERAPEUTIC DEVICES

The following is a list of systems in micro- and nanotherapeutic delivery devices:

1. oral drug delivery
2. injection-based drug delivery
3. transdermal drug delivery
4. bone marrow infusion
5. organ-system-specific drug delivery
   a. pulmonary drug delivery
   b. nasal delivery to central nervous system
   c. cardiovascular system (CV)
   d. genito-urinary tract
   e. gastrointestinal tract
   f. ocular drug delivery
6. controlled release system
7. novel packaging and formulation
   a. fast dissolving system
   b. chewable tablets
   c. solubility enhancement
8. target drug delivery
   a. polymer and collagen system
   b. particle-based system
      i) therapeutic monoclonal antibodies
      ii) liposomes
      iii) microparticles

    c. modified blood cells
    d. nanoparticles
    e. viral-assisted intracellular gene delivery, and
    f. nonviral intracellular gene delivery
9. implant drug-delivery system

Some of the above delivery systems are obvious from the title. Some do need certain explanations and examples. The targeted drug delivery is just one of the cases. Poly(amino) amine dendrimers (28,29) are one of the polymer systems. Block copolymer has potential to encapsulating large numbers of guest molecules within the cavity for therapeutic applications. Nanoparticles engineered with specific binding power can be suspended in body fluids or even injected into the circulation system. Nanoparticles can be used both quantitatively and qualitatively for in vivo detection of tumor cells. At the present time, most nanotherapeutic devices and drug-delivery systems are concentrated on oncology for detection and curing tumor cells. In particular, nanotherapeutic systems can reach tumor cells much easier than other cells. Tumor tissue is usually different from normal tissue. This phenomenon provides the so-called "enhanced permeability and retention (EPR) effect" (30). Antitumor agent delivery with EPR will be more effective. The application of nanoparticles to CVs has two purposes: detection and targeted drug delivery. Recently, a report by Corie Lok in the May 2005 Issue of the *Technology Review* described a new diagnostic tool called "metabolomics" which can be used to detect diseases at an earlier stage and can cure the diseases as well. The principles involved in metabolomics are the analysis of a large number of small molecules, such as sugar and fats to reveal abnormal behaviors. This will lead to metabolic fingerprints to give an earlier and more accurate diagnosis for diseases. Implantable devices consisting of sealed arrays of reservoirs can be used for in vivo and in vitro drug analysis and delivery. These devices are filled with chemicals that can be released on demand and can check the efficacy of drug released over a long period of time. Implantable brain probes have been studied for neural activities. The results can be used in the treatment of various mental and other brain disorders. Another example is the nanorobots injected into the human body to work in patients' bloodstreams. In future, medical nanodevices can routinely be implanted or even injected into the bloodstream to monitor wellness and to participate in the repair of the system that deviates from the normal state. Implantable sensors could be used in the detection of glucose for diabetes. Regulation of glucose metabolism in the human body by insulin can be achieved by the design described by Gouch (31). The device can be programmed to warn of hypoglycermia (low blood glucose) or hyperglycermia (high blood glucose). Such indication can guide diabetics to adjust insulin injection or even could be coupled to an implanted pump to deliver insulin correctly. The principle of operation is based on glucose oxidase, which catalyzes the reaction:

$$\text{Glucose} + O_2 + H_2O \longrightarrow \text{gluconic acid} + H_2O_2$$

Oxygen is used for the reaction. The unreacted oxygen will be detected in the form of electric current. Thus, the amount can be calibrated in relation to the current of a system without the presence of the enzyme, the oxidase. Another biosensor developed recently is to measure the level of H_2O_2 using Pt electrode (32). One more method mentioned here is the measurement of glucose concentration for diabetes by direct electrochemistry of glucose oxidase absorbed on a colloidal gold-modified carbon paste electrode (33). Castillo et al. (34) have measured glucose concentration based on enzyme-based amperometric biosensor.

The search for nanotherapeutic applications is mainly due to the limitation of current therapeutics, especially chemotherapies and radiotherapies. These therapeutics have a high degree of toxicity. They also produce many invasive side effects; not only do they give unfavorable therapeutic effects, but they also cause damages during administrations of such drugs or radiation treatments. There are many advantages of nanotherapeutic systems over the traditional drug administration. For any drug delivery, the penetrations of strong acids/bases depend on the permeability of cell membrane. Penetration of drug with nanodevices into mitochondria follows the same principle as cell membrane. Also pH value between intracellular and extracellular fluids is small (pH of 7.0–7.4). The gradient of drug across the plasma membrane is small. In general, weak bases are slightly concentrated inside cells, whereas weak acids are less concentrated inside cells. Lowering pH value, or increasing the concentration of H^+ ion of the extracellular fluids, will cause an increase in the intracellular concentration.

REQUIREMENTS FOR NANOTHERAPEUTIC APPLICATIONS

1. Transit and penetration properties of nanoscale particles: Nanoparticles of size less than 20 nm can transit through blood vessel wall. They can also penetrate blood–brain barrier or stomach epithelium.
2. Interaction: the nanoscale size of nanoparticles can interact with biomolecules on the cell surfaces, but will not change the biological properties of the molecules. They also have the ability to interact with receptors, nucleic acids, and proteins at the molecular scale.
3. Intracellular imaging: Nanoparticles, such as quantum dots, can be used for intracellular imaging as they can accommodate large numbers of atoms, or molecules of imaging agent, such as gadolinium, to increase the sensitivity for detection.
4. Surface chemistry: modifying or altering the surface of nanoparticles to form covalency with chemical and biological species results in the increase of the solubility and biocompatibility. For example, attaching a hydrophilic polymer to the nanoparticle surface will increase hydration. As absorption depends on solubility, it eventually increases the absorption. They can also be used to encapsule insoluble compounds.
5. Coating and uncoating: nanoparticles coated with hydrophilic polymers have longer half-life; uncoated nanoparticles used in intravenous injection can be cleared from bloodstream by reticuloendothelial system.
6. Ionic attachments: Attaching the surface with ionic cation or anion species can influence the biocompatibility of nanoparticles and the ability to traverse biological barriers. An example is dendrimers with amine, a cationic group on the surface was more cytotoxic than carboxylic-terminated dendrimers.
7. Liposomes used as drug-delivery vehicles. They were developed in early 1960s. Liposomes are vesicles enclosed by lipid bilayer from self-assembly process of amphiphilic molecules. They have been used to study membranes, also as vesicles for controlled drug delivery, catalysis, nonviral gene delivery, and diagnostic devices. The disadvantage of liposomes application is due to the

TABLE 2 Applications of Nanoparticles in Therapeutics

Nanoparticle	Descriptions	References
Nanospheres	Drug is uniformly dispersed	(36,37)
Nanocapsules	Drug is enclosed by polymer membrane in a vesicular system	(38)
Micelles	Amphiphilic blood-copolymer that can self-associate in aqueous solution	(39,40)
Ceramic nanoparticles	Nanosphere of $17Y_2O_3$–$19Al_2O_3$–$64SiO_2$ (mol%) composition, 20–30 μm diameter for targeted radiotherapy of liver cancer (nonradioactive [89]Y can be activated by neutron bombardment to ^{90}Y, a μ-emitter ($t_{1/2} = 64.1$ hr)	(41)
Liposomes	Artificial spherical vesicles from natural phospholipids and cholesterol	(43)
Dendrimers	Micromolecules consisting of a number of branches around the inner core	(44)
TNT system	Developed by Triton BioSystem with the U.S. Army Lab attacking cancer in three steps: (*i*) patient receiving a single infusion containing trillions of magnetic biosphere, bound to vantibodies; (*ii*) the biosphere will seek and attach to cancer cells in bloodstream; (*iii*) switch on the magnetic field in the cancer region will cause the biospheres to heat up to kill the cancer cells in minutes	(45)

Abbreviation: TNT, targeted nano therapeutics.

TABLE 3 Some Nanoparticles Used in Biological Research

Nanoparticle	Application	References
Dendrimers	Targeting of cancer cells, drug delivery, imaging, boron neutron capture therapy	(44,46)
Ceramic nanoparticle	Passive targeting of cancer cells	(47)
Lipid-encapsulated perfluorocarbon nanoemulsions	Passive targeting of cancer cells	(48)
Magnetic nanoparticles	Specific targeting of cancer cells, tissue imaging	(49,50)
LH–RH-targeted silica-coated lipid micelles	Specific targeting of cancer cells	(49)
Thiamine-targeted nanoparticles	Directed transfer across Caco-2 cells	(51)
Liposomes	Specific targeting of cancer cells, gene therapy, drug delivery	(52–54)
Nanoparticle-aptamer bioconjugate	Targeting of prostate cancer cells	(55)
Anti-Flk antibody-coated ^{90}Y nanoparticles	Antiangiogenesis therapy	(56)
Gold nanoshells	Tissue imaging, thermal ablative cancer therapy	(57–59)
Anti-HER2 antibody-targeted gold/silicon nanoparticles	Breast cancer therapy	(59)
CLIO paramagnetic nanoparticles	Imaging of migrating cells	(60)
Quantum dots	Tissue imaging	(61–63)
Silicon-based nanowires	Real-time detection and titration of antibodies, virus detection, chip-based biosensors	(64–66)
Carbon nanotubes	Electronic biosensors	(67)
Transfersomes	Noninvasive vaccine delivery, drug delivery	(68,69)

Abbreviation: CLIO, cross linked iron oxide.

biological instability, so they have a short lifetime. This has been improved from research on the synthesis of the polymeric nanocontainers.
8. Targeted drug delivery of nanoparticles can be achieved by binding monoclonal antibodies on the surfaces of the targeted cells.

Various nanoparticles have been tried in imaging tumors in animal and human trials. Samples are shown in Table 2 from McNeil (35). Studies of biological effects of chemical and medical devices on immunological, inflammatory, and proliferate effects of nanomaterials, and the interactions of nanomaterials as applied in medical devices and toxicological risks have been carried out at various laboratories (Table 3).

REFERENCES

1. Banghman AD. Diffusion of univalent ions across the lamellae of swollen phospholipids. J Mol Biol 1965; 13:238.
2. Sibylle K, Koller-Lucae M, Schott H, Schwendener RA. Interactions with human blood in vitro and pharmacokinetic properties in mice of liposomal N^4-octadecyl-1-β-D-arabino-furanosylcytosine, a new anticancer drug. J. Pharm Exp Ther1997; 282(3):1572.
3. Xu S. Liquid-Phase Synthesis and Modification of Colloidal Particles, M. S. Thesis. Tsinghua University, 2005.
4. Sun Xiao-ming. Solution-Based Synthesis, Characterization and Property Investigation of Low-Dimensional Functional Nanomaterials, Ph.D. Thesis. Tsinghua University, 2005.
5. Piner RD, Zhu J, Xu F, Hong SH, Mirkin CA. Dip-pen nanolithography. Science 1999; 283:661.
6. Hong SH, Zhu J, Mirkin CA. Multiple ink nanolithography toward a multiple pen nano-plotter, 7. A nano-plotter with both parallel and serial writing capabilities. Science 1999; 286:523.
7. Hong SH, Mirkin CA. A nano–plotter with both parallel and serial writing capabilities. Science 2000; 288:1808.
8. Weinberger DA, Hong, SH, Mirkin CA, Wessels BW, Higgins TB. Combinatorial generation and analysis of nanometer-and micrometer-scale silicon features via dip-pen nanolithography and wet chemical etching. Adv Mater 2000; 12:1600.
9. Zhang H, Li Z, Mirkin CA. Dip-pen nanolithography-based methodology for preparing arrays of nanostructures functionalized with oligonucleotides. Adv Mater 2002; 14:1472.
10. Zhang H, Chung SW, Mirkin CA. Fabrication of sub-50-nm solid state nanostructures, based on dip-pen nanolithography. Nano Lett 2003; 3:43.
11. Ivanisevic A, McCumber KV, Mirkin CA. Site-directed exchange studies with combinatorial libraries of nanostructures. J Am Chem Soc 2002; 124:11997.
12. Maynor BW, Filocamo SF, Grinstaff MW, Liu J. Nano-direct writing of polymer nanostructures: poly(thiophene)nanowires on semiconducting and insulating surfaces. J Am Chem Soc 2002; 124:522.
13. Lim JH, Mirkin CA. Electrostatically driven dip-pen nanolithography of conducting polymers. Adv Mater 2002; 14:1474.
14. Noy A, Miller AE, Klare JE, Weeks BL, Woods BW, DeYoreo JJ. Fabrication of luminescent nanostructures and polymer nanowires using dip-pen nanolithography. Nano Lett 2002; 2:109.
15. Wilson DL, Martin R, Hong S, Cronin-Golomb M, Mirkin CA, Kaplan DL. Nanopatterning collagen by dip-pen nanolithography. Proc Natl Acad Sci USA 2001; 98:13660.
16. Demers LM, Ginger DS, Park SJ, Li Z, Chung SW, Mirkin CA. Direct patterning of modified oligonucleotide on metals and insulators by dip-pens. Science 2002; 296:1836.
17. Ben Ali B, Ondarcuhu T, Brust M, Joachim C. AFM tip nanoprinting of gold nanoclusters. Langmuir 2002; 18:872.
18. Liao JH, Huang L, Gu N. Fabrication of nanoparticle pattern through atomic force tip-induced deposition on modified siliconsurfaces. Chin Phys Lett 2002; 19:134.

19. Garno JC, Yang YY, Amro NA, Cruchon-Dupeyrat S, Chen S, Liu GY. Precise positioning of nanoparticles on surfaces using scanning probe lithography. Nano Lett 2003; 3:389.

20. Li Y, Maynor BW, Liu J. Electrochemical AFM "dip-pen" nanolithography. J Am Chem Soc 2001; 123:2105.

21. Maynor BW, Li Y, Liu J. "Ink" for AFM "dip pen" nanolithography. Langmuir 2001;17:2575.

22. Porter LA Jr, Choi HC, Schmeltzer JM, Ribbe AE, Elliott LCC, Buriak JM. Electroless nanoparticle film deposition compatible with photolithography, microcontact printing, and dip-pen nanolithography patterning technologies. Nano Lett 2002; 2:1368.

23. Itoh H, Utampanya S, Stark JV, Klabunde KJ, Schlup JR. Nanoscale metal oxide particles as chemical reagent. intrinsic effects of particle size on hydroxyl content and on reactivity and acid/base properties of ultrafine magnesium oxide. Chem Mater 1993; 5:71.

24. Palkar VR. Sol–gel derived nanostructure γ-alumina porous spheres as an adsorbent in liquid chromatography. Nanostruct Mater 1999; 11(3):369.

25. Interrante LV, Hampden-Smith MJ, eds. Chemistry of Advanced Materials: An Overview. New York: Wiley-VCH, 1998.

26. Wasserman SR, Tao YT, Whiteheades GM. Structure and reactivity of alkylsiloxane monolayers formed by reaction of alkyltrichlorosilanes on silicon substrates. Langmuir 1989; 5:1074.

27. Bain CD, Evall J, Whitesides GM. Formation of monolayers by the coadsorption of thiols on gold: variation in the head group, tail group, and solvent. J Am Chem Soc 1989; 111:7155.

28. Hawker CJ, Frechet JMJ. Preparation of polymers with controlled molecular architecture, a new convergent approach to dendrite macromolecules. J Am Chem Soc 1990; 112:7638.

29. Tomalia DA. Dendrimer molecules. Sci Am 1995; May:62.

30. Duncan R. Drug targeting: where are we now and where are we going? J Drug Targeting 1997; 5(1):1.

31. Gouch D. In: Fung YC, ed. Introduction to Bioengineering. Singapore: World Scientific, 2001.

32. Kim L, Parris NA, Potts RO, Tierney MJ. Biosensor, iontophoretic sampling system, and methods of use thereof. United States Patent 6,736,777, 2004.

33. Liu B, Ju J. Reagentless glucose biosensor based on direct electron transfer of glucose oxidase immobilized on colloidal gold modified carbon paste electrode. Biosens Bioelectron 2003; 19(3):1773.

34. Castillo J, Gaspar S, Soukharev V, Domeanu A, Ryabov A, Csregi E. Biosensors for life quality design development and applications. Sens Actuators B 2004; 102:179.

35. McNeil SE. Nanotechnology for the biologist. J Leukoc Biol 2005; 78.

36. Santhi K, Dhanaraj SA, Joseph V, Ponnusankar S, Suresh B. A study on the preparation and anti-tumor efficacy of bovine serum albumin nanospheres containing 5-fluorouracil. Drug Dev Ind Pharm 2002; 28:1171.

37. Walsh S, Rubenstein R, Zeitlin P, Leong KW. Therapeutic nanospheres. US Patent No. 6,207,195, 1998.

38. Velinova MJ, Staffhorst RWHM, Mulder WJM, et al. Preparation and stability of lipid-coated nanocapsules of cisplatin: anionic phospholipid specificity. Biochim Biophys Acta 2004; 1663:135.

39. Kwon GS. Polymeric micelles for delivery of poorly water-soluble compounds. Crit Rev Therap Drug Carrier 2003; 20(5).

40. Ehrhardt GJ, Day DE. Therapeutic use of ^{90}Y microspheres. Int J Rad Appl Instrum B 1987; 14(3):233.

41. Kokubo T. In: Ben-Nissan B, Sher D, Walsh W, eds. Bioceramics. Vol. 15. Uetikon-Zurich: Trans Tech Publications, 2003:523.

42. Ikenaga M, Ohura K, Yamamura T, Koyoura Y, Oka M, Kobuko T. Localized hyperthermic treatment of experimental bone tumors with ferromagnetic ceramics. J Orthop Res 1993; 11:849.

43. Geng L, Osusky K, Konjeti S, Hallahan FA. Radiation-guided drug delivery to tumor blood vessels results in improved tumor growth delay. J Control Release 2004; 99:369.

44. Quintana A, Raczka E, Piehler, et al. Design and function of dendrimer-based herapeutic nanodevice targeted to tumor cells through the folate receptor. Pharm Res 2002; 19:1310.

45. Triton BioSystem. www.siliconiron.com/magazine/cover_story/index.shtme.

46. Baker JR, Jr. The synthesis and testing of anti-cancer therapeutic devices. Biomed Microdev 2001; 3:61.
47. Roy I, Ohulchanskyy TY, Pudavar HE, et al. Ceramic-based Nanoparticles entrapping water soluble photosensitizing anti-cancer drugs. J Am Chem Soc 2003; 125:7860.
48. Lanza GM, Winter P, Caruthers S, et al. Novel paramagnetic contrast agents for molecular imaging and targeted drug delivery. Pharm Biotechnol 2004; 5:495.
49. Bergey EJ, Wang XP, Krebs LJ et al. DC magnetic field induced magnetocytolysis of cancer cells targeted by L11-R11 magnetic nanoparticless in vitro. Biomed Microdev 2002; 4:293.
50. Jirak D, Kriz J, Herynek V, et al. MRI of transplanted pancreatic islets. Magn Reson Med 2004; 52:1228.
51. Russwll-Jones GJ, Arthur L, Walker H. Vitamin B12-medicated transport of nanoparticless across Caco-2 cells. Int Pharm 1999; 179:247.
52. Dubey PK, Mishra V, Jain S, Mahor S, Vyas SP. Liposomes modified with cyclic RGD peptide for tumor targeting. J Drug Target 2004; 12:257.
53. Reszka RC, Jacobs A, Voges J. Liposomes mediated suicide gene therapy in humans. Methods Enzymol 2005; 391:200.
54. Ten Hagen TL. Liposomal cytokines in the treatment of infectious disease and cancer. Methods Enzymol 2005; 391:125.
55. Farokhzad OG, Jon S, Khademhosseini A, Tran TN, Lavan DA, Langer R. Nanoparticle-aptamer bioconjugates: a new approach for targeting prostate cancer Cells. Cancer Res 2004; 64:7668.
56. Li L, Warchow CA, Danthi SN, et al. A novel antiangiogenesis therapy using an integrin antagonist or anti-flk antibody-coated 90Y-labeled nanoparticle. Int J Radiat Oncol Biol Phys 2004; 58:1215.
57. Sokolov A, Aaron J, Hsu B, et al. Optical system for in vivo molecular imaging of Cancer. Technol Cancer Res Treat 2003; 2:491.
58. Wang G, Huang T, Murray RW, Menard L, Nuzzo RG. Near-IR luminescence of monolayer-protected metal clusters. J Am Chem Soc 2005; 127:812.
59. Hirsch LR, Stafford RJ, Bankkson JA, et al. Nanoshel-mediated near-infrared thermal therapy of tumors under magnetic resonance guidance. Proc Natl Acad Sci USA 2003; 100:13549.
60. Kirscher MF, Allport JR, Graves EE, et al. In vivo high resolution three-dimensional imaging of antigen specific cytotoxic T-lymphocyte trafficking to tumor. Cancer Res 2003; 63:6838.
61. Voura EB, Jaiswal JK, Mattoussi H, Simon SM. Tracking metastatic tumor cell extravasation with quantum nanocrystals and fluorescence emission-scanning microscopy Nat Med 2004; 10:993.
62. Wu X, Bruchez MP. Labeling cellular targets with semiconductor quantum dot conjugates. Methods Cell Biol 2004; 75:171.
63. Hirsch LR, Jacobson JB, Lee A, Halas NJ, West JL. A whole blood immunoassay using gold nanoshells. Anal Chem 2003; 75:2377.
64. Cui Y, Wei Q, Park H, Lieber CM. Nanowire nanosensors for highly sensitive and selective detection of biological and chemical species. Science 2001; 293:1289.
65. Bunimovich YL, Ge G, Beverly KC, Ries RS, Hood L, Heath JR. Electrochemically programmed spatially selective biofunctionzlization of silicon wires. Langmuir 2004; 20:10630.
66. Patolsky F, Zheng G, Hayden O, Lakadamyali M, Zhuang X, Lieber CM. Electrical detection of single viruses. Proc Natl Acad Sci USA 2004; 101:14017.
67. Chen RJ, Bangsaruntip S, Drouvalakis KA, et al. Non-covalent functionalization of carbon nanotubes for highly specific electronic biosensors. Proc Natl Acad Sci USA 2003; 100:4984.
68. Gupta PN, Mishra V, Rawat A, et al. Non-invasive vaccine delivery in transfersomes noisome, and liposomes: a comparative study. Int J Pharm 2005; 293:73.
69. Simoes SL, Degado TL, Lopes RM, et al. Developments in the rat adjuvanr arthritis model and its use in therapeutic evaluation of novel non-invasive treatment by SOD in transfersomes. J Control Release 2005; 103:419.

12 Role of Nanobiotechnology in the Development of Nanomedicine

K. K. Jain
Jain PharmaBiotech, Basel, Switzerland

INTRODUCTION

Given the inherent nanoscale functional components of living cells, it was inevitable that nanotechnology would be applied in biotechnology giving rise to the term "nanobiotechnology," which will be used in this chapter and indicates biotechnology as the main field. A less recognized and less frequently used term, almost synonymously, is "bionanotechnology," which implies application in life sciences of nanotechnology as the main discipline. An up-to-date description of nanobiotechnologies and their applications in healthcare are given in a special report on this topic (1). The topic of this book is the nanoparticulate drug-delivery systems. This chapter will provide an integrated overview of application of nanobiotechnology-based molecular diagnostics, drug discovery, and drug delivery in the development of nanomedicine with the relationships as shown in Figure 1.

ROLE OF NANOBIOTECHNOLOGY IN MOLECULAR DIAGNOSTICS

Nanomolecular diagnostics is the use of nanobiotechnology in molecular diagnostics and can be termed "nanodiagnostics" (2). In contrast to drug delivery which uses mainly nanoparticles, nanodiagnostics uses both particulate and nonparticulate technologies, which are described in detail in a book on this topic (3). Some examples of the use of nanoparticles for molecular diagnosis are given here and described here as they can be combined with drug delivery and therapeutics.

Nanoparticles for Molecular Diagnostics

Nanoparticles that are commonly used for diagnostics are

- gold particles
- magnetic and supramagnetic nanoparticles
- quantum dot (QD) technology
- nanoparticle probes
- DNA–protein and nanoparticle conjugates

Gold Nanoparticles

Bits of DNA and Raman-active dyes can be attached to gold particles no larger than 13 nm in diameter. The gold nanoparticles assemble onto a sensor surface only in the presence of a complementary target. If a patterned sensor surface of multiple DNA strands is used, the technique can detect millions of different DNA sequences simultaneously. Nanoparticle-based DNA detection systems are 10 times more sensitive and 100,000 times more specific than current genomic detection systems. ClearRead® (Nanosphere, Inc.), a nanoparticle technology, enables microarray-based

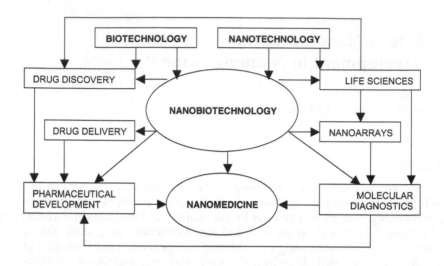

© Jain PharmaBiotech

FIGURE 1   Integration of nanobiotechnologies for the development of nanomedicine.

multiplex single nucleotide protein (SNP) genotyping of human genomic DNA without the need for target amplification (4). This direct SNP genotyping method requires no enzymes and relies on the high sensitivity of the gold nanoparticle probes. A "spot-and-read" colorimetric detection method for identifying nucleic acid sequences is based on the distance-dependent optical properties of gold nanoparticles without the need for conventional signal or target amplification (5).

Quantum Dots

There is considerable interest in the use of QDs as inorganic fluorophores, owing to the fact that they offer significant advantages over conventionally used fluorescent markers. For example, QDs have fairly broad excitation spectra – from ultraviolet to red – that can be tuned depending on their size and composition. Potential applications of QDs in molecular diagnostics are

- cancer
- genotyping
- whole blood assays
- multiplexed diagnostics
- DNA mapping
- immunoassays and antibody tagging
- detection of pathogenic microorganisms

Magnetic Nanoparticles

Magnetic nanoparticles are a powerful and versatile diagnostic tool in biology and medicine. It is possible to incorporate sufficient amounts of superparamagnetic iron oxide nanoparticles into cells, enabling their detection in vivo using magnetic resonance imaging (MRI) (6). Bound to a suitable antibody, magnetic nanoparticles are used to label specific molecules, structures, or microorganisms.

ROLE OF NANOBIOTECHNOLOGY IN DRUG DISCOVERY

The postgenomic era is revolutionizing the drug-discovery process. The new challenges in the identification of therapeutic targets require efficient and cost-effective tools. Label-free detection systems use proteins or ligands coupled to materials the physical properties of which are measurably modified following specific interactions. Among the label-free systems currently available, the use of metal nanoparticles offers enhanced throughput and flexibility for real-time monitoring of biomolecular recognition at a reasonable cost. Some nanotechnologies will accelerate target identification, whereas others will evolve into therapeutics. This is closely related to drug delivery, another important pharmaceutical aspect of nanobiotechnology.

Nanoparticles for Drug Discovery

Nanocrystals (QDs) and other nanoparticles (gold colloids, magnetic nanoparticles, nanobarcodes, nanobodies, dendrimers, fullerenes, and nanoshells) have received considerable attention recently with their unique properties for potential use in drug discovery.

Use of Gold Nanoparticles for Drug Discovery

Gold nanoparticles can emit light so strongly that it is readily possible to observe a single nanoparticle at laser intensities lower than those commonly used for multiphoton absorption-induced luminescence (7). Moreover, gold nanoparticles do not blink or burn out, even after hours of observation. These observations suggest that metal nanoparticles are a viable alternative to fluorophores or semiconductor nanoparticles for biological labeling and imaging. Other advantages of the technique are that the gold nanoparticles can be prepared easily, have very low toxicity, and can readily be attached to molecules of biological interest. In addition, the laser light used to visualize the particles is a wavelength that causes only minimal damage to most biological tissues. This technology could enable tracking of a single molecule of a drug in a cell or other biological samples.

Use of Quantum Dots for Drug Discovery

The use of QDs for drug discovery has been explored extensively. Both advantages and drawbacks have been investigated (8). Advantages of the use of QDs for drug discovery are as follows:

- Enhanced optical properties as compared with organic dyes. QDs offer great imaging results that could not be achieved by organic dyes.
- Multiple leads can be tested on cell culture simultaneously. Similarly, the absorption of several drug molecules can be studied simultaneously for a longer period of time.
- Using the surface functionalization properties of QDs, targeting capabilities can be added as well.
- Due to the inorganic nature of QDs, their interaction with their immediate environment at in vivo states can be minimal compared with their organic counterparts.

    Drawbacks of QDs for drug discovery are as follows:

- Size variation during the synthesis of single color dots is 2% to 4% and for applications such as capillary electrophoresis or gel electrophoresis, it could create false results. Therefore, QD synthesis techniques need to have improved quality control with respect to size distribution before they can be seriously utilized in drug-discovery research.

- For absorption, distribution, metabolism and excretion (ADME) purposes, blue QDs (diameter of 3.7 nm) are the smallest class of the QD family but they are considerably larger than organic dyes. Hence, the use of QDs for this purpose might not be desirable in special cases.
- Similarly, the number of functional groups attached to an organic dye is usually 1, or it can be controlled very precisely.
- The transport of a large volume (due to multiple attachments of drug molecules to a single QD) across the membrane will be more difficult than a single molecule itself.
- The "blinking" characteristics of QDs when they are excited with high-intensity light could be a limiting factor for fast scan systems such as flow cytometry.

Other Nanotechnologies for Drug Discovery

None of the nanoparticles available is ideal for all requirements of drug discovery. The choice may depend on the needs. Nanodevices such as nanobiosensors and nanobiochips are being used to improve drug discovery and development. Nanoscale assays can significantly contribute to cost-saving in screening campaigns. In addition, some nanosubstances may be potential drugs of the future. These include dendrimers, fullerenes, and nanobodies (9).

Dendrimers are a novel class of three-dimensional nanoscale, core-shell structures that can be precisely synthesized for a wide range of applications. They are most useful in drug delivery and can also be used for the development of new pharmaceuticals with novel activities. Polyvalent dendrimers interact simultaneously with multiple drug targets. They can be developed into novel-targeted cancer therapeutics (10).

A key attribute of the fullerene molecules is their numerous points of attachment, allowing for precise grafting of active chemical groups in three-dimensional orientations. This attribute, the hallmark of rational drug design, allows for positional control in matching fullerene compounds to biological targets. In concert with other attributes, namely the size of the fullerene molecules, their redox potential and their relative inertness in biological systems, it is possible to tailor requisite pharmacokinetic characteristics to fullerene-based compounds and optimize their therapeutic effect (11).

Nanobodies are the smallest available intact antigen-binding fragments harboring the full antigen-binding capacity of the naturally occurring heavy-chain antibodies. Nanobodies have the potential of a new generation of antibody-based therapeutics as well as diagnostics for diseases such as cancer (12).

ROLE OF NANOBIOTECHNOLOGY-BASED DRUG DELIVERY IN DEVELOPMENT OF NANOMEDICINE

Several nanoparticle-based technologies for drug delivery are described in various chapters of this book. This section will briefly describe the relevance of these technologies for practical human therapeutics.

An important clinical aspect of nanoparticle-based therapeutics is targeted drug delivery. When nanoparticles are used in the treatment of cancer, their powerful targeting ability and potential for large cytotoxic payload dramatically enhance the efficacy of conventional pharmaceuticals as well as novel therapeutic approaches, such as gene therapy, radioimmunotherapy, and photodynamic therapy.

There are particular advantages of drug delivery for the treatment of various diseases by nanoscale devices. There are several requirements for developing a device small enough to efficiently leave the vasculature and enter cells to perform multiple, smart tasks. However, the major requirement involves size. Vascular pores limit egress of therapeutics to materials less than approximately 50 nm in diameter, and cells will not internalize materials much greater than 100 nm. As a result, the only currently available technology that fulfills these criteria consists of synthetic nanodevices. These are designed, synthetic materials with structures less than 100 nm in size. Unlike fictional mechanical nanomachines, based on devices that have been "shrunken" to nanometer dimensions, several true nanomolecular structures have now been synthesized and applied to drug delivery, gene transfer, antimicrobial therapeutics, and immunodiagnostics.

Nanoparticles are important for delivering drugs intravenously so that they can pass safely through the body's smallest blood vessels, for increasing the surface area of a drug so that it will dissolve more rapidly, and for delivering drugs via inhalation. Porosity is important for entrapping gases in nanoparticles, for controlling the release rate of the drug, and for targeting drugs to specific regions. Owing to their small size, lipid nanocapsules might be promising for an injectable as well as for an oral drug-delivery system, providing sufficient drug solubility to avoid embolization in blood after intravenous injection as well as a positive effect of drug absorption after oral administration. A drug-delivery system for intravenous administration of ibuprofen has been developed which exhibits sustained-release properties by either oral or intravenous route and may be useful for the treatment of postoperative pain.

NANOMEDICINE

Besides nanoparticles, various nanotechnologies and other nanomaterials that are currently under investigation in medical research and diagnostics will soon find a practical application in practice of medicine. Nanobiotechnologies are being used to create and study models of human disease, particularly immune disorders. Introduction of nanobiotechnologies in medicine will not create a separate branch of medicine but simply implies improvement of diagnosis as well as therapy and can be referred to as nanomedicine. This broad term covers various therapeutic areas including treatments that may require surgical intervention. Applications of nanobiotechnology in medicine are shown in Table 1.

Clinical Nanodiagnostics

Application of nanotechnology in molecular diagnostics will have a tremendous impact on the practice of medicine. Biosensor systems based on nanotechnology could detect emerging disease in the body at a stage that may be curable. This is extremely important in management of infections and cancer. Some of the body functions and responses to treatment will be monitored without cumbersome laboratory equipment. Some examples are a radiotransmitter small enough to put into a cell and acoustical devices to measure and record the noise a heart makes. Nanodiagnostics will also be integrated with nanotherapeutics.

Nanoendoscopy

Endoscopic microcapsules that can be ingested and precisely positioned are being developed. A control system will enable the capsule to attach to the digestive tract

TABLE 1   Nanomedicine in the Twenty-First Century

Nanodiagnostics
Molecular diagnostics
Nanoendoscopy
Nanoimaging
Nanotechnology-based drugs
Drugs with improved methods of delivery
Regenerative medicine
Tissue engineering with nanotechnology
Transplantation medicine
Exosomes from donor dendritic cells for drug-free organ transplants
Nanorobotic treatments
Vascular surgery by nanorobots introduced into the vascular system
Nanorobots for detection and destruction of cancer
Implants
Bioimplantable sensors that bridge the gap between electronic and neurological circuitry
Durable rejection-resistant artificial tissues and organs
Implantations of nanocoated stents in coronary arteries to elute drugs and to prevent reocclusion
Implantation of nanopumps for drug delivery
Minimally invasive surgery using catheters
Miniaturized nanosensors implanted in catheters to provide real-time data to surgeons
Nanosurgery by integration of nanoparticles and external energy

Source: From Ref. 1.

and move within it. Precisely positioned microcapsules would allow physicians to view any part of the inside lining of the digestive tract in detail, resulting in more efficient, accurate, and less invasive diagnoses. In addition, these capsules could be modified to include treatment mechanisms as well, such as the release of a drug or chemical near a diseased area.

PillCam™ capsule (Given Imaging Ltd., Yoqneam, Israel), an endoscope to visualize small intestine abnormalities, was approved in 2001. Other companies are now producing ingestible capsules for this purpose. The patient ingests the capsule, which contains a tiny camera, and intestinal peristalsis propels the capsule for approximately eight hours. During this time, the camera snaps the pictures and images that are transmitted to a data recorder worn by the patient. The physicians can review the images later on to make the diagnosis, but some abnormalities may be missed as this method has only a 50% success rate in detection of diseases. Controlling the positioning and movement on a nanoscale will greatly improve the accuracy of this method. Similar nanorobots are under development for other parts of the body.

Nanobiotechnology for Developing Stem-Cell-Based Therapies
Stem-cell-based therapies are one of the most promising areas of development in human therapeutics. Nanobiotechnology can be applied to delivery of gene therapy using geneti-cally modified stem cells and further applied in tracking stem cells introduced into the human body.

Nanofibrous scaffolds are being developed for stem cells to mimic the nanometer-scale fibers normally found in that matrix (13). They are being used to grow stem cells derived from adipose tissue. They can conceivably be used for tissue repair.

Application of Nanobiotechnology in Various Therapeutic Areas

Nanobiotechnology has been applied in almost every area of human healthcare. Some examples are given of applications in important therapeutic areas: cancer, neurological disorders, cardiovascular diseases, and infections.

Oncology

Nanoparticles can deliver chemotherapy drugs directly to tumor cells and then give off a signal after the cells are destroyed. Drugs delivered this way are several times more potent than standard therapies. Combination of gold nanoparticles followed by X-ray treatment reduces the size of the tumors, or completely eradicates them in mice (14). The technique works because gold, which strongly absorbs X rays, selectively accumulates in tumors. This increases the amount of energy that is deposited in the tumor compared with nearby normal tissue. Gold nanoparticle radiotherapy for patients is under consideration for clinical trials.

Nanoshells may be combined with targeting proteins and used to ablate target cells. This procedure can result in the destruction of solid tumors or possibly metastases not otherwise observable by the oncologist. In addition, nanoshells can be utilized to reduce angiogenesis present in cancer. Experiments in animals, in vitro and in tissue demonstrate that specific cells (e.g., cancer cells) can be targeted and destroyed by an amount of infrared light that is otherwise not harmful to surrounding tissue. This procedure may be performed using an external (outside the body) infrared laser. Prior research has indicated the ability to deliver the appropriate levels of infrared light at depths of up to 15 cm, depending upon the tissue. Photothermal tumor ablation in mice has been achieved by using near-infrared-absorbing nanoparticles (15). Nanoshells enable a seamless integration of cancer detection and therapy.

It is within the realm of possibility to use molecular tools to design a miniature device that can be introduced in the body, locate and identify cancer cells, and finally destroy them. The device would have a biosensor to identify cancer cells and a supply of anticancer substance that could be released on encountering cancer cells. A small computer could be incorporated to program and integrate the combination of diagnosis and therapy and provide the possibility to monitor the in vivo activities by an external device. As there is no universal anticancer agent, the computer program could match the type of cancer to the most appropriate agent. Such a device could be implanted as a prophylactic measure in persons who do not have any obvious manifestations of cancer. It would circulate freely and could detect and treat cancer at the earliest stage. Such a device could be reprogrammed through remote control and enable change of strategy if the lesion encountered is other than cancer.

Disorders of the Central Nervous System

Applied nanobiotechnology aimed at the regeneration and neuroprotection of the central nervous system (CNS) will significantly benefit from basic nanotechnology research conducted in parallel with advances in cell biology, neurophysiology, and neuropathology (16). QD technology is used to gather information about how the CNS environment becomes inhospitable to neuronal regeneration following injury or degenerative events by studying the process of reactive gliosis. Glial cells, housekeeping cells for neurons, have their own communication mechanisms that can be triggered to become reactive following injury. QDs, with added bioactive molecules, might spur growth of neurites in a way that provides a medium that will encourage this growth in a directed way.

Nanoparticles can be used as an aid to neurosurgery. Iron oxide nanoparticles can outline not only brain tumors under MRI, but also other lesions in the brain that may otherwise have gone unnoticed (17).

Cardiovascular Diseases

The diagnosis and treatment of unstable plaque is an area in which nanotechnology could have an immediate impact. Nanoprobes can be targeted to plaque components for noninvasive detection of patients at risk. Targeted nanoparticles, multifunctional macromolecules, or nanotechnology-based devices could deliver therapy to a specific site, localized drug release being achieved either passively (by proximity alone) or actively (through supply of energy as ultrasound, near-infrared, or magnetic field). Targeted nanoparticles or devices could also stabilize vulnerable plaque by removing material, for example, oxidized low-density lipoproteins. Devices able to attach to unstable plaques and warn patients and emergency medical services of plaque rupture would facilitate timely medical intervention.

Restenosis after percutaneous coronary intervention continues to be a serious problem in clinical cardiology. Recent advances in nanoparticle technology have enabled the delivery of NK911, an antiproliferative drug, selectively to the balloon-injured artery for a longer time (18). NK911 is a core-shell nanoparticle of polyethylene glycol-based block copolymer encapsulating doxorubicin. It accumulates in vascular lesions with increased permeability. In a balloon injury model of the rat carotid artery, intravenous administration of NK911 significantly inhibited the neointimal formation. The effect of NK911 was due to inhibition of vascular smooth muscle proliferation but not to enhancement of apoptosis or inhibition of inflammatory cell recruitment. NK911 was well tolerated without any adverse systemic effects. These results suggest that nanoparticle technology is a promising and safe approach to target vascular lesions with increased permeability for the prevention of restenosis after balloon injury. A novel approach to prevention of restenosis involves incorporation of nitric oxide (NO)-eluting nanofibers into stents for antithrombogenic action. NO has vasodilating action as well, which may be beneficial in ischemic heart disease.

Infections

An important role of nanotechnology in the management of infections is use of formulations which improve the action of known bactericidal agents. The bactericidal properties of some agents are manifest only in nanoparticulate form. Certain formulations of nanoscale powders possess antimicrobial properties. These formulations are made of simple, nontoxic metal oxides such as magnesium oxide (MgO) and calcium oxide (CaO, lime) in nanocrystalline form, carrying active forms of halogens, for example, $MgO.Cl2$ and $MgO.Br2$. When these ultrafine powders contact vegetative cells of *Escherichia coli*, *Bacillus cereus*, or *Bacillus globigii*, over 90% are killed within a few minutes. Likewise, spore forms of the *Bacillus* species are decontaminated within several hours. Dry contact with oflatoxins and contact with MS2 bacteriophage (surrogate of human enterovirus) in water also cause decontamination in minutes. A nanopowder of MgO can scour contaminated rooms of anthrax spores (19). Unlike antibacterial gases and foams which are messy, corrosive, and ruin electrical equipment, the powder can be sprayed into rooms and swept or vacuumed up. The chemical specks attract oppositely charged spores. The particles then cut open and chemically break down the spores' tough outer shell.

Silver powder with particle size ranging from 50 to 100 nm has a homogeneous distribution of nanoparticles in the material and antiinfective properties.

Silver nanoparticles have been incorporated in commercial preparations for wound care to prevent infection.

A simple molecule from a hydrocarbon and an ammonium compound has been used to produce a unique nanotube structure with antimicrobial capability (20). The quaternary ammonium compound is known for its ability to disrupt cell membranes and causes cell death, whereas the hydrocarbon diacetylene can change colors when appropriately formulated; the resulting molecule would have the desired properties of both a biosensor and a biocide.

Antimicrobial nanoemulsions, containing water and soybean oil with uniformly sized droplets in the 200 to 400 nm range, can destroy microbes effectively without toxicity or harmful residual effects (21). The nanoparticles fuse with the membrane of the microbe and the surfactant disrupts the membrane, killing the microbe. The classes of microbes eradicated are viruses (e.g., HIV, herpes), bacteria (e.g., *E. coli, Salmonella*), spores (e.g., anthrax), and fungi (e.g., *Candida albicans, Byssochlamys fulva*).

ROLE OF NANOBIOTECHNOLOGY IN THE DEVELOPMENT OF PERSONALIZED MEDICINE

Personalized medicine simply means the prescription of specific therapeutics best suited for an individual. It is usually based on pharmacogenetic, pharmacogenomic, and pharmacoproteomic information, but other individual variations in patients are also taken into consideration (22,23). Personalized medicine is beginning to be recognized and is expected to become a part of medical practice within the next decade. Molecular diagnostics is an important component of personalized medicine. Improvement of diagnostics by nanotechnology has a positive impact on personalized medicine. Nanotechnology has potential advantages in applications in point-of-care diagnosis, for example, on patient's bedside or the outpatient clinic, self-diagnostics for use in the home, and integration of diagnostics with therapeutics. All of these will facilitate the development of personalized medicines. Cancer is a good example of advantages of personalized management. In cases of cancer, the variation in behavior of cancer of the same histological type from one patient to another is also taken into consideration. Personalization of cancer therapies is based on a better understanding of the disease at the molecular level, and nanotechnology will play an important role in this area (24).

CONCLUDING REMARKS AND FUTURE PROSPECTS

Disease and other disturbances of function are caused largely by damage at the molecular and cellular level, but current surgical tools are large and crude. Even a fine scalpel is a weapon more suited to tear and injure than heal and cure. It would make more sense to operate at the cell level to correct the cause of disease, rather than chop off large lesions as a result of the disturbances at cell level.

Nanotechnology will enable construction of computer-controlled molecular tools that are much smaller than a human cell and built with the accuracy and precision of drug molecules. Such tools will be used for interventions in a refined and controlled manner at the cellular and molecular levels. They could remove obstructions in the circulatory system, kill cancer cells, or take over the function of subcellular organelles. Instead of transplanting artificial hearts, a surgeon of the future would be transplanting artificial mitochondrion.

Nanotechnology will also provide devices to examine tissue in minute detail. Biosensors that are smaller than a cell would give us an inside look at cellular function. Tissues could be analyzed down to the molecular level, giving a completely detailed "snapshot" of cellular, subcellular, and molecular activities. Such a detailed diagnosis would guide the appropriate treatment.

An increasing use of nanobiotechnology by the pharmaceutical and biotechnology industries is anticipated. Nanotechnology will be applied at all stages of drug development – from formulations for optimal delivery to diagnostic applications in clinical trials.

It is expected that within the next few years, we will have a better understanding of how to coat or chemically alter nanoparticles to reduce their toxicity to the body, which will allow us to broaden their use for disease diagnosis and for drug delivery. Biomedical applications are likely to be some of the earliest. The first clinical trials are anticipated for cancer therapy.

REFERENCES

1. Jain KK. Nanobiotechnology: applications, markets, and companies. Basel: Jain Pharma Biotech Publications, 2007.
2. Jain KK. Nanodiagnostics: application of nanotechnology in molecular diagnostics. Expert Rev Mol Diagn 2003; 4:153–161.
3. Jain KK. Nanobiotechnology in Molecular Diagnostics. Norwich, UK, Norwich: Horizon Scientific Press, 2006.
4. Bao YP, Huber M, Wei TF, et al. SNP identification in unamplified human genomic DNA with gold nanoparticle probes. Nucleic Acids Res 2005; 33:e15.
5. Storhoff JJ, Lucas AD, Garimella V, Bao YP, Müller UR. Homogeneous detection of unamplified genomic DNA sequences based on colorimetric scatter of gold nanoparticle probes. Nat Biotechnol 2004; 22: 883–887.
6. Bulte JW, Arbab AS, Douglas T, et al. Preparation of magnetically labeled cells for cell tracking by magnetic resonance imaging. Methods Enzymol 2004; 386:275–299.
7. Farrer RA, Butterfield FL, Chen VW, Fourkas JT. Highly efficient multiphoton-absorption-induced luminescence from gold nanoparticles. Nano Lett 2005; 5:1139–1142.
8. Ozkan M. Quantum dots and other nanoparticles: what can they offer to drug discovery? Drug Discov Today 2004; 9:1065–1071.
9. Jain KK. The role of nanobiotechnology in drug discovery. Drug Discov Today 2005; 10:1435–1442.
10. Kukowska-Latallo JF, Candido KA, Cao Z, et al. Nanoparticle targeting of anticancer drug improves therapeutic response in animal model of human epithelial cancer. Cancer Res 2005; 65:5317–5324.
11. Wilson SR. Nanomedicine: fullerene and carbon nanotube biology. In: Osawa E, ed. Perspectives in Fullerene Nanotechnology. Kluwer Academic Publishers, 2002.
12. Revets H, De Baetselier P, Muyldermans S. Nanobodies as novel agents for cancer therapy. Expert Opin Biol Ther 2005; 5:111–124.
13. Kang X, Xie Y, Kniss DA. Adipose tissue model using three-dimensional cultivation of preadipocytes seeded onto fibrous polymer scaffolds. Tissue Eng 2005; 11:458–468.
14. Hainfeld J, Slatkin DN, Smilowitz HM. The use of gold nanoparticles to enhance radiotherapy in mice. Phys Med Biol 2004; 49:N309–N315.
15. O'Neal DP, Hirsch LR, Halas NJ, et al. Photo-thermal tumor ablation in mice using near infrared-absorbing nanoparticles. Cancer Lett 2004; 209:171–176.
16. Silva GA, Czeisler C, Niece KL, et al. Selective differentiation of neural progenitor cells by high-epitope density nanofibers. Science 2004; 303:1352–1355.
17. Neuwelt EA, Varallyay P, Bago AG, et al. Imaging of iron oxide nanoparticles by MR and light microscopy in patients with malignant brain tumours. Neuropathology and Applied Neurobiology 2004; 30:456–471.

18. Uwatoku T, Shimokawa H, Abe K, et al. Application of nanoparticle technology for the prevention of restenosis after balloon injury in rats. Circ Res 2003; 92:e62–e69.
19. Stoimenov PK et al. Metal oxide nanoparticles as bactericidal agents. Langmuir 2002; 18:6679–6696.
20. Lee SB, Koepsel R, Stolz DB, et al. Self-assembly of biocidal nanotubes from a single-chain diacetylene amine salt. J Am Chem Soc 2004; 126:13400–13405.
21. Hamouda T, Myc A, Donovan B, et al. A novel surfactant nanoemulsion with a unique non-irritant topical antimicrobial activity against bacteria, enveloped viruses and fungi. Microbiological Research 2001; 156: 1–7.
22. Jain KK. Personalised medicine. Curr Opinion Mol Ther 2002; 4:548–558.
23. Jain KK. Personalized Medicine: Scientific and & Commercial Aspects. Basel: Jain Pharma Biotech Publications, 2007.
24. Jain KK. Role of nanobiotechnology in developing personalized medicine for cancer. TCRT 2005; 4:645–650.

13

Pharmaceutical Applications of Nanoparticulate Drug-Delivery Systems

Yashwant Pathak
UCB Manufacturing, Inc., Rochester, New York, U.S.A.

Deepak Thassu
UCB Pharma, Inc., Rochester, New York, U.S.A.

Michel Deleers
*Global Pharmaceutical Technology and Analytical Development (GPTAD),
UCB, Braine l'Alleud, Belgium*

INTRODUCTION

The successful introduction of the first drug-delivery system (DDS) brought about tremendous interest in the research and application of these systems, especially for the entry of drugs in the systemic circulation of the body. The goal of any DDS is to provide a therapeutic amount of drug to the proper site in the body while achieving it rapidly and maintaining desired drug concentrations in the body circulation. Most drugs are delivered to patients using a systemic approach, the belief being that if you flood the body with enough active compounds, there will be a desired therapeutic effect on the body. The DDSs are supposed to deliver the drug at a rate dictated by the needs of the body over a specified period of the treatment. The idealized objective for the DDS points to two major aspects, namely spatial placement and temporal delivery of the drug. Spatial placement relates to targeting a drug to a specific organ or tissue. Temporal delivery refers to controlling the rate of delivery to the target tissues (1). Hundreds of drug-delivery products have been introduced in the market and many are now in different stages of development.

Lately, in the field of pharmaceutical research, a plethora of drug-delivery groups and companies have emerged, partly as a result of surging interest in generic drug development and continued technological advances. The drug-delivery technology can enhance the therapeutic as well as the commercial value of the healthcare products. It takes into consideration the carrier, the route, and the target, and develops a strategy of processes or devices designed to increase the therapeutic efficacy of the drug and in many cases reduce the side effects of the drug.

The drug-delivery sector has evolved from being simply a part of the pharmaceutical production process to a driving force for innovation and profits. Industry and commercial interests in drug-delivery continue to build steadily. The benefits to the patients can be seen in improved compliance and medical outcomes. The pharmaceutical industry is able to extend the patent protection through novel DDSs and bring new therapies to the market. U.S. demands for DDSs will grow nearly 9% annually to more than $82 billion by 2007. Growth opportunities extend into all therapeutic classes of pharmaceuticals: respiratory, central nervous system (CNS), and cardiovascular agents will remain the top three applications based on the special formulating needs of medicines for conditions such as asthma, arthritis, and hypertension. The other areas such as anticancer drugs, hormones, and vaccines will also follow the track.

NANOPARTICULATE DRUG-DELIVERY SYSTEMS

Nanoparticulate drug-delivery systems (NPDDSs) are being explored for the purpose of solving the challenges of drug delivery. Coming in many shapes and sizes, most carriers are less than 100 nm in diameter. NPDDSs provide methods for targeting and releasing therapeutic compounds in very defined regions. These vehicles have the potential to eliminate or at least ameliorate many problems associated with drug distribution. As many drugs have a hydrophobic component, they often suffer from problems of precipitation in high concentration, and there are many examples of toxicity issues with excipients designed to prevent drug aggregation. To combat these issues, many NPDDSs provide both hydrophobic and hydrophilic environments, which facilitate drug solubility. Alternatively, many drugs suffer from rapid breakdown and/or clearance in vivo. Encapsulating the drugs in a protective environment, NPDDSs increase their bioavailability, thereby allowing the clinicians to prescribe lower doses.

With recent advances in polymer and surface conjugation techniques as well as microfabrication methods, perhaps the greatest focus in drug-delivery technology is in the design and applications of NPDDSs. Ranging from simple metal–ceramic core structure to complex lipid–polymer matrices, these submicron formulations (2) are being functionalized in numerous ways to act as therapeutic vehicles for a variety of conditions (Fig. 1).

NPDDSs can be defined as the DDSs where nanotechnology is used to deliver the drug at nanoscale. Below 100 nm, materials exhibit different, more desirable physical, chemical, and biological properties. Given the enormity and immediacy of the unmet needs of therapeutic areas such as CNS disorders, this can lead to drugs that can extend life and save untimely deaths (2).

Advantages of Nanoparticulate Drug-Delivery Systems

The nanoparticles (NPs) may offer some advantages such as protection of drugs against degradation, targeting the drugs to specific sites of action, organ or tissues,

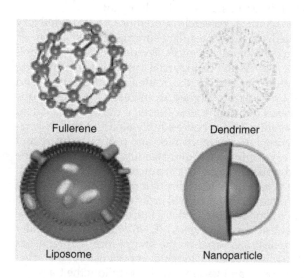

Fullerene   Dendrimer

Liposome   Nanoparticle

FIGURE 1 (*See color insert.*) Different types of nanoparticulate structures.

and delivery of biological molecules such as proteins, peptides, and oligonucleotides. A number of different strategies have been proposed in order to modify the physico-chemical characteristics of the NPs, and thus their interactions within the biological systems. For example, it is possible to change the chemical nature of the polymeric matrix of the NPs and thereby alter certain biological phenomena such as biorecognition, biodistribution, bioadhesion, biocompatibility, and/or biodegradation. Some polymeric materials used for this purpose are gelatin, chitosan (CS), sodium alginate, poly(alkyl)cynoacrylates, poly(lactic acid) (PLA), poly(lactic-co-glycolic acid) (PLGA), poly(ethylene glycol-co-(lactic-glycolic acid), poly(caprolactone), and polymethyl methacrylate (3–5). Another approach to modify the biological response is based on the incorporation of suitable adjuvants in the NPs, like proteins such as albumin, invasins, and lectins, and polymers such as poloxamers and poloxamines (6). Different manufacturing methods can also enable modifications of the physico-chemical characteristics of NPs such as size, shape, structure, morphology, texture, and composition (3).

Manufacturing Techniques for Nanoparticulate Drug-Delivery Systems
Conventionally, two groups of manufacturing techniques have been reported for producing NPs. The first involves polymerization of the monomers, whereas the second one is based on dispersion of the performed polymers. The salting-out (7), emulsification-diffusion (8), and nanoprecipitation (9) can be cited as typical examples of the second method. NP is a collective term used to describe the nanospheres and nanocapsules (NCs). The difference between these forms lies in the morphology and the architecture. NCs are composed of a liquid core (generally an oil) surrounded by polymeric membrane, whereas nanospheres are formed by a dense polymeric matrix (10). NCs are pharmaceutically attractive due to their oil-based central cavities, which allow a high encapsulation level for lipophilic substances, enabling improved drug delivery. It is possible to avoid drug precipitation during preparation and subsequent stability problems caused by the presence of the drug on the surface of the NPs. Two techniques are widely used to prepare a biodegradable NC.

Interfacial Polymerization of Alkylcyanoacrylate Monomers
In this process, the cyanoacrylate monomer and the lipophilic drug are dissolved in a mixture of oil and ethanol. This organic solution is then added slowly to water or a buffer solution (pH 3–9) containing surfactants such as poloxamers or phospholipids. NCs are formed spontaneously by anionic polymerization of the cyanoacrylate in the oily phase after contact with hydroxyl ions which act as initiators.

Interfacial Deposition of Performed Polymers
In this process, the lipophilic drug, oil polymer, and optionally phospholipids are dissolved in a water-miscible solvent (e.g., acetone). This solution is then poured while stirring into an aqueous solution containing a nonionic surfactant (e.g., poloxamer 188). NCs are instantly formed by the fast diffusion of solvent into water, which provokes the spontaneous emulsification of the oily solution in the form of nanodroplets where the dissolved polymer will form a film around the droplets that contain the drug (11).

The method of interfacial polymerization is not ideal for three reasons: (*i*) the probable presence of the residual, (*ii*) potentially toxic monomers or oligomers, and the possibility of cross-reaction with the drug, and (*iii*) the difficulty in predicting the molecular weight of the resulting polymer (12). The principal drawback of this method is the polymer aggregation that is frequently observed when working with high polymer concentration or low organic solvent/water ratio. Guerrero et al. (13) have described a new process based on an emulsification-diffusion technique, over-coming these drawbacks. This study demonstrated that the emulsification-diffusion technique represents a viable alternative for preparing biodegradable NCs starting from performed polymers. It is simple and versatile, and permits high efficiency of entrapment of lipophilic drugs (13).

It is important to note that a deeper understanding of the physicochemical phenomena involved during the NPs formation is also necessary. Specifically, the relationship between physicochemical parameters and their quantitative effects on NP features could be an invaluable tool in the controlled engineering of particles. Knowledge of these fundamental relationships would allow NPs to be designed with defined size and surface characteristics for delivery to specific cells or organs without requiring exhaustive experimental procedures. Rodriguez et al. (3) studied the influence of certain physicochemical properties of the aqueous and organic phases used during NP preparation and the effects on the characteristics of NPs produced by salting-out, emulsification-diffusion, and nanoprecipitation methods, and concluded that the mean size of the NPs could be narrowed, using different methods. For example, salting-out offered NP mean size range between 123 and 710 nm. Emulsification method gave 110 to 715 nm mean size, whereas nanoprecipi-tation gave a very narrow size range distribution of 147 to 245 nm (3).

The water–solvent interaction and diffusion motion of the solvent play an important role in explaining the variation of the NP size during NP preparation by the nanoprecipitation method. Common disadvantages of solid–lipid nanoparticles (SLNs) include: particle growing, unpredictable gelation tendency, unexpected dynamics of polymorphic transitions, and inherent low incorporation rates resulting from the crystalline structure of the solid lipids (14).

NANOPARTICULATE DRUG-DELIVERY SYSTEM APPLICATIONS

NPDDSs have been utilized for their therapeutic applications over a wide range, from cancer treatments to some over the counter (OTC) preparations. Many drugs have been used as model drugs for specific spatial and temporal applications. Table 1 enumerates various drugs which have been used in NPDDSs. In the pharmaceutical formulations, NPDDSs can be used with advantages. Table 2 shows applications of NPDDSs to address various formulations issues.

Nanoparticulate Drug-Delivery Systems for Proteins and Peptides

Large numbers of new therapeutic proteins and peptides are being discovered, thus protein drug-delivery technologies are of ever increasing importance. Traditionally, the protein is delivered parenterally via solutions that are injected subcutaneously, intramuscularly, and intravenously. Although such injections bene-fit from high bioavailability, they fail to provide sustained plasma concentrations and suffer from poor patient compliance due to the required frequency of injec-tions. NPDDSs are designed to provide the drug release over an extended period of time, thereby minimizing the need for frequent injections. These can be used for systemic or oral delivery, and the biodegradable nature of the nanoparticulate materials alleviates the need for surgical removal.

TABLE 1   Drugs Used for Nanoparticulate Drug Delivery Systems

Name of the drug	Carrier	References
Aclacinomycin	PBCA NPs	(15)
Adriamycin	PBCA NPs	(16)
Antifungal drugs	Submicronized emulsion	(17)
Atovaquone	SLN	(18)
Betamethasone	CaCo3 NPs	(19)
Bifonazole	B Cyclodextrin NPs	(20)
Brimonidine	Polyacrylic NPs	(21)
Budesonide	Polylactic acid NPs nanosuspension	(22)
Camptothecin	SLN	(23)
Cephalosporin	Nanoconjugates	(24)
Cisplatin	Polymeric micelles	(25)
Clotrimazole	B Cyclodextrin NPs	(20)
Clobetasol	SLN	(26)
Clozapine	SLN	(27)
Curdlan derivative: anticancer drugs	SLN	(28)
B-Cyclodextrin	Nanosphere	(29)
Cyclosporine	SLN	(30)
Cyclosporine	Stearic acid NPs	(31)
Cyclosporine	HPMCP	(32)
Cyclophosphamide	PBCA NCs	(33)
Diclofenac	Inorganic microparticles	(34)
	Polylactide	(35)
	Polylactide	(36)
	Caprolactone	(37)
Danazol	Lipid-based emulsion	(35,38)
Darodipine	SLN	(36,39)
Delargin	PBCA NPs	(37)
Dexamethasone	Supercritical carbon dioxide—PLGA	(38)
Diminazine	Lipid-based	(39)
Diminazenediaceturate	Lipid drug conjugate	(40)
Gadolinium	Lipid-based NPs	(41)
5-Fluouracil	Colloidal NPs	(42)
Flurbiprofen	Nanosuspension	(43)
Halofantrine	Lipid-based emulsion	(44)
Heparin	Methacrylate polymers	(45)
Hydrocortisone	SLN	(46)
Idarubicin	SLN	(47)
Indomethacin	SLN	(48)
Isoniazid	PL glycolide polymer	(49)
Ketoprofen	Polycaprolactone and Eudragit S 100	(50)
Kytorphin	PBCA NPs	(51)
Loperamide	Polysorbate 80-coated PBCA NPs	(52)
Methotrexate	Colloidal carriers	(42)
Mitoxantrone	Magnetic NPs	(53)
Nifedipine	SLN nanocrystals	(54–56)
Ontazolost	Lipid-based delivery	(57)
Paclitaxel	SLN	(58)
	Cetyl alcohol/polysorbate NPs	(59)
	Gelatin NCs	(60)
	PLGA	(61)
Phenothiazine	SLN	(54)
Pilocarpine	PLGA	(62)
Praziquantel	PLGA NC	(63)
Prednisolone	SLN	(64)

(Continued)

TABLE 1 Drugs Used for Nanoparticulate Drug Delivery Systems (*Continued*)

Name of the drug	Carrier	References
Porpofol	Lipid-free NC	(65)
Progesterone	SLN	(45)
Protamine phosphorothioate	NP complexes	(66)
Pyrazinamide	PL glycolide	(48)
Retinal	SLN	(67)
Rifabutine	SLN	(18)
Rifamycin	PL glycolide	(48)
Tamoxifen	Polycaprolactone NPs	(68)
Tarazepide	Cyclodextrin	(69)
Thiamine	Lipid	(70)
Tobramycin	SLN	(71)
Tretinoin	SLN	(72)
Triclosan	Submicron emulsion and NCs	(73)
Tubocurarine	Polysorbate 80-coated PBCA NPs	(74)
Ubidecarone	SLN	(75)
UCB-35440-3	Nanocrystals	(76)
Vincristine	Colloidal carriers	(42)
Vitamin A	SLN	(77)
Xanthone	PLGA	(78)

Abbreviations: HPMCP, hydroxypropyl methyl cellulose phthalate; NC, nanocapsules; NPs, nanoparticles; PBCA; polybutylcyno acrylate; PLGA, poly-lactic-co-glycolic acid; SLN, solid–lipid nanoparticles.

Biodegradable nanoparticulate delivery for protein must satisfy several technical requirements. Among these: the proteins should be encapsulated with a high loading efficiency, and remain stable throughout the manufacturing process and the course of their intended dosing period. NPs need to be less than 125 μm in diameter and form a free flowing powder so that they can be resuspended in an injectable vehicle and passed through a needle. The release profile of the drug needs to be

TABLE 2 Nanoparticulate Drug Delivery Systems: Formulation Applications

Addressing the drug-delivery problems
  Solving the issues related to solubility
  Overcoming the poor bioavailability of the drugs
  Issues with fed/fasted variability
  Pharmacokinetic variability
Finding solutions with nanoparticulate drugs
  Technology advances
  Reduction in particle size of the poorly water-soluble drugs
  Increased active agent surface area
Benefits for faster dissolution
  Greater bioavailability
  Smaller drug doses
  Diminished toxicity
  Decreased dosing variability
Pharmacodynamic factors: applicable to peptides and other drugs
  These can be formulated as receptor-specific
  These can be more resistant to unspecific degradation
  They can deliver the drug in encapsulated form to delay the degradation, set a depot form for
    prolonged signaling, and increase the treatment efficacy as compared to substitution of the
    natural form of peptide

reproducible and therapeutically effective and pose no pharmacological or toxicological risks due to rapid early release or burst.

Macromolecules such as proteins and DNA play an increasingly important role in our arsenal of therapeutic agents. Delivery of these molecules to their site of action at the desired rate is a challenge because their transport through compartmental barriers, for example, endothelium and epithelium in the body, is inefficient and/or they are readily metabolized. For controlled release or site-specific delivery of such macromolecules, delivery systems are required which need to be more sophisticated than our present day strategies. These systems must be custom-made, taking into account both molecular size and specific characteristics of these molecules. One has to build a platform of different delivery strategies that use input from technical, pharmaceutical, and biomedical disciplines to meet these challenges.

The development of appropriate DDSs for new macromolecules coming out of the biotech industry is a meaningful challenge to pharmaceutical scientists. Proteins, peptides, oligonucleotides, and genes are very unstable compounds that need to be protected from degradation in the biological environment. Their efficacy is highly limited by their inability to cross biological barriers and to reach the target sites. They are vulnerable to harsh conditions in the gastrointestinal tract, leading to chemical and enzymatic degradation. The future of these molecules solely depends on the delivery systems and appropriate carriers.

There are three possible pathways for protein and peptide drug absorption through the GI tract. The first is via the M-cells of Payer's patches, the second via a transcellular route involving enterocytes, and the third via paracellular avenues through tight junctions (6,79). The nanosystems are providing a viable alternative for these drugs such as liposomes, polymeric micelles, and NPDDSs. One of the crucial and pervasive troubles in human therapy is to achieve a balance between toxicity and therapeutic effect of the drugs. Therefore, the site-specific delivery could reduce such side effects at nontarget sites and increase the efficacy. Rodrigues et al. (80) have reported an interesting work on lectin nanocarrier conjugate. They used dextran/poly(e-caprolactone) polyester polymers and conjugated with three different proteins, lectins from leaves of Bauhinia monandra and Lens culinaris, and bovine serum albumin (BSA). The NPs having a size around 200 nm could be used for delivering proteins (80).

A polypeptide hormone consisting of 32 amino acids plays a crucial role in both bone remodeling and calcium homeostasis. Yoo and Park (81) formulated salmon calcitonin (sCT) into biodegradable PLGA NPs using sCT oleate complexes. The sCT oleate complexes were prepared by hydrophobic ion pairing. SCT NPs were readily taken up by Caco-2 cells and sCT was transported across the Caco-2 monolayer in vitro. In vivo experiments showed sCT was orally absorbed. Vranckx et al. (82) also reported similar results where they used an NC formulation with hydrophilic core for delivering salmon calcitonin in rats.

A study by Alphandary et al. (83) has shown the crossing of insulin through the intestinal epithelial barrier to the blood compartment where it was absorbed by portions of the M-cell-free epithelium. The insulin was incorporated in biodegradable poly (alkylcynoacrylate) NCs (83).

An excellent review discusses the strategies of enhancing the immunostimulatory effects of CpG oligonucleotides and outlines the latest development in the application of liposomes and NPDDSs for the delivery of oligonucleotides with an extensive literature survey (84). Leach et al. (85) demonstrated that excipient-free protein NPs prepared by spray-freezing into liquid technology (86) can be dispersed into PLGA and PLA microparticles and the burst effect can be prevented. The uniform encapsulation of the stable proteins at high loading was achieved with minimal burst effect. NPs based on hydrogels are being developed for the delivery of macromolecules.

An interesting mechanistic study reported by Mo and Lim (87) exhibited uptake of wheat germ agglutinin-conjugated NPs by A549 cells. In this study, they prepared the PLGA NPs by solvent diffusion method (88) and later surface modified with wheat germ agglutinin through a two-step carbodiimide method. Cellular uptake was studied using confluent A549 cells as an in vitro model of the type II alveolar epithelial cells. Uptake of the WGA-conjugated PLGA NPs was compared to that of NPs similarly modified with the bovine serum albumin (BSA) to demonstrate the specificity of the surface WGA in enhancing the cellular uptake of the NPs. The mechanism of uptake was studied by performing the uptake experiments under several inhibiting conditions. They concluded that the grafting of WGA on PLGA NPs has increased the uptake by five to eight times, hence this method can be exploited for the intracellular delivery of therapeutic and diagnostic agents (87).

Targeted delivery of proteins and DNA requires a carrier system in submicron size or nanosize. This carrier needs to be target site (cell or tissue)-specific. Often, the actual target site location is intracellular, and the delivery of the carrier payload at this intracellular target site is a prerequisite for therapeutic success. For example, plasmid DNA needs to be delivered inside the nucleus of the target cell before the cell can express the desired therapeutic protein. A very good example of this system is the immunoliposomes, where liposomes carrying the drug with monoclonal antibodies or monoclonal antibody fragments are covalently attached to the bilayer for targeting purposes. A selection of monoclonal antibodies, with induced endocytic uptake, can lead to the entrance of immunoliposomes (Fig. 2) into tumor cells (84,89).

Another application of liposome-dependent drug is diphtheria toxin A (DTA) chain. Liposome dependent means that the drug as such cannot reach its target site of action inside the cell without a carrier, as it cannot pass the cytoplasmic membrane

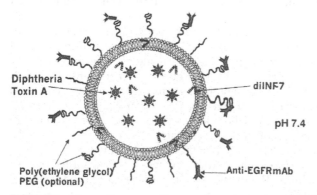

FIGURE 2 Immunoliposomes: the use of nanotechnology to build a carrier system for site-specific delivery of a protein. The anti-EGFR antibody permits endocytosis helping the immunoliposomes to enter the target cells after cell binding. The peptide di INF-7 induces the release of liposome-entrapped diphtheria toxin A chain from immunoliposomes. *Abbreviation*: EGFR, epidermal growth factor receptor. *Source*: From Ref. 89.

without help (a carrier). Such a drug will show neither the desired nor the unde-sired pharmacological effects. Diphtheria toxin, a protein consisting of an A chain coupled with a B chain, can readily enter cells through the transporter B chain. Upon entering the cell, the A chain causes the cell kill with exceptional efficiency by blocking ribosomal activity. Thus DTA (lacking B chain) alone needs a cell-specific transport system, that is, a system that transports it into the desired target cells, for example, tumor cells (90).

The design of a custom-made carrier at the nanometer level is a targeted delivery system for plasmid DNA to efficiently transfer only to target cells. The cat-ionic polymer pDMAEMA (poly-(2)-(dimethylamino)ethyl methacrylate) condenses plasmid DNA effectively into 100 nm NPs (polyplexes). In vitro transfection is very efficient but in vivo was ineffective. Polyplexes were subsequently coated with lipids yielding lipopolyplexes, which demonstrated target cell-specific binding characteris-tics, and were able to transfect the cells with hardly any cell toxicity (91).

Ocular Applications of Nanoparticulate Drug-Delivery System
Topical ophthalmic drugs have generally poor absorption in the eye due to the cor-nea's low permeability to drugs and noncorneal factors such as rapid tear turnover, nasolacrimal drainage, and systemic absorption. One of the major problems in ocular delivery is providing and maintaining an adequate concentration of the ther-apeutic agent in the precorneal area. Topical drop administration of ophthalmic drugs in aqueous solutions results in extensive drug loss due to tear fluid and eyelid dynamics (21,92,93). Most noninvasive approaches for enhancing ocular drug absorption involve the use of prodrugs, the use of viscosity agents designed to pro-long the drug residence time, and colloidal systems (94,95). Polymeric NPs are attractive colloidal systems because they demonstrate increased stability and have a longer elimination half-life in tear fluid (up to 20 min), than do conventional drugs applied topically to the eye, which have half-lives of just one to three minutes.

NPDDSs have been evaluated for ocular applications to enhance absorption of thera-peutic drugs, improve bioavailability, reduce systemic side effects, and sustain intraocular drug levels (96). NPDDSs have shown potential in the treatment of external eye diseases (97). PLGA has been evaluated and proved to be a very useful biodegradable polymer for NPDDS formulation due to its medical use, biocompatibility, and safety (98). Qaddoumi et al. (95) have studied the characteris-tics and mechanism of uptake of PLGA-based NPDDSs for ophthalmic application. They suggested that PLGA-based NPDDSs could be used for the enhancement of drug absorption in the eye and the controlled release of proteins and drugs. Some reports in ocular applications are very novel approaches involving periocular routes for retinal drug delivery of Celecoxib and Aldose reductose inhibitors (99–101). Salgueiro et al. (33) demonstrated ophthalmic application of cyclophosphamide-loaded polybutylcyanoacrylate (PBCA) nanosphere as an immunosuppressive agent. The morphometrical properties such as average particle size and polydisparity index of these DDSs are adequate for ophthalmic application without induced corneal or conjunctival irritation (33).

Nanoparticulate Drug-Delivery Systems for Pulmonary Treatment
Pulmonary drug delivery for both systemic and local treatments has many adv-antages over other delivery routes because the lungs have a large surface area (43–102 m²), thin absorption barrier, and low enzymatic activity. In addition, the

alveoli of the lungs have a slower mucociliary clearance than the airways, and the lung epithelia are thinner and more permeable. There is a potential for possible systemic absorption of the peptides and proteins through the alveolar region of the lungs. Several studies have exhibited the absorption of high-molecular-weight drugs such as insulin, heparin, and GCSF (recombinant human granulocyte colony-stimulating factor) through pulmonary DDSs (102–104,104a). As these peptides have a short life, the development of delivery systems with sustained pharmacological action would be very useful.

Innovative, noninvasive, inhalable DDSs for peptides are being explored for lung disease therapy with the vasoactive intestinal peptide (VIP) being used in the treatment of severe lung diseases. Owing to its known antiinflammatory and vasodilative properties, it has been demonstrated to possess a high therapeutic potential for other lung diseases, which are common in industrialized countries. VIP unfortunately reveals a variety of bifunctions mediated by at least two different receptors on the cell surface. The ways thought to deal with this situation are to develop a receptor-specific system to make it more specific in function. These need to be protected by licensing, and allow for superior treatment compared to natural VIP. It can be achieved by designing, engineering, and production of analog peptides, which will be very useful. By modifying the peptide, VIP in the amino acid sequence become more receptor-selective and more resistant to unspecific degradation. It can deliver the new peptides in nanoencapsulated form (NPDDS) to delay the degradation, and to set in depot form for prolonged signaling, increasing the treatment efficacy as compared to substitution of the natural form of the peptide.

An enormous diversity of therapeutic agents is currently administered to the patients via aerosol inhalation, and the number of potential drug candidates for pulmonary application increase daily. The major areas of research and therapeutic applications are asthma (105), cystic fibrosis (106), lung cancer (107), tuberculosis (108–109), pulmonary hypertension (110), and diabetes (111). Nanostructured drug delivery and targeting systems are tools to overcome the limitations of lung delivery by stabilizing and protecting the release in the bronchi and make lung therapy through inhalation possible and effective. Some of the polymers such as PLGA, protamine, thiomer, and lipid-based particles can be loaded by VIP or new designed analogs. The parameters, which need to be tested, will be improved by in vitro enzymatic stability, in vitro long-term drug release, and retarding properties and bioavailability of the carrier.

Insulin-loaded PBCA NPs were studied by Zhang et al. (112); they demonstrated that the pulmonary administration of these NPs could significantly prolong the hypoglycemic effect of insulin. It was reported that the bioavailability of insulin NPs was relatively higher than that of solution when administered by pulmonary route to normal rats, but when NPs were administered subcutaneously the bioavailability was comparatively lower compared to solution administered the same way (112). Another study using PLGA NPs to deliver insulin by nebulization also showed the usefulness of NPDDSs for insulin (113). An interesting study was reported by Liu et al. (114,115) incorporating estradiol and colloidal gold NPs in PLGA NPs to be used as a model for the pulmonary DDSs. They proposed that large porous NPs can be used as delivery systems for the pulmonary tract.

Several issues complicating the development of aerosol formulation include: compound loss during inhalation, dosing difficulties, enzymatic degradation within the lungs, and the high cost of production. Nanoparticulate-controlled release DDS has the potential to overcome many of these problems. Such formulation may be incorporated in aerosol form, remaining stable against forces of degradation during aerosolization. It can target a specific site or cell population in the lung, protect the drug-aggressive elements in the pulmonary tract, and release the compound in a predetermined manner concurrently. It can be inert to the surrounding tissues and contains no irritant or toxic additives and degrades when applicable within an acceptable period of time, producing no toxic byproducts (116). Polymeric nanoparticulate systems show promise in fulfilling the stringent requirements of the pulmonary DDSs.

An interesting study is reported by Dailey et al. (116) using short-chain PLGA grafted onto an amine-substituted poly(vinyl alcohol) backbone (3-diethyl amino-1-propylamine (8%)–poly(vinyl alcohol)-grafted poly(lactide-co-glycolide) (DEAPA–PVAL-g-PLGA) polymer. This polymer has amphiphilic properties and is highly suited for the pulmonary delivery system. It was also reported that by adding varying amounts of polyanion such as carboxymethyl cellulose, dextran sulfate, or even DNA to the polymer ring during NPs formation, NPs of variable physicochemical properties could be generated enable. This can high loading of various drugs along with greater stability. However, these polymer derivatives were found to degrade from 24 hours to within a week. Some related studies have described these aspects in detail (117,114).

NPs may be very effective DDSs for various pulmonary therapeutic schemes. The study by Dailey et al. (118) investigated the effect of nebulization technology and NP characteristics on the features of aerosol generation. They concluded that biodegradable NPs contained in the suspensions did not affect the aerosol droplet size in a clinically relevant manner; however, both NP characteristics and the technique of aerosolization influence NP aggregation occurring during the aerosolization (118). Vila et al. (119) have shown that polyethylene glycol (PEG) coating of the PLA NPs increased the absorption of drug in nasal mucosa. Pandey et al. (49) demonstrated the application of NPDDSs for the treatment of experimental tuberculosis using poly(D,L-lactide-co-glycolide) as a polymer. They used an inhalable system using the NPs and three anti-TB drugs Rifampicin, Isoniazid, and Pyrazinamide (49).

Nanoparticulate Drug-Delivery Systems for Central Nervous System

The entry of a drug molecule into the brain is limited by one of the most challenging barriers, the blood–brain barrier (BBB). The BBB consists of a continuous layer of endothelial cells joined together by tight junctions (Zonulae occludens), which severely restrict paracellular transport across the barrier. The BBB allows passive diffusion of small lipid-soluble molecules, whereas hydrophilic substances or molecules with high molecular weight have minimal passive permeation. The mechanism of permeability regulation includes macrovascular endothelial tight junctions, enzymatic regulation, and active brain efflux. Transport across BBB is additionally regulated by a number of transporters including very effective efflux transporters such as multidrug resistance-associated protein or p-glycoprotein. Several strategies have been tried to cross the BBB; one alternative strategy is to use drug-carrier systems such as liposomes, antibodies, and NPs (120). Numerous studies have shown the applications of NPs for brain targeting (51,52,121,122). Hexapeptide Dalargin, a Leu encephalin analogue with no BBB permeability adsorbed to the surface of PBCA NPs, caused central analgesia after IV administration (123). Other drugs Tubocurarine (72), Doxorubicin (124), Kytorphin (51), and Loperamide (52) were also used as model drugs for these purposes. Brain uptake of NPs in these studies was suggested based on the fact that the drugs adsorbed to PBCA NPs caused a resultant pharmacologic effect in the CNS (51,72,123). Brain

distribution of drugs delivered on the surface of NPs was also confirmed by quantification of the drug in the brain tissue itself (124). Studies have also shown the intact
presence of NPs in brain cells in vivo (125). Koziara et al. (120) tried to quantify the
presence of the NPs in brain in situ and studied the impact on BBB parameters (126).
Another study from the same laboratories showed the effectiveness of using microemulsions as precursors to engineer NPs. The advantages with the microemulsions
were simplistic production of the NPs approximately 100 nm in diameter, possible
incorporation of hydrophobic drugs in oil droplets, and inclusion of site-specific
ligands. They also reported the kinetic modeling of brain uptake, and their data
suggested the probable mechanism of brain entry (70).

Nanoparticulate Drug-Delivery Systems for Enzymes

Many scientists attempted application of nanocarriers for delivery of therapeutic
enzymes (127,128). A catalase-delivery system seems to be an ideal testing model for
evaluating the key aspects of enzyme delivery by nanocarriers. There is a fascinating study describing the loading and protection of an active enzyme catalase into a
poly-nanocarrier composed of diblock PEG–PLGA copolymers (127). It showed
nanocarriers in the size range of 200 to 500 nm protecting at least 25% of the loaded
proteases. Figure 3 demonstrates the method of formulation of PLGA–PLA NPs

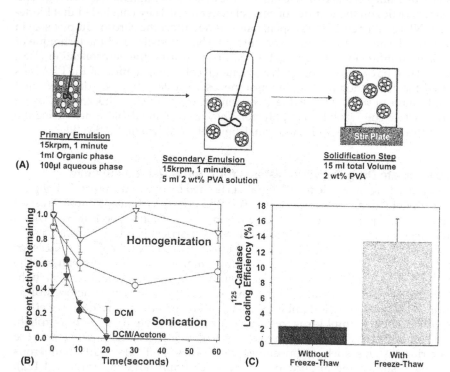

FIGURE 3 Formulation of PLGA–PEG nanoparticles: (**A**) scheme with the double emulsion synthesis procedure and (**B**) by sonication in DCM/acetone mixture. (**C**) The loading efficiency was
determined by tracing the amount of radiolabelled catalase contained inside either the micro particles
(i.e., pellet obtained after centrifuging for 15 minutes at 1000 X g) or nanoparticles fractions (2nd pellet
obtained by centrifuging for 30 minutes at 22,000 X g). Loading efficiency was greatly enhanced
(eightfold) when a freeze thaw cycle (*grey bar*) was included in the primary emulsion step. The data
in this figure is presented as M ± S.E.M. (*n* = 3). *Source*: From Ref. 127.

carrying the enzymes (127). Nanocapsulation helps to lengthen the therapeutic window by designing biodegradable polymeric nanocarriers, which protect encapsulated catalase from lysosomal proteolysis, thus prolonging the duration of the desired effects. They hypothesized that the poly-nanocarriers formation, sizing, and loading should a potential basis for a more general framework for the formulation of NPDDSs, especially for enzymes. Many enzymes using small substrates diffusing through polymer shells such as sugars, amino acids, and glutathione may be amenable to loading into protecting poly-nanocarriers. The study recommended testing of the delivery vehicles in cell culture and animal studies, as a new strategy for a prolonged protection against vascular oxidative stress (127).

Weissenbock et al. (129) showed the application of wheat germ agglutinin to enhance the absorption of PLGA NPs. The wheat germ agglutinin has cyto-adhesive and cyto-invasive properties. This process of surface engineering the PLGA NPs by wheat germ agglutinin promises high versatility of application in the search for biorecognitive ligands enhancing the cyto-adhesion, cyto-invasion, and probably transcellular transport of colloidal carriers after peroral administration (129). Gref et al. (130) and Lochner et al. (131) reported novel surface engineering of the NPDDS.

Proticles: Protamine Nanoparticles as Drug-Delivery Systems

Proticles are novel NPs composed of protamine, a peptide used in many pharmaceutical formulations with DNA, proteins such as albumin and other therapeutically active substances. Junghans et al. (132) reported the use of proticles as delivery systems for oligonucleotides. The stability of the particles and the oligonucleotides bound to the proticles was examined in fetal calf serum and cell culture medium. Proticles significantly decreased cellular growth in a cell proliferation assay using oligonucleotides against the c-myc proto-oncogene. Proticles can also be used for diagnostics. NPs can bind large amounts of substances on their surface by adsorption, and so they can be used as an absorber. Proticles with ligand-specific as amyloid-beta can bind the neurotoxic amyloid-beta protein. The neuro-protective effects of this delivery system may find a novel therapy for Alzheimer's disease. Amyloid-binding peptide depot system is aimed at developing therapy for Alzheimer's disease. Amyloid-binding peptides are substances which can disintegrate amyloid plaques. These are hidden in the interior of proticles to cross the BBB and for slow controlled release to achieve a high concentration of amyloid-binding peptides in the brain over a long period. This can be further studied using the MRI with gadolinium as a contrast substance. VIPs, which are used in the treatment of severe lung diseases, can be packaged in proticles and can be used to create a pulmonary depot for the treatment for 12 to 24 hours. Antigens are bound to the surface of proticles for efficient composition of the proticles that might further boost the immune response. Some recent reports show the application of proticles as DDSs (133–135).

Mucoadhesive Nanoparticulate Drug-Delivery Systems

Mucosal surfaces are the most common and convenient routes for delivering drugs to the body. However, macromolecular drugs such as peptides and proteins are unable to overcome the mucosal barrier and are degraded before reaching the bloodstream. NPDDSs show a promising strategy for delivering drugs through mucosa. Polysaccharide Chitosan (CS) is mucoadhesive and CS NPs, CS-coated oil nanodroplets (nanocapsules), and CS-coated lipid NPs have shown interesting possibilities for this purpose (136). CS-coated systems have exhibited an important capacity to enhance the intestinal absorption of the peptide salmon calcitonin and in vivo, a long-lasting decrease in the calcemia levels observed in rats (137).

Takeuchi et al. (138) have written a review on mucoadhesive NPDDSs for peptide drugs. They discussed the preparation and methods for evaluation of muco-adhesive nanoparticulate systems. Mucoadhesive properties were conferred on the systems by coating with mucoadhesive polymers such as CS and Carbapol. The feasibility of this surface adhesion was confirmed by measuring the zeta potential. They suggested that these delivery systems could be used for delivery of peptides by oral and pulmonary administration. Nanoprecipitation techniques using PLGA and PLA polymers were found to be useful for nanoparticulate delivery of proteins and have shown more versatility and flexibility in the formulation for protein delivery (139). Takeuchi et al. (140) described mucoadhesive PLGA nanospheres prepared by surface modification with CS for oral peptide delivery. CS-modified nanospheres were applied to improve the pulmonary delivery of peptides by nebulization. The particle average diameter of 650 nm of the aqueous dispersion of the nanospheres was an important factor to enclose the particles in the aerosolized aqueous droplets produced with the nebulizer. The elimination rate of CS-modified nanospheres from the lungs was decreased significantly due to their mucoadhesive property after pulmonary administration compared to that of the unmodified nanospheres, and as a result the pharmacological action was significantly prolonged. It is also confirmed that the CS on the surface of the nanospheres enhanced the absorption by opening the intercellular tight junctions in the lung epithelium (104).

Nanoparticulate Drug Delivery in Cancer Treatment

Several NPDDSs are reported for the application in cancer therapy, transferring con-jugated paclitaxel-loaded NPs (141), nanovaccines (142), adriamycin-loaded NPs for hepatoma treatment (143), magnetic PBCA nanospheres with aclacinomycin A in gastric cancer (15), near-infrared absorption nanospheres (144), polypropylenimine dendrimer NPs for oligonucleotides (145), lytic-peptide-bound magnetite NPs for breast cancer treatment (146), ceramic-based NPs entrapping water-insoluble photo-sensitizing anticancer drugs (147), and poly(epsilon-caprolactone) NPs for the delivery of Tamoxifen for breast cancer treatment (148,149).

Yoo and Park (150) have reported a study of folate receptor targeted antican-cer therapy using Doxorubicin-PEG folate nanoconjugates. Doxorubicin and folate were, respectively, conjugated to alpha and omega terminal of the PEG chain. The conjugates assisted formation of Doxorubicin nanoaggregates with average size of 200 nm in diameter when combined with an excess amount of depronated Doxorubicin in an aqueous phase. In vivo studies have shown significant reduction in the tumor volume in a human tumor xenograft nude mouse model. Controlled release of paclitaxel through submicroemulsion with particle size of 45 to 270 nm was evaluated in vitro and in vivo for their antitumor activity by Kang et al. (151). They used PLGA polymer for formulating self-emulsifying DDSs and showed the effectiveness of the system.

Nanoparticles in the Treatment of Vascular Thrombosis

The formation of blood clots in the circulatory system is associated with a range of serious medical conditions, including heart attacks, pulmonary embolisms, strokes, and deep vein thrombosis. The main component of the clot is the insoluble protein fibrin. Treatment of vascular thrombosis involves the use of thrombolytic drugs that break up the fibrin, allowing the clot to disperse. Biocompatible NPs are used to develop such delivery systems, which can carry the thrombolytic drugs. Chellini (152) explained that the thrombolytic drugs are powerful agents, with serious side effects like causing hemorrhage if they are given systemically. However, orally they are less efficient. If they can be incorporated in NPs, they can be delivered directly to the specific site, using less drug materials, and the treatment will be cost-effective with less side effects. The drug will be released from the NPs by diffusion, degradation, or erosion. A sustained release NP formulation may be more helpful (152).

Nanoparticulate Drug-Delivery Systems for Gene Therapy

Intracellular gene delivery involves changing the expression of genes in order to prevent, cure, or treat a disorder or a disease. Therefore, this treatment method alters the expression of a gene and corrects a defective gene that may be the cause of a disease or a disorder. Nonviral vectors for gene therapy have inherent advantages of safety and flexibility over viral vectors, although they are less efficient. Serious issues of integration with the host genome to permanently alter its genetic structure, self-replication capability, recombination potential, and the possibility of complement activation (immunogenicity) of the otherwise transfection efficient viral vectors limit their use for gene delivery. In the last decade, the focus of development is on nonviral gene-delivery systems. Specific characteristics that must be included in nonviral vectors include small size and stability against aggregation in blood, serum, and extracellular fluid, the ability to be efficiently internalized by the target cells and the ability to disassemble and release the payload into the cell nucleus once internalized.

Gene therapy has attracted considerable interest for the treatment of life-threatening diseases. Several viral and nonviral vectors (transporting devices) are under investigation (153,154). One of the common disadvantages of both types is rapid clearance from the blood circulation to first-pass organs such as liver and lungs. A frequently applied strategy to circumvent this rapid elimination is to coat the outer surface of the complexes with hydrophilic uncharged polymers by which the positive charge of these lipo/polyplexes is shielded (155–157). Several polymers such as poly-L-lysine, CS (158) polyamidoamine dendrimers (159), polyethylenimine (PEI) (160), poly(4 aminobutyl-L-glycolic acid) (161), poly-L-glutamic acid (162), poly(β-amino esters) (163), poly(2(dimethylamino)ethyl methacrylate), plasmid-lipid particles have been used for this purpose with PEG coating (161,162,164). Funhoff et al. (165) have reported the use of PEG-shielded double-layered micelles for gene delivery. Zhang et al. (166) reported galactosylated ternary DNA/poly-phosphoramidate NPs as hepatocyte-targeted gene carriers. Zhao et al. (167–170) wrote an excellent review on polyphosphoesters in drug and gene delivery. A report described the application of PLGA:poloxamer and PLGA:poloxamine blend NPs as new carriers for the gene delivery: plasmid DNA (171). They developed several formulations and found that all NP formulations provided continuous and controlled release of the plasmid with minimal burst effect. In addition, the release rate and duration were dependent on the composition of the particle matrix. Zahr et al. (72) have created a layer-by-layer stepwise self-assembly of the polyelectrolytes poly(allylamine hydrochloride). Poly(styrenesulfonate) was used to create a macromolecular nanoshell around drug NPs (approximately 150 nm in diameter). Dexamethasone was chosen as a model drug. The polymeric nanoshell on the surface of the drug NPs provides a template upon which surface modifications can be made to create stealth or targeted DDSs (172).

Kaul et al. (173) in their study used PEG-modified gelatin NPs as long-circulating intracellular delivery systems with a mean particle size of 300 nm. They could efficiently encapsulate hydrophilic macromolecules including plasmid DNA. These particles were internalized by tumor cells and were found near the nucleus after 12 hours. The PEGylated gelatin NPs were also very efficient in expressing GEP. Drug loading and drug-release rates from NPs are important parameters for the formulation of NPDDSs to optimize the therapeutic efficacy of the encapsulated drug (174–178). Panyam et al. (178) showed that solid-state solubility of the drug in polymer could be an important determinant that could influence the drug loading in NPs as well as release characteristics of the encapsulated drug. In a recent study by Kaul et al., plasmid DNA was formulated with gelatin and PEGylated gelatin with average diameter of 200 nm for targeted systemic delivery to solid tumors. The results showed 61% transfection efficiency, which was attributed to a biocompatible, biodegradable long-circulating carrier system (179).

Dendrimers are emerging as a new generation of nonviral vectors for gene delivery because of two distinctive features: their structures can be controlled and their chemistry can be adapted for various requirements such as drug or gene delivery (180,181). They also belong to the polyamine group of nonviral vectors, which includes poly-L-lysine, polyethylenimine, and polyamidoamine. The versatility of these vectors has been exploited to attach various ligands such as transferrin, sugars, and antibodies for receptor-targeting dendrimers. A new family of composite dendrimers with lipidic amino acids was synthesized by Bayle et al. and used for transporting DNA both single- and double-stranded as well as RNA (182). Polyamidoamine dendrimer (PAMAM) represents one of the most efficient polymeric gene carriers. Zhang et al. (183) have shown their utility for gene delivery.

Xia et al. (177) report a novel DDS recently by preparing monodispersed NPs consisting of interpenetrating polymer networks (IPNs) of polyacrylic acid (PAAc) and isopropylacrylamide by a seed and feed method. The aqueous dispersion of IPN NPs was found to be a unique NPDDS due to its abrupt inverse thermoreversible gelation at around 33°C. The IPN and drugs were thoroughly mixed as an aqueous solution at room temperature and formed a drug-delivery gel at body temperature. The drug-delivery model was found very useful because such a dispersion and drug was mixed without chemical reaction and the liquid can be injected into a body to form in situ a gelled drug depot to release the drug slowly (177).

Benita et al. (184) described the application of PLGA–PEI NPs for gene delivery to pulmonary epithelium. Diwan et al. (185) have shown that antigen delivery in biodegradable NPs can facilitate induction of strong T-cell response, particularly of the TH1 type, at an extremely low dose of CPG oligonucleotides. Such reduction in dose would be advantageous for minimizing the potential side effects of these novel adjuvants (185).

Rhaese et al. (186) reported NPs consisting of DNA, human serum albumin, and polyethylenimine to be a carrier for the nonviral gene delivery. They could achieve optimum transfection efficiency, and displayed a low cytotoxicity when tested in cell culture. They recommended these carriers for delivering DNA for IV administration.

An interesting strategy for the treatment of various vascular diseases uses poly (methylidene malonate 2.1.2) NPs which is a biocompatible polymer that enhances the peri-adventitial adenoviral gene delivery (187).

Gene therapy strategies have been proposed for a vast and diverse range of disorders for which currently available treatments are deemed unsatisfactory. Effective delivery of genes into cells has been considered a major hurdle in achieving successful gene therapy. A number of delivery systems based on viral (188) or nonviral vectors (189,190) have been devised; none of them have proven to be completely satisfactory. Viral vectors can only introduce genes, not other macromolecules such as siRNA or antisense nucleotide. Furthermore, side reactions such as host immune response and insertional mutagenesis leading to death, carcinogenesis, or germline alternations have led to serious concerns about the use of viruses as gene transfer vectors (191–194). Several analytical techniques were reported to be useful for the characterization and establishing the structure/function relationship of polyamido-amine/DNA dendrimers as nanoparticulate drug/gene-delivery systems. Braun et al. (195) used dynamic and electrophoretic light scattering technique for particle size, and phase analysis light scattering for zeta potential. Ethium bromide displacement assay has been utilized for determining the interaction between the dendrimer and DNA, and extent of gene uptake. Circular dichroism spectroscopy was used for characterizing helical structure of DNA within dendrimer DNA complexes. Fourier transform infrared spectroscopy was used as a complimentary technique to further investigate the secondary structure of DNA component complexes. Isothermal titration calorimetry was employed to investigate the thermodynamics of binding of dendrimers and DNA complexes. Differential scanning calorimetry was applied to evaluate the thermal stability of DNA/dendrimer complexes (195). Zaitsev et al. (96) used a strategy based on the formation of polyelectrolyte NPs and later deposition of negatively charged polyelectrolytes onto a DNA core. They showed that these negatively charged particles exhibited colloidal stability and high transfection efficiency in an in vivo model (196).

The mechanistic pathways for gene expression are limited by at least five major barriers: in vivo stability, cell entry, endosome escape, cytosolic transport, and nuclear entry. The nuclear membrane restricts the transport of the plasmid DNA and the efficiency of the DNA transfer from the cytoplasm to the nucleus has been estimated to be about 10^{-4}. In order to obtain the high gene expression, the genes introduced into the cells must be reduced to a compact size which can pass through nuclear pores. The collapsing of the DNA into NPs of reduced negative or increased positive charges (i.e., DNA condensation) has received considerable interest due to its biological importance in DNA packaging in virus heads (197).

Gene delivery usually takes advantage of the endocytic pathway of the cell. The cells continually ingest a part of their plasma membrane via endocytosis to form endocytic vesicles. The cells can take up solvent and solute by the endocytosis activity later. Endocytic vesicles incorporating DNA-bearing particles are transferred to endosomes and then to lysomes, where liberation of DNA somehow takes place. However, the plasma membrane is directly linked to and functionally integrated with the underlying cytoskeleton; the endocytosis at the membrane would require the rearrangement of actin and tubulin.

Nonviral vectors hold several advantages over modified virus employed for gene delivery, in terms of improved and predictable safety profile, a high DNA-carrying capacity, increased versatility, the ease of large-scale production, and quality control. Nevertheless, their efficiency lags behind that of viral systems. Those nonviral vectors efficient in transfection are often toxic because of their nondegradable property (189). The gene transfer efficiency of nontoxic vectors, for example, biodegradable cationic polymers, is often not satisfactory (198). Li et al.

have reported the synthesis, characterization of poly(D,L-lactide-co-4-hydroxy-L-porline) polymer for the purpose of gene delivery, and they studied degradation, cytotoxicity, as well as pDNA release kinetics and sustained gene expression of this polymer-based system. They showed the usefulness of these polymers with multiple advantages (190).

Gupta and Gupta (191) have shown the application of the Pullulan, a water-soluble, neutral linear polysaccharide for gene delivery. They showed that these NPs had high transfection potential, could release DNA efficiently, and were stable against degradation by DNAse. As specific ligands can be bound to the NP surface, these particles offer the possibility for additional targeting strategies.

Kabanov et al. (199) suggested an interesting approach using polymer genomics in their recent publication. Pluronic, the A-B-A amphiphilic block copolymers of poly(ethylene oxide), can upregulate the expression of selected genes in cells and alter the genetic response to antineoplastic agents in cancer. They reported that these block copolymers alone as well as in combination with polyethylenimine can upregulate the expression of the reporter genes in stably transfected cells. This underscores the ability of selected synthetic polymers to enhance transgene expression through a mechanism that augments improved DNA delivery into cell. Pluronic is genetically benign when combined with an antineoplastic agent Doxorubicin. It drastically alters pharmacogenomic responses to this agent and prevents the development of multi-drug resistance in breast cancer cells. They proposed the need for a thorough assessment of pharmacogenomic effects of polymer therapeutics to maximize the clinical outcomes and understand the pharmacological and toxicological effects of polymer-based drugs and delivery systems (199).

Tabatt et al. (200) compared the cationic SLN and liposomes for gene transfer as a carrier. They found that DNA binding differed only marginally in these two systems. They concluded that cationic lipid composition seems to be more dominant for the in vitro transfection performance than the kind of arranged colloidal structure. Hence, cationic SLN extends the range of highly potent nonviral transfection agents by one with favorable and distinct technological properties (200). Wissing et al. (201) published a review which describes the use of NPs based on solid lipid for the parenteral application of drugs. Different types of NPs based on solid lipids such as SLNs, nanostructured lipid carriers, and lipid drug nanoconjugates are introduced and structural differences are pointed out. Different production methods including the suitability for large-scale production are described along with the stability issues, and drug-incorporation mechanisms into the particles are discussed in detail. The biological activity of parenterally applied SLNs and biopharmaceutical aspects such as pharmacokinetic profiles as well as toxicity aspects are reviewed (201).

NANOPARTICULATE SYSTEMS: KNOWN AND UNKNOWN RISKS

An excellent review was recently published by Hoet et al. (202) with an extensive literature survey in which they suggested that the particles in the nanosize range could certainly enter into the human body through lungs, gastrointestinal system, mucosa, and the skin. It is possible that some particles penetrate deep in the dermis and gradually may be taken up by the body. The chances of penetration depend on the size and surface properties of the particles and also point of contact. The distribution of particles in the body systems is also a function of the surface characteristics of the NPs. There might be a critical size involved beyond which the movement of the particles might be restricted. The pharmacokinetic behavior of different types of the nanosystems requires a detailed investigation and a database of health risks associated with different NPs needs to be created. The increased risk of cardiopulmonary disease requires specific measures to be taken for every newly developed nanoparticulate product. There is no universal NP to fit all the cases; each NP system needs to be treated individually when a health risk is expected. The tests currently used to verify safety of materials should be applicable to identify hazardous NPs, and more stringent and efficient testing procedures are needed to evaluate the nanoparticulate systems, especially when used as a food component or as DDSs (119,203–206). A study reported by Bilati et al. (207) discussed the processing and formulation issues related to PLGA protein-loaded NPs prepared by double-emulsion method. They evaluated the effect of some typical formulation factors and processing conditions on the mean size and the drug entrapment efficiency of PLGA NPs. They found that the parameters that generally increase the entrapment efficiency are (*i*) high molecular weight of the polymer, (*ii*) the presence of uncapped carboxylic end groups when PLGA is used, (*iii*) the use of methylene chloride instead of ethyl acetate, and (*iv*) an increased nominal drug loading. An interesting study regarding the GI uptake and transport of SLN to the lymphatic system was reported by Bargoni et al. (208). They showed that particle size is a critical determinant of the fate of NPs administered orally; larger particles may be retained for longer time in Peyer's patches, whereas smaller particles are transported to the thoracic duct. Another study by Passirani et al. (209) reported that NPs bearing heparin or dextran covalently bound to polymethylmethacrylate was found to be in the circulation for a long time. The potent capacity for opsonization of the polymethylmethacrylate core was hidden by the protective effect of either polysaccharide. In the case of heparin NPs, the stealth effect was probably increased by its inhibiting properties against complement activation. Silveira et al. (210) reported a new type of NPs where they used polyisobutylcyanoacrylate and cyclodextrin combination as polymeric carrier. Owing to the presence of many lipophilic sites belonging to the cyclodextrins which were firmly anchored to the structure of the NPs, these types of carriers were very useful to enhance and increase the loading of the lipophilic drugs with probable less side effects. But, the risks involved need to be verified and established by appropriate sensitive methods to ensure the safety of the NPDDS.

REFERENCES

1. Gennaro AR, ed. Remington's: The science and practice of pharmacy. 20th ed. USA: Lippincott Williams and Wilkins, 2000:903.
2. Willis RC. Good things in small packages. Modern Drug Discov 2004; 7:1.
3. Rodriguez SG, Allemann E, Fessi H, Doelker E. Physicochemical parameters associated with nanoparticles formation in the salting out, emulsification–diffusion and nanoprecipitation methods. Pharm Res 2004; 21:1428.
4. Couvreur P, Barratt G, Fattal E, Legrand P, Vauthier C. nanocapsule technology: a review. Crit Rev Ther Drug Carrier Syst 2002; 19:99.
5. Hans ML, Lowman AM. Biodegradable nanoparticles for drug delivery and targeting. Curr Opin Solid State Mater Sci 2002; 6:319.
6. Florence AT. The oral absorption of micro and nano particulates: neither exceptional nor unusual. Pharm Res 1997; 14:259.
7. Bindschaedler C, Gurny R, Doelker E. Process for preparing a powder of water insoluble polymer which can be redispersed in a liquid phase, the resulting powder and utilization thereof. Patent WO 88/08011, 1988.
8. Leroux JC, Allemann E, Doelker E, Gurny R. New approach for the preparation of nanoparticles by an emulsification–diffusion method. Eur J Pharm Biopharm 1995; 41:14.

9. Fessi H, Puisieux F, Devissaguet JP, Ammoury N, Benita S. Nanocapsule formation by interfacial polymer deposition following solvent displacement. Int J Pharm 1989; 55:R1.

10. Puglisi G, Fresta M, Giammona G, Ventura CA. Influence of the preparation conditions on polyethyl cyanoacrylate nanocapsule formation. Int J Pharm 1995; 125:283.

11. Kreuter J. Nanoparticles. In: Kreuter J, ed. Colloidal Drug Delivery Systems. New York: Marcel Dekker, 1994:219.

12. Guterres SS, Fessi H, Barratt G, Devissaguet JP, Puisieux F. Poly(D,L-lactide) nanocapsules containing diclofenac. I. Formulation and stability studies. Int J Pharm 1995; 113:57.

13. Guerrero DQ, Allmann E, Doelker E, Fessi H. Preparation and characterization of nanocapsules from performed polymers by a new process based on emulsification-diffusion technique. Pharm Res 1998; 15:1056.

14. Mehnert W, Mader K. Solid–lipid nanoparticles: production, characterization and applications. Adv Drug Deliv Rev 2001; 40:165.

15. Gao H, Wang JY, Shen XZ, Deng YH, Zhang W. Preparation of magnetic polybutylcyanoacrylate nanospheres encapsulated with aclacinomycin A and its effect on gastric tumor. World J Gastroenterol 2004; 10:2010.

16. Chen JH, Ling R, Yao Q, et al. Enhanced antitumor efficacy on hepatoma bearing rats with adriamycin loaded nanoparticles administered into hepatic artery. World J Gastroenterol 2004; 10:1989.

17. Piemi MPY, Korner D, Benita S, Marty JP. Positively and negatively charged submicron emulsions for enhanced topical delivery of antifungal drugs. J Control Release 1999; 58:177.

18. Dalencon F, Amjaud Y, Lafforgue C, Derouin F, Fessi H. Atovaquone and Rifabutine loaded nanocapsules: formulation studies. Int J Pharm 1998; 153:127.

19. Ueno Y, Futagawa H, Takagi Y, Ueno A, Mizushima Y. Drug incorporating calcium carbonate nanoparticles for a new delivery system. J Control Release 2005; 103:93.

20. Memisoglu E, Bochot A, Ozalp M, Sen M, Duchene D, Hincal AA. Direct formation of nanospheres from amphiphilic beta cyclodextrin inclusion complexes. Pharm Res 2003; 20:117.

21. De TK, Rodman DJ, Holm BA, Prasad PN, Bergey EJ. Brimonidine formulation in polyacrylic acid nanoparticles for ophthalmic delivery. J Microencapsul 2003; 20:361.

22. Jacobs C, Muller RH. Production and characterization of a Budesonide nanosuspension for pulmonary administration. Pharm Res 2002; 19:189.

23. Yang S, Zhu J, Lu Y, Liang B, Yang C. Body distribution of camptothecin solid–lipid nanoparticles after oral administration. Pharm Res 1999; 16:751.

24. Cortez RV, Backmann N, Senter PD, et al. Efficient cancer therapy with a nanobody based conjugate. Cancer Res 2004; 15:2853.

25. Cabral H, Nishiyama N, Okazaki S, Koyama H, Kataoka K. Preparation and biological properties of dichloro(1,2-diaminocyclohexane) platinum (II) (DACHPt) loaded polymeric micelles. J Control Release 2005; 101:223.

26. Hu FQ, Yuan H, Zhang HH, fang M. Preparation of solid–lipid nanoparticles with Clobetasol propionate by a novel solvent diffusion method in aqueous system and physicochemical characterization. Int J Pharm 2002; 239:121.

27. Venkateswarlu V, Manjunath K. Preparation, characterization and in vitro release kinetics of Clozapine solid–lipid nanoparticles. J Control Release 2004; 95:627.

28. Kun N, Keun-Hong P, Sung WK, You HB. Self assembled hydrogel nanoparticles from curdlan derivatives: characterization, anticancer drug release and interaction with a hepatoma cell line (Hep G2). J Control Release 2000; 69:225.

29. Geze A, Putaux JL, Choisnard L, Jehan P, Wouessidjewe D. Long term shelf stability of amphiphilic B-cyclodextrin nanospheres suspensions monitored by dynamic light scattering and cryo-transmission electron microscopy. J Microencapsul 2004; 21:607.

30. Olbrich C, Kayser O, Muller RH. Lipase degradation of Dynasan 114 and 116 solid–lipid nanoparticles—effect of surfactants, storage time and crystallinity. Int J Pharm 2002; 237:119.

31. Zhang Q, Yie G, Li Y, Yang Q, Nagai T. Studies on the cyclosporine A-loaded stearic acid nanoparticles. Int J Pharm 2000; 200:153.

32. Wang X, Dai J, Chen Z, et al. Bioavailability and pharmacokinetics of cyclosporine A-loaded pH sensitive nanoparticles for oral administration. J Control Release 2004; 97:421.
33. Salgueiro A, Egea MA, Espina M, Valls O, Garcia ML. Stability and ocular tolerance of cyclophosphamide loaded nanospheres. J Microencapsul 2004; 21:213.
34. Beck RCR, Pohlman AR, Guterres SS. Nanoparticles-coated microparticles: preparation and characterization. J Microencapsul 2004; 21:499.
35. Porter CJH, Kaukonen AM, Boyd BJ, Edwards GA, Charman WN. Susceptibility to lipase mediated digestion reduces the oral bioavailability of Danazol after administration as a medium chain lipid based microemulsion formulation. Pharm Res 2004; 21:1405.
36. Hubert B, Atkinson J, Guerret M, Hoffman M, Devissaguet JP, Maincent P. The preparation and acute antihypertensive effects of a nanoparticle form of Darodipine, a dihydropyridine calcium entry blocker. Pharm Res 1991; 8:734.
37. Schroeder U, Sommerfield P, Sabel BA. Efficacy of oral Delargin loaded nanoparticles delivery across blood–brain barrier. Peptides 1998; 19:777.
38. Thote AJ, Gupta RB. Formation of nanoparticles of a hydrophilic drug using supercritical carbon dioxide and microencapsulation for sustained release, nanomedicine: nanotechnology. Biol Med 2005; 1:85.
39. Olbrich C, Gessner A, Schroder W, Kayser O, Muller RH. Lipid–drug conjugate nanoparticles of the hydrophilic drug diminazene-cytotoxicity testing and mouse serum absorption. J Control Release 2004; 96:425.
40. Olbrich C, Gessner A, Kayser O, Muller RH. Lipid drug conjugate nanoparticles as novel carrier system for the hydrophilic antitrypanosomal drug diminazenediaceturate. J Drug Targeting 2002; 10:387.
41. Oyewumi MO, Yokel RA, Jay M, Coakley T, Mumper RJ. Comparison of cell uptake, bio-distribution and tumor retention of folate coated and PEG coated Gadolinium nanoparticles in tumor bearing mice. J Control Release 2004; 95:613.
42. Moutardier V, Tosini F, Vlieghe P, Cara L, Delpero JR, Clerc T. Colloidal anticancer drugs bioavailability in oral administration. Int J Pharm 2003; 260:23.
43. Castelli F, Messina C, Sarpietro MG, Pignatello R, Puglisi G. Flurbiprofen release from Eudragit RS and RL aqueous nanosuspensions: a kinetic study by DSC and dialysis experiments. AAPS Pharm Sci Tech 2002; 3:9.
44. Khoo SM, Humberstone AJ, Porter CJH, Edwards GA, Chapman WN. Formulation design and bioavailability assessment of lipidic self emulsifying formulations of Halofantrine. Int J Pharm 1998; 87:164.
45. Dufresne MH, Leroux JC. Study of the micellization behavior of different order amino block copolymers with heparin. Pharm Res 2004; 21:160.
46. Cavalli R, Peira E, Caputo O, Gasco MR. Solid–lipid nanoparticles as carriers of hydrocortisone and progesterone complexes with beta cyclodextrins. Int J Pharm 1999; 182:59.
47. Zara GP, Bargoni A, Cavelli R, Fundaro A, Vighetto D, Gasco MR. Pharmacokinetics and tissue distribution of Idarubicin loaded solid–lipid nanoparticles after duodenal administration to rats. J Pharm Sci 2002; 91:1324.
48. Calvo P, Alonso MJ, VilaJato JL, Robinson JR. Improved ocular bioavailability of Indomethacin by novel ocular drug carriers. J Pharm Pharmacol 1996; 48:1147.
49. Pandey R, Sharma A, Zahoor A, Sharma S, Khuller GK, Prasad B. Poly(D,L-lactide-co-glycolide) nanoparticles based inhalable sustained drug delivery system for experimental tuberculosis. J Antimicrob Chemother 2003; 10:1093.
50. Palmiri GF, Bonacucina G, Martino DP, Martelli S. Gastroresistant microspheres containing Ketoprofen. J Microencapsul 2002; 19:111.
51. Schroder U, Sommerfield P, Urlich S, Sable B. Nanoparticle technology for delivery of drugs across the blood–brain barrier. J Pharm Sci 1998; 78:1305.
52. Alyautidin RN, Petrov VE, Langer K, Berthold A, Kharkievich DA, Kreuter J. Delivery of Loperamide across the blood–brain barrier with polysorbate 80 coated nanoparticles. Pharm Res 1997; 14:325.
53. Alexiou C, Jurgons R, Schmid RJ, et al. Magnetic drug targeting biodistribution of the magnetic carrier and the chemotherapeutic agent Mitoxantrone after loco-regional cancer treatment. J Drug Target 2003; 11:139.

54. Cavalli R, Caputo O, Carlotti ME, Trotta M, Scarnecchia C, Gasco MR. Study by X ray diffraction and differential scanning calorimetry of two model drugs, Phenothiazine and Nifedipine, incorporated into lipid nanoparticles. Eur J Pharm Biopharm 1995; 41:329.
55. Hecq J, Deleers M, Fanara D, Vranckx H, Amighi K. Preparation and characterization of nanocrystals for solubility and dissolution rate enhancement of nifedipine. Int J Pharm 2005; 299:167.
56. Hecq J, Nollevaux G, Deleers M, et al. In vitro transport studies of nifedipine nanoparticles across caco-2 HT 29-5M21 culture and cocultures. Eur J Pharm Biopharm. In press.
57. Hauss DJ, Fogal SE, Ficorilli JV, et al. Lipid based delivery systems for improving the bioavailability and lymphatic transport of a poorly water soluble LTB4 inhibitor. J Pharm Sci 1998; 87:164.
58. Chen DB, Yang TZ, Lu WL, Zhang Q. In vitro and in vivo study of two types of long circulating solid–lipid nanoparticles containing Paclitaxel. Chem Pharm Bull 2001; 49:1444.
59. Koziara JM, Lockman PR, Allen DD, Mumper RJ. Paclitaxel nanoparticles for the potential treatment of brain tumors. J Control release 2004; 99:259.
60. Yeh TK, Lu Z, Woentjes MG, Au JLS. Formulating Paclitaxel in nanoparticles alters its disposition. Pharm Res 2005; 22:867.
61. De S, Miller DW, Robinson DH. Effect of particle size of nanospheres and microspheres on the cellular association and cytotoxicity of Paclitaxel in 4T1 cells. Pharm Res 2005; 22:766.
62. Yoncheva K, Vandervoort J, Ludwig A. Influence of process parameters of high pressure emulsification method on the properties of Pilocarpine loaded nanoparticles. J Microencapsul 2003; 20:449.
63. Mainerdes RM, Evangelista RC. Praziquantel loaded PLGA nanoparticles: preparation and characterization. J Microencapsul 2005; 22:13.
64. Muhlen AZ, Mehenert W. Drug release and release mechanisms of prednisolone loaded solid–lipid nanoparticles. Pharmazie 1998; 53:552.
65. Chen H, Zhang Z, Almarsson O, Marier JF, Berkovitz D, Gardner CR. A novel lipid free nanodispersion formulation of Propofol and its characterization. Pharm Res 2005; 22:356.
66. Lochmann D, Vogel V, Weyermann J, et al. Physicochemical characterization of protamine-phosphorothioate nanoparticles. J Microencapsul 2004; 21:625.
67. Muller RH, Dobrucki R, Radomska A. Solid–lipid nanoparticles as a new formulation for Retinal. Acta Pol Pharm Drug Res 1999; 56:117.
68. Shenoy DB, Amiji MM. Poly(ethylene oxide)-modified poly(varepsilon-caprolactone) nanoparticles for targeted delivery of Tamoxifen in breast cancer. Int J Pharm 2005; 293:261.
69. Jacobs C, Kayser O, Muller RH. Nanosuspensions as a new approach for the formulation for the poorly soluble drug Tarazepide. Int J Pharm 2000; 196:161.
70. Lockman PR, Oyewumi MO, Kozira JM, Roder KE, Mumper RJ, Allen DD. Brain uptake of thiamine coated nanoparticles. J Control Release 2003; 93:271.
71. Bargoni A, Cavalli R, Zara GP, Fundaro A, Caputo O, Gasco MR. Transmucosal transport of Tobramycin incorporated in solid–lipid nanoparticles after duodenal administration to rats. Part II. Tissue distribution. Pharmacol Res 2001; 43:497.
72. Maria M, Chiara S, Donatella V, Giuseppe L, Anna MF. Niosomes as carriers for Trentinoin: preparation and properties. Int J Pharm 2002; 234:237.
73. Maestrell F, Mura P, Alonso MJ. Formulation and characterization of Triclosan submicron emulsions and nanocapsules. J Microencapsul 2004; 21:857.
74. Alyautidin RN, Tezikov EB, Ramage P, Kharkevich DA, Begly DJ, Kreuter J. Significant entry of Tubocurarine into the brain of rats by adsorption to polysorbate 80 coated poly(butyl cyanoacrylate) nanoparticles: an in situ brain perfusion studies. J Microencapsul 1998; 15:67.
75. Bunjes H, Drechsler M, Koch MHJ, Westesen K. Incorporation of the model drug Ubidecarone in to solid–lipid particles. Pharm Res 2001; 18:287.
76. Hecq J, Deleers M, Fanara D, et al. Preparation and in vitro/in vivo evaluation of nanosized crystals for dissolution rate enhancement of UCB-35440-3, a highly dosed poorly water soluble weak base. Eur J Pharm Biopharm. 2006; 64:360.

77. Jennings V, Korting MS, Gohla S. Vitamin A loaded solid–lipid nanoparticles carrier system for topical use: drug release properties. J Control Release 2000; 66:115.

78. Teixeira M, Alonso MJ, Pinto MM, Barbosa CM. Development and characterization of PLGA nanospheres and nanocapsules containing Xanthone and 3-methoxy xanthone. Eur J Pharm Biopharm 2005; 59:491.

79. Delie F. Evaluation of nano and micro particles uptake by the gastrointestinal tract. Adv Drug Deliv Rev 1998; 34:221.

80. Rodrigues JS, Magalhaes NSS, Coelho LCBB, Couvreur P, Ponchel G, Gref R. Novel core (polyester)-shell (polysaccharide) nanoparticles: protein loading and surface modification with lectins. J Control Release 2003; 92:103.

81. Yoo HS, Park TG. Biodegradable nanoparticles containing protein–fatty acid complexes for oral delivery of salmon calcitonin. J Pharm Sci 2004; 93:488.

82. Vranckx H, Demoustier M, Deleers, M. New nanocapsule formulation with hydrophilic core: Application to the oral administration of salmon calcitonin in rats. Eur J Pharm Biopharm 1996; 42:346.

83. Alphandary HP, Aboubaker M, Jaillard D, Couvreur P, Vauthier C. Visualization of insulin loaded nanocapsules: in vitro and in vivo studies after oral administration to rats. Pharm Res 2003; 20:1071.

84. Mutwiri GK, Nichani AK, Babiuk S, Babiuk LA. Strategies for enhancing the immunostimulatory effects of CpG oligodeoxynucleotides. J Control Release 2004; 97:1.

85. Leach WT, Simpson DT, Val TN, et al. Uniform encapsulation of stable protein nanoparticles produced by spray freezing for the reduction of burst release. J Pharm Sci 2005; 94:56.

86. Yu Z, Rogers TL, Hu J, Johston KP, Williams RO. Preparation and characterization of microparticles containing peptide produced by a novel process: spray freezing into liquid. Eur J Pharm Biopharm 2002; 54:221.

87. Mo Y, Lim LY. Mechanistic study of the uptake of wheat germ agglutinin-conjugated PLGA nanoparticles by A549 cells. J Pharm Sci 2004; 93:20.

88. Murakami H, Kobayashi M, Takeuchi H, Kawashima Y. Preparation of poly(d,l-lactide-co-glycolide) nanoparticles by modified spontaneous emulsification solvent diffusion method. Int J Pharm 1999; 187:143.

89. Crommelin DJA, Storm G, Jiskoot W, Stenekes R, Mastrobattista E, Hennink WE. Nanotechnological approaches for the delivery of macromolecules. J Control Release 2003; 87:81.

90. Nassander UK, Steerenberg PA, Poppe H, et al. In vivo targeting of OV-TL3 immunoliposomes to ovarian carcinoma ascetic cells (OVCAR-3) in anthymic nude mice. Cancer Res 1992; 52:646.

91. Mastrobattista E, Kapel RHG, Eggenhuizen MH, et al. Lipid coated polyplexes for targeted gene delivery to ovarian carcinoma cells. Cancer Gene Ther 2001; 8:405.

92. De TK, Hoffman AS. A reverse microemulsion polymerization method for preparation of bioadhesive polyacrylic acid nanoparticles for mucosal drug delivery: loading and release of timolol maleate. Artif Cells Blood Subst Immobil Biotech 2001; 29:31.

93. De TK, Hoffman AS. An ophthalmic formulation of beta adrenoreceptor antagonist, levobetaxolol, using polyacrylic acid nanoparticles as carriers, loading and release studies. J Bioactive Compatible Polym 2001; 16:20.

94. Bourlais CL, Acar L, Zia H, Sado PA, Needham T, Leverge R. Ophthalmic drug delivery systems: recent advances. Prog Retin Eye Res 1998; 17:33.

95. Qaddoumi MG, Ueda H, Yang J, Davda J, Labhasetwar V, Lee VHL. The characteristics and mechanisms of uptake of PLGA nanoparticles in rabbit conjunctival epithelial cell layers. Pharm Res 2004; 21:641.

96. Zimmer A, Chetoni P, Saettone M, Zerbe H, Kreuter J. Evaluation of pilocarpine loaded albumin nanoparticles as controlled drug delivery systems for the eye. II. Coadministration with bioadhesive and viscous polymers. J Control Release 1995; 33:31.

97. Diepold R, Kreuter J, et al. Comparison of different models for the testing of pilocarpine eye drops using conventional eye drops and a novel depot nanoparticles formulation. Graefes Arch Clin Exp Ophthalmol 1989; 227:188.

98. Gilding DK, Reed AM. Biodegradable polymers for use in surgery: polyglycolic/poly lactic acid homo and copolymers. Polymers 1979; 20:1459.

99. Raghava S, Hammond M, Kompella UB. Periocular routes for retinal drug delivery. Exp Opin Drug Deliv 2004; 1:99.
100. Ayalasomayajula SP, Kompella UB. Retinal delivery of celecoxib is several-fold higher following subconjunctival administration compared to systemic administration. Pharm Res 2004; 21:1797.
101. Sunkara G, Ayalasomayajula SP, Cheruku RS, Vennerstrom JL, De Ruiter J, Kompella UB. Systemic and ocular pharmacokinetics of N-4-benzoylaminophenylsulfonylglycine (BAPSG), a novel aldose reductase inhibitor. J Pharm Pharmacol 2004; 56:351.
102. Contreras LG, Morcol T, Bell SJ, Hickey AJ. Evaluation of novel particles as pulmonary delivery systems for insulin in rats. AAPS Pharm Sci 2003; 5:E9.
103. Yamamoto A. Improvement of transmucosal absorption of biologically active peptide drugs. Yakugaku Zasshi 2001; 121:929.
104. Yamamoto H, Kuno Y, Sugimoto S, Takeuchi H, Kawashima Y. Surface modified PLGA nanospheres with chitosan improved pulmonary delivery of calcitonin by mucoadhesion and opening of the intercellular tight junctions. J Control Release 2005; 102:373.
104a. Courrier HM, Butz N, Vandamme TF. Pulmonary drug delivery systems: recent developments and prospects. Crit Rev Ther Drug Carrier Syst 2002; 19:425.
105. Pahl A, Szelenyi I. Asthma therapy in the new millennium. Inflamm Res 2002; 51:273.
106. Contreras LG, Hickey AJ. Pharmaceutical and biotechnological aerosols for cystic fibrosis in therapy. Adv Drug Deliv Rev 2002; 54:1491.
107. Sharma S, White D, Imondi AR, Placke ME, Vail DM, Kris MG. Development of inhalational agents for oncological use. J Clin Oncol 2001; 19:1839.
108. Suarez S, O'Hara P, Kazantseva M, et al. Airways delivery of rifampicin microparticles for the treatment of tuberculosis. J Antimicrob Chemother 2001; 48:431.
109. Sharma R, Saxena D, Dwivedi AK, Misra A. Inhalable microparticles containing drug combinations to target alveolar macrophages for treatment of pulmonary tuberculosis. Pharm Res 2001; 18:1405.
110. Zwissler B. Inhaled vasodilators. Anaesthesist 2002; 51:603.
111. Owens DR. New horizons-alternative routes for insulin therapy. Nat Rev Drug Discov 2002; 1:529.
112. Zhang Q, Shen Z, Nagai T. Prolonged hypoglycemic effect of insulin loaded polybutylcyanoacrylate nanoparticles after pulmonary administration to normal rats. Int J Pharm 2001; 218:75.
113. Kawashima Y, Yamamoto H, Takeguchi H, Fujioka S, Hino T. Pulmonary delivery of insulin with nebulized d,l-lactide/glycolide copolymer, nanospheres to prolong hypoglycemic effect. J Control Release 1999; 62:279.
114. Tsapis N, Bennett D, Jackson B, Weitz DA, Edwards DA. Trojan particles: large porous carriers of nanoparticles for drug delivery. Proc Natl Acad Sci USA 2002; 99:12001.
115. Liu Y, Tsapis N, Edwards DA. Investigating sustained-release nanoparticles for pulmonary drug delivery. Cambridge, MA: Harvard University Press, 2003.
116. Dailey LA, Kleemann E, Wittmar M, et al. Surfactant free biodegradable nanoparticles for aerosol therapy based on the branched polyesters, DEAPA-PVAL-g-PLGA. Pharm Res 2003; 20:2011.
117. Jung T, Kamm W, Breitenbach A, Klebe G, Kissel T. Loading of tetanus toxoid to biodegradable nanoparticles from branched poly (sulfobutyl-polyvinyl alcohol)-g-(lactide-c0-glycolide) nanoparticles by protein adsorption: a mechanistic study. Pharm Res 2002; 19:1105.
118. Dailey LA, Schmehl T, Gessler T, et al. Nebulization of biodegradable nanoparticles: impact of nebulizer technology and nanoparticles characteristics on aerosol features. J Control Release 2003; 86:131.
119. Vila A, Gill H, McCallion O, Alonso MJ. Transport of PLA–PEG particles across the nasal mucosa: effect of particle size and PEG coating density. J Control Release 2004; 98:231.
120. Koziara JM, Lockman PR, Alen DD, Mumper RJ. In situ blood–brain barrier transport of nanoparticles. Pharm Res 2003; 20:1772.
121. Lockman PR, Mumper RJ, Khan MA, Allen DD. Nanoparticle technology for drug delivery across the blood–brain barrier. Drug Dev Ind Pharm 2002; 28:1.

122. Kreuter J. Nanoparticulate systems for brain delivery of drugs. Adv Drug Deliv Rev 2001; 47:65.
123. Schroder U, Sable BA. Nanoparticles: a drug carrier system to pass the blood–brain barrier, permit central analgesic effects of i.v. dalargin injections. Brain Res 1996; 710:121.
124. Gulyaev A, Gelperina SE, Skidan IN, Antorpove AS, Kivman GY, Kreuter J. Significant transport of Doxorubicin into the brain with polysorbate 80 coated nanoparticles. Pharm Res 1999; 16:1564.
125. Kreuter J, Alyautdin RN, Kharkevich DA, Ivanov AA. Passage of peptides through the blood–brain barrier with colloidal polymer particles (nanoparticles). Brain Res 1995; 674:171.
126. Lockman PR, Koziara J, Roder KE, Allen DD. In vivo and in vitro assessment of baseline blood–brain barrier parameters in the presence of novel nanoparticles. Pharm Res 2003; 20:705.
127. Dziubla TD, Karim A, Muzykantov VR. Polymer nanocarriers protecting active enzyme cargo against proteolysis. J Control release 2005; 102:427.
128. Allen TM, Cullis PR. Drug delivery systems: entering the mainstream. Science 2004; 303:1818.
129. Weissenbock A, Wirth M, Gabor F. WGA grafted PLGA nanospheres preparation and association with Caco-2 single cells. J Control Release 2004; 99:383.
130. Gref R, Couvreur P, Barratt G, Mysiakine E. Surface engineered nanoparticles for multiple ligand binding. Biomaterials 2003; 24:4529.
131. Lochner N, Pittner F, Wirth M, Gabor F. Wheat germ agglutinin binds to the epidermal growth factor of artificial Caco-2 membranes as detected by silver nanoparticles enhanced fluorescence. Pharm Res 2003; 20:833.
132. Junghans M, Kreuter J, Zimmer A. Antisense delivery using protamine–oligonucleotide particles. Nucleic Acid Res 2000; 28:e45.
133. Vogel V, Lochmann D, Weyermann J, et al. Oilgonucleotide-protamine albumin nanoparticles, preparation, physical properties and its distribution. J Control Release 2004; 103:99.
134. Mayer G, Vogel V, Weyermann J, et al. Oligonucleotide–protamine–albumin nanoparticles: protamine sulfate causes drastic size reduction. J Control Release 2005; 106:181.
135. Weyermann J, Lochmann D, Zimmer A. Comparison of antisense oligonucleotides drug delivery systems. J Control Release 2004; 100:411.
136. Vila A, Sanchez A, Tobio M, Calvo P, Alonso MJ. Design of biodegradable particles for protein delivery. J Control Release 2002; 78:15.
137. Prego C, Garcia M, Torres D, Alonso MJ. Transmucosal macromolecular drug delivery. J Control Release 2005; 101:151.
138. Takeuchi H, Yamamoto H, Kawashima Y. Mucoadhesive nanoparticulate systems for peptide drug delivery. J Control Release 2004; 98:1.
139. Bilati U, Allemann E, Doelker E. Development of a nanoprecipitation method intended for the entrapment of hydrophilic drugs into nanoparticles. Eur J Pharm 2005; 24:67.
140. Takeuchi H, Yamamoto H, Kawashima Y. Mucoadhesive nanoparticulate systems for peptide drug delivery. Adv Drug Deliv Rev 2001; 47:39.
141. Sahoo SK, Ma W, Labhasetwar V. Efficacy of transferring conjugated paclitaxel loaded nanoparticles in a murine model of prostate cancer. Int J Cancer 2004; 112:335.
142. Fifis T, Gamvrellis A, Crimeen-irwin B, et al. Size dependent immunogenicity: therapeutic and protective properties of nano vaccines against tumors. J Immunol 2004; 173:3148.
143. Chen JH, Wang L, Ling R, et al. Body distribution of nanoparticles containing adriamycin injected into the hepatic artery of hepatoma bearing mice. Dig Dis Sci 2004; 49:1170.
144. O'Neal DP, Hirsch LR, Halas NJ, Payne JD, West JL. Photo thermal tumor ablation in mice using near infra red absorbing nanoparticles. Cancer Lett 2004; 23:2406.
145. Santhakumaran LM, Thomas T, Thomas TJ. Enhanced cellular uptake of a triplex-forming oligonucleotides by nanoparticles formation in the presence of polypropylenimine dendrimers. Nucleic Acid Res 2004; 15:2102.
146. Kumar CS, Leuschner C, Doomes EE, Henry L, Juban M, Hormes J. Efficacy of lytic peptide bound magnetite nanoparticles in destroying breast cancer cells. J Nanosci Nanotechnol 2004; 4:245.

147. Roy I, Ohulchanskyy TY, Pudavar HE, et al. Ceramic based nanoparticles entrapping water soluble photosensitizing anticancer drugs a novel drug carrier system for photodynamic therapy. J Am Chem Soc 2003; 125:7860.

148. Chawla JS, Amiji MM. Cellular uptake and concentrations of tamoxifen upon administration in poly(epsilon-caprolactone) nanoparticles. AAPS Pharm Sci 2003; 5:E3.

149. Chawla JS, Amiji MM. Biodegradable poly(epsilon-caprolactone) nanoparticles for tumor targeted delivery of Tamoxifen. Int J Pharm 2005; 249:127.

150. Yoo HS, Park TG. Folate receptor targeted delivery of Doxorubicin nano aggregates stabilized by Doxorubicin PEG-folate conjugate. J Control Release 2004; 100:247.

151. Kang BK, Chon SK, Kim SH, et al. Controlled release of paclitaxel from microemulsion containing PLGA and evaluation of anti tumor activity in vitro and in vivo. Int J Pharm 2004; 286:147.

152. Chellini E. Nanotechnologies and nanosciences, knowledge-based multifunctional materials and new production processes and devices, TATLYS project. Italy: University of Pisa, 2003.

153. Wagner E. Strategies to improve DNA polyplexes for in vivo gene transfer: will artificial viruses be the answer? Pharm Res 2004; 21:8.

154. Pichon C, Gonsalves C, Midoux P. Histidine rich peptides and polymers for nucleic acids delivery. Adv Drug Deliv Rev 2001; 53:75.

155. Verbaan FJ, Ousorren C, Snel CJ, et al. Steric stabilization of poly(2(dimethyl amino) ethyl methacrylate) based polyplexes mediates prolonged circulation and tumor targeting in mice. J Gen Med 2004; 6:64.

156. Ogris M, Walker G, Blessing T, Kirchesis R, Wolschek M, Wagner E. Tumor targeted gene therapy: Strategies for the preparation of ligand polyethylene glycol-polyethylenimine/DNA complexes. J Control Release 2003; 91:173.

157. Oupicky D, Ogris M, Howard PR, Dash K, Ulbrich K, Seymore LW. Importance of lateral and steric stabilization of polyelectrolyte gene delivery vectors for extended systemic circulation. Mol Ther 2002; 5:463.

158. Borchard G. Chitosan for gene delivery. Adv Drug Deliv Rev 2001; 52:145.

159. Ohsaki M, Okuda T, Wada A. In vitro gene transfection using dendritic poly(l-lysine). Bio Conjug Chem 2002; 13:510.

160. Forrest ML, Koerber JT, Pack DW. A degradable polyethylenimine derivative with low toxicity for highly efficient gene delivery. Bioconjug Chem 2003; 14:934.

161. Lim YB, Han SO, Kong HU. Biodegradable polyester, poly(alpha-(4-aminobutyl)-l-glycolic-acid) as a nontoxic gene carrier. Pharm Res 2000; 17:811.

162. Dekie L, Toncheva V, Dubruel P. Poly-l-glutamic acid derivatives as vectors for gene therapy. J Control release 2000; 65:187.

163. Akinc A, Anderson DG, Lynn DM. Synthesis of poly-(beta-amino esters) optimized for highly effective gene delivery. J Am Chem Soc 2000; 122:10761.

164. Bettinger T, Remy JS, Erbacher P. Size reduction of galactosylated PEI/DNA complexes improves lectin mediated gene transfer into hepatocytes. Bioconjug Chem 1999; 10:558.

165. Funhoff AM, Monge S, Teeuwen R, Koning GA, Nieuwenbrock NMES, Crommelin DJA, Haddleton DM, Hennik WE, van Nostrum CF. PEG shielded polymeric double layered micelles for gene delivery. J Control Release 2005; 102:711.

166. Zhang XQ, Wang XL, Zhang PC, et al. Galactosylated ternary DNA/polyphosphoramidate nanoparticles mediate high gene transfection efficiency in hepatocytes. J Controlled Release 2005; 102:749.

167. Zhao Z, Wang J, Mao HQ. Polyphosphoesters in drug and gene delivery. Adv Drug Deliv Rev 2003; 55:483.

168. Li Y, Wang J, Li CG. CNS gene transfer mediated by a novel controlled release system based on DNA complexes of degradable polycation PPE-EA: a comparison with polyethylenimine/DNA complexes. Gene Ther 2004; 11:109.

169. Wang J, Gao SJ, Zhang PC. Polyphosphoramidate gene carriers: Effect of charge group on gene transfer efficiency. Gene Ther 2004; 11:1001.

170. Wang J, Zghang PC, Lu HF. New polyphosphoramidate with a spermidine side chain as a gene carrier. J Control Release 2002; 83:157.

171. Csaba N, Caamano P, Sanchez A, Dominguez F, Alonso MJ. PLGA: Poloxamer and PLGA; poloxamine blend nanoparticles, new carriers for gene delivery. Biomacro Mol 2005; 10:271.
172. Zahr AS, deVillers M, Pishko MV. Encapsulation of drug nanoparticles in self assembled macromolecular nano-shells. Langmuir 2005; 21:403.
173. Kaul G, Parsons CL, Amiji M. Poly(ethylene glycol) modified gelatin nanoparticles for intracellular delivery. Pharm Eng 2003; 23:1.
174. Panyam J, Labhasetwar V. Biodegradable nanoparticles for drug and gene delivery to cells and tissues. Adv Drug Deliv Rev 2003; 55:329.
175. Panyam J, Labhasetwar V. Sustained cytoplasmic delivery of drugs with intracellular receptors using biodegradable nanoparticles. Mol Pharm 2004; 1:77.
176. Moghimi SM, Hunter AC, Murray JC. Long circulating and target specific nanoparticles, theory and practice. Pharmacol Rev 2001; 53:283.
177. Xia X, Hu Z, Marquez M. Physically bonded nanoparticles networks: a novel drug delivery system. J Control Release 2005; 103:21.
178. Panyam J, Williams D, Dash A, Pelecky DL, Labhasetwar V. Solid state solubility influences encapsulation and release of hydrophobic drugs from PLGA/PLA nanoparticles. J Pharm Sci 2004; 93:1804.
179. Kaul G, Amiji M. Tumor targeted gene delivery using poly (ethylene glycol) modified gelatin nanoparticles: in vitro and in vivo studies. Pharm Res 2005; 22:951.
180. Esfand R, Tomalia DA. Poly(amidoamine) PAMAM dendrimers: from biomimetic to drug delivery and biomedical applications. Drug Discov Today 2001; 6:427.
181. Toth I, Salthivel T, Wilderspin AF, et al. Novel cationic lipidic peptide dendrimer vectors: in vitro gene delivery. STP Pharm Sci 1999; 9:93.
182. Bayele HK, Salthivel T, O'Donnell M, et al. Versatile peptide dendrimers for nucleic acid delivery. J Pharm Sci 2005; 94:446.
183. Zhang XQ, Wang XL, Huang SW, et al. In vitro gene delivery using polyamidoamine dendrimers with a trimesyl core. Biomacromolecules 2005; 6:341.
184. Benita BM, Romejin S, Jungingger HE, Borchard G. PLGA–PEI nanoparticles for gene delivery to pulmonary epithelium. Eur J Pharm Biopharm 2004; 85:1.
185. Diwan M, Elamanchilli P, Cao M, Samuel J. Dose sparing of CpG oligodeoxynucleotide vaccine adjuvants by nanoparticles delivery. Curr Drug Deliv 2004; 1:405.
186. Rhaese S, Briesen HV, Waigmann HR, Kreuter J, Langer K. Human serum albumin-polyethylenimine nanoparticles for gene delivery. J Control Release 2003; 92:199.
187. Quiang B, Segev A, Beliard I, Nili N, Strauss BH, Sefton MV. Poly(methylidene malonate 2.1.2) nanoparticles: a biocompatible polymer that enhances peri adventitial adenoviral gene delivery. J Control Release 2004; 98:447.
188. Lee HC, Kim S, Kim K, Shin H, Yoon J. Remission in models of type 1 diabetes by gene therapy using a single chain insulin analogue. Nature 2000; 408:483.
189. Godbey WT, Wu KK, Mikos AG. Tracking the intracellular path of poly(ethylenimine)/DNA complexes for gene delivery. Proc Natl Acad Sci USA 1999; 96:5177.
190. Li Z, Huang L. Sustained delivery and expression of plasmid DNA based on biodegradable polyester, poly(d,l-lactide-co-4-hydroxy-l-proline). J Control Release 2004; 98:437.
191. Gupta M, Gupta AK. Hydrogel pullulan nanoparticles encapsulating pBUDLacZ plasmid as an efficient gene delivery carrier. J Control Release 2004; 99:157.
192. Marshall E. Gene therapy death prompts review of adenovirus vector. Science 2000; 286:2244.
193. Boyce N. Trial halted after gene shows up in semen. Nature 2001; 414:677.
194. Check E. Gene therapy, a tragic setback. Nature 2002; 420:116.
195. Braun CS, Vetro JA, Tomalia DA, Koe GS, Middaugh CR. Structure/function relationships of polyamidoamine/DNA dendrimers as gene delivery vehicles. J Pharm Sci 2005; 94:423.
196. Zaitsev S, Cartier R, Vyborov O, et al. Polyelectrolyte nanoparticles mediate vascular gene delivery. Pharm Res 2004; 21:1656.
197. Montigny WJ, Houchens CR, Illenye S, et al. Condensation by DNA looping facilities transfer of large DNA molecules into mammalian cells. Nucleic Acid Res 2001; 29:1982.

198. Lim Y, Kim C, Kim K, Park J. Development of a safe gene delivery system using biodegradable polymer, poly(4-aminobutyl)-l-glycolic acid). J Am Chem Soc 2000; 122:6524.
199. Kabanov AV, Batrakova EV, Sriadibhatla S, Yang Z, Kelly DL, Alakov VY. Polymer genomics: Shifting the gene and drug delivery paradigms. J Control Release 2005; 101:259.
200. Tabatt K, Kneuer C, Sameti M, et al. Transfection with different colloidal systems: comparison of solid–lipid nanoparticles and liposomes. J Control release 2004; 97:321.
201. Wissing SA, Kayser O, Muller RH. Solid–lipid nanoparticles for parenteral drug delivery. Drug Deliv Rev 2004; 56:1257.
202. Hoet P, Hohlfeld IB, Salata OV. Nanoparticles-known and unknown health risks. J Nanobiotechnol 2004; 2:12.
203. Service RF. Nanomaterials show signs of toxicity. Science 2003; 300:243.
204. Brown JS, Zeman KL, Bennett WD. Ultrafine particle deposition and clearance in the healthy and obstructed lung. Am J Respir Crit Care Med 2002; 166:1240.
205. Kreilgaard M. Influence of microemulsions on cutaneous drug delivery. Adv Drug Deliv Rev 2002; 54:S77.
206. Davda J, Labhasetwar V. Characterization of nanoparticles uptake by the endothelial cells. Int J Pharm 2002; 233:51.
207. Bilati U, Allemann E, Doelker E. Polu(d-l lactide-co-glycolide) protein loaded nanoparticles prepared by the double emulsion method-processing and formulation issues for enhanced entrapment efficiency. J Microencapsul 2005; 22:205.
208. Bargoni A, Cavalli R, Caputo O, Fundaro A, Gasco MR, Zara GP. Solid–lipid nanoparticles in lymph and plasma after duodenal administration to rats. Pharm Res 1998; 15:745.
209. Passirani C, Barratt G, Devissaguet JP, Labarre D. Long circulating nanoparticles bearing heparin or dextran covalently bound to poly (methyl methacrylate). Pharm Res 1998; 15:1046.
210. Silveira AM, Ponchel G, Puisieux F, Duchene D. Combined poly (isobutylcyanoacrylate) and cyclodextrins nanoparticles for enhancing the encapsulation of lipophilic drugs. Pharm Res 1998; 15:1051.

14

Lipid Nanoparticles (Solid Lipid Nanoparticles and Nanostructured Lipid Carriers) for Cosmetic, Dermal, and Transdermal Applications

Eliana B. Souto and Rainer H. Müller
Department of Pharmaceutical Technology, Biotechnology, and Quality Management, Freie Universität Berlin, Berlin, Germany

INTRODUCTION

The skin, together with the mucosal tissues of the digestive, respiratory, and urogenital tracts, forms the frontier of the body, separating the external environment from internal organs. The epidermis forms the barrier between those "worlds," that is, between the most varied conditions of temperature and humidity of the external environment, in contrast to the very stable internal environment of the living tissues and body fluids. Thus, epidermis behaves as the protective organ showing functions of physical protection of the body, sensation, and temperature control, as well as physical barrier against the exchange of chemical substances into and out of the human organism.

These days, the pharmaceutical industry supplies the costumer with many physicochemically different dosage forms intended for skin application, ranging from powders to liquids, as well as semisolid formulations. When developing such formulations, the pharmaceutical technologists must have in mind many concerns, such as stability, compatibility, and costumer acceptability of the vehicle and active ingredient, as well the bioavailability of this latter in cases of dermal and transdermal treatment (1).

It is a fact that preparations for topical, dermal, and transdermal use have the unique feature that their physical properties are almost as important as any pharmacologically active ingredient that they contain. The composition of the vehicle and active compounds deserves special emphasis, particularly because the intimate contact with the skin is always accompanied by possible risks of adverse reactions. The treatment of skin lesions is often conducted conservatively, mainly intended to soothe the skin during the progress of natural tissue repair. The principles of formulation closely resemble those applicable to cosmetic products and in both cases a good deal of caution is necessary to ensure the success of the therapy.

Concerning dermatological and transdermal therapy, the precise quantity of active ingredient which is necessary to achieve a given response cannot be predicted with certainty. This lack of precision is largely due to variability of skin penetration by the active ingredient, which is related to the thickness of the epidermis and its keratin layer, as well as to mechanical removal of the applied formulation if the affected area is not covered by a dressing.

To overcome many of these above-mentioned drawbacks, attempts have been made to introduce lipid nanoparticles into the cosmetic and pharmaceutical fields.

Solid lipid nanoparticles (SLNs) (2) and nanostructured lipid carriers (NLC) (3) are novel colloidal delivery systems with many cosmetic and dermatological features, such as adhesive properties when applied to the skin (4). These properties bring many other advantages such as occlusion and skin hydration, absorption-increasing effects, active penetration enhancement, and controlled-release properties (4,5). SLN and NLC systems differ because SLNs were developed by exchanging the liquid lipid (oil) of oil-in-water (o/w) emulsions by a solid lipid (6), which can bring many advantages in comparison to a liquid core (7). The concept of NLC was developed by nanostructuring the lipid matrix, in order to give more flexibility for modulation of drug release, increasing the drug loading and preventing its leakage. This approach was accomplished by mixing solid lipids with liquid lipids (NLC concept), instead of highly purified lipids with relatively similar molecules (SLN concept). The result is a less ordered lipid matrix with many imperfections, which can accommodate a higher amount of drug (5,8–10). The mixture obtained with solid and liquid lipids needs to be solid at least at 40°C to make sure that it does not melt at room and body temperature if used for drug delivery.

Advantages of using lipids as carrier systems for skin administration are related to their physiological and well-tolerated nature, which reduces the risk of toxicological problems and local irritancy (5,6,11). A range of very different lipids with generally recognized as safe status has been used to produce SLNs and NLCs, ranging from highly purified lipids, for example, tristearin (12) in SLNs, to mixtures of mono-, di-, and triacylglycerols in NLCs, including monoacid and polyacid acylglycerols.

When transforming the bulk lipid into a nanoparticulate form (i.e., SLNs or NLCs), a melting point depression is, in general, observed. This melting point depression is described in the Thomson equation which itself is derived from the Kelvin equation (13). An additional melting point depression occurs when a foreign compound (active ingredient or surfactant molecule) is dissolved in the lipid matrix, for example, surfactant will partition from the water phase to the lipid phase, and active-loaded lipid nanoparticles show a melting point depression when a molecular-dispersed active ingredient is present.

When comparing the lipid materials as bulk and as nanoparticulate systems, melting and recrystallization temperatures can be different, especially in chemically polydispersed lipids. When producing lipid nanoparticles, the difference can be between 10°C to 20°C or even more. For example, lipids, such as trilaurin (C_{12}), which has an original melting point of 43°C to 47°C, show a very pronounced super-cooling when formulated as lipid nanoparticles. In such compounds, crystallization will not take place anymore at room temperature, and it will only happen if cooled down to freezing temperatures (14).

Lipid molecules show different three-dimensional structures, that is, polymorphic forms: unstable α, metastable β', and as the most stable the β modification (Table 1).

In cases of mixtures of acylglycerols, polymorphic transitions occur from β' to βi and then to β, which means that another intermediate polymorph form is present. Most bulk lipids are obtained in β modification or at least predominantly in β modification. In many cases, the production of lipid nanoparticles leads to a change in the relative fraction of the polymorphic forms. Depending on the chemical nature of the lipid and on the parameters established for the production of lipid nanoparticles, different fractions of α and β' modification will be obtained. This can lead again to a reduction of the melting point, or more precisely change in form and shift of the

TABLE 1 Three-Dimensional Structure of the Crystal Order in the Three Main Polymorphs from Monoacid Triacylglycerols

	α modification	β' modification	β modification
Crystal system	Hexagonal	Monoclinical	Triclinical
Subcell	Orthorhombic	Orthorhombic	Triclinical

Source: From Refs. 15, 16.

melting peak. In contrast, it might be that the created polymorphic forms are not long-term stable, that is, there is a gradual transformation to more stable modifications, which means increasing the content of β'/βi and finally β. This phenomenon is not desired and the changes in lipid structure can cause drug expulsion during storage and changes in the release profile of the incorporated active molecules. To avoid such undesired effects, lipid mixtures should be chosen which transform relatively fast to more stable modifications directly after particle production (i.e., within one to three days). It is also perfectly acceptable or it can even be planned to trigger drug release, when the generated fractions of the different polymorphic forms remain unchanged during storage and do not transform back to the β modification of the bulk lipid.

Drug expulsion from lipid matrices is a well-known phenomenon from suppositories (17). Concerning the different possibilities for how the active ingredients can be incorporated within the lipid nanoparticle matrix, one can mention: (*i*) the replacement of host molecules in the lattice by a guest molecule or (*ii*) its incorporation in between the host molecules. However, for this latter hypothesis the guest molecule needs to have a size less than 20% of the host molecule. Active molecules can be localized in between the lipid lamellae which then results in an increase of the lattice spacing d (i.e., interatomic distance defined by the Bragg's equation; see Ref. 18). There is also the possibility that the active ingredient is present in the form of amorphous clusters, mainly localized in the imperfections of the crystal. In general, the accommodation of the active molecules is improved with the increase of the number of imperfections in the lipid crystals (19). Active loading can be increased by using rather crude lipid mixtures, such as the ones used in cosmetic products. An even further improvement of active loading can be achieved by controlled nanostructuring of the lipid matrix, that is, creating as many imperfections as possible. Depending on the nature of the lipids used for blending and the lipid matrix, different types of NLCs will be obtained. The crystalline nature of the lipid matrix is, therefore, the dominant factor determining the active loading, the release profile pattern, and also the long-term stability of SLNs and NLCs regarding the release and subsequent bioavailability of the active ingredient. Thus, the crystalline status needs to be closely monitored when developing a SLN or NLC formulation.

HISTORICAL BACKGROUND AND PRODUCTION OF SOLID LIPID NANOPARTICLES AND NANOSTRUCTURED LIPID CARRIERS

The first lipid particles were produced by the research group of Speiser, the father of the nanoparticles, in Zurich (20) (J. Paris Match). High-speed stirring was applied for the production of an o/w emulsion between a melted lipid phase and a hot aqueous surfactant solution. The obtained emulsion was then cooled and the inner lipid phase formed solid particles. However, in general, the use of stirring techniques has some drawbacks, such as the relatively broad size distribution of particles and the fact that relatively high concentrations of surfactant molecules are usually required to obtain a mean particle diameter in the nanometer range. The product developed by Speiser was called "lipid nanopellets" and was intended for oral delivery. The patent obtained by Speiser was not followed up by the owner Rentschler, and patent protection no longer exists in a number of countries.

A similar process was developed and patented by Domb, who prepared particle dispersions applying a sonication procedure. The product developed by Domb was called "liposphere" (21), and they also found no broad application in pharmaceutical products.

In 1991, the patent application of the first generation of lipid nanoparticles—SLNs—was submitted describing the nanoparticle production by high-pressure homogenization (HPH) (22) and also via microemulsion technique (23).

HPH is a technique broadly used in different research areas, and it is also established in pharmaceutical production, for example, for the production of emulsions for parenteral nutrition (Intralipid®, Lipofundin®, Lipovenoes®) (24–26). Using this technique, the problems of other nanoparticles (polymeric nanoparticles), such as the lack of scaling up and large-scale production lines, has been overcome. In addition, HPH leads to a product being relatively homogeneous in size, that is, possessing a higher physical stability of the aqueous dispersion; in general, polydisperse dispersions show a greater tendency to aggregate or coalesce. Furthermore, it is a simple and very cost-effective production technique. There are basically two different production methods: the hot and the cold HPH techniques.

For the hot HPH technique, the lipid is melted at approximately 5°C to 10°C above its melting point, the active ingredient is dissolved or finely dispersed in the melt and then the active-ingredient containing lipid melt is dispersed by stirring in a hot surfactant solution. The obtained preemulsion is homogenized applying a pressure between 200 and 500 bar and two to three homogenization cycles. After the homogenization, a hot nanoemulsion is obtained; cooling leads to recrystallization of the lipid and formation of lipid nanoparticles.

For the cold HPH technique, the lipid melt containing the active ingredient is cooled, and after solidification is ground using a mortar mill. The obtained lipid microparticles are further dispersed in a cold aqueous surfactant solution. The resulted presuspension is homogenized in the solid state at or below room temperature by cooling the high-pressure homogenizer. The sheer forces and cavitation forces in the homogenizer are strong enough to break the microparticles directly into lipid nanoparticles.

For the production of lipid nanoparticles via the microemulsion technique, the lipid is melted, the surfactant, cosurfactant, and water are added in such concentrations that a microemulsion results (27). The size of the microemulsion region in the phase diagram is a function of temperature, that is, the microemulsion can be converted to a different system when, for example, reducing the temperature. Therefore, for particle production, the microemulsion needs to be kept at the elevated temperature during the process. The hot microemulsion is diluted into cold water, leading to a "breaking" of the microemulsion and subsequent formation of an ultrafine nanoemulsion. The dilution with water and the reduction of temperature narrowing the microemulsion region are the reasons for breaking of the microemulsion (28). One disadvantage of this procedure is the dilution of the particle suspension by water, obtaining concentrations usually below 1% of particle content. When processing to a final dosage form, a very large amount of water needs to be removed.

Other approaches for the production of lipid nanoparticles have been adapted from polymeric nanoparticle production procedures, for example, the solvent emulsification-evaporation method described by Sjöström and Bergenståhl (29), the solvent displacement method described by Fessi et al. (30), and the emulsification-diffusion technique patented by Quintanar-Guerrero et al. in 1999 (31). The novel phase-inversion-based technique has been described by Heurtault et al. (32,33) for the production of SLNs.

The solvent emulsification-evaporation is a method analogous to the production of polymeric nanoparticles and microparticles by solvent evaporation in o/w emulsions. The lipid is dissolved in an organic solvent which shows no miscibility with water [e.g., cyclohexane (29,34), chloroform (34), or methylene chloride (35,36)]. The organic solution is dispersed in aqueous surfactant phase, the solvent is then removed by evaporation (34). It can be applied for the incorporation of hydrophilic molecules such as peptides and proteins, which must be previously dissolved into a water phase preparing in this case a water-in-oil-in-water (w/o/w) emulsion (36).

In the solvent displacement method, an organic solvent which is miscible with water is used. In this case, the lipid material is previously dissolved in a semipolar water-miscible solvent, such as ethanol, acetone, or methanol (37–40).

In the emulsification-diffusion technique, benzyl alcohol (41) or tetrahydrofuran (42), which is previously saturated with water, is used to ensure the initial thermodynamic equilibrium between the two liquids (water and solvent). Then, the water-saturated organic solvent is used to dissolve the lipid, and after this an o/w emulsion is prepared. Owing to the saturation of the organic solvent with water, no solvent diffuses from the droplets into the external water phase from the o/w emulsion. Removal of solvent from the droplets and particle formation is achieved by adding additional water to the emulsion and extracting the solvent (41).

A very interesting approach based on the physics behind it is the phase-inversion-based technique, which is a two-step method. First, all components are placed on a magnetic stirrer using a temperature program from room temperature to, for example, 85°C. This is followed by progressive cooling to 60°C. Three temperature cycles (85–60–85–60–85°C) are applied to reach the inversion process defined by temperature range. In step 2, an irreversible shock is induced by dilution with cold water. This fast cooling–diluting process leads to the formation of stable nanoparticles (43).

MORPHOLOGY AND STRUCTURE OF SOLID LIPID NANOPARTICLES AND NANOSTRUCTURED LIPID CARRIERS

Different models have been described in the literature for how active molecules can be incorporated into SLNs and NLCs (4). For each of the carriers, three basic types are described (Fig. 1).

The type of SLNs depends on the chemical nature of the active ingredient and lipid, the solubility of actives in the melted lipid, nature and concentration of surfactants, type of production (hot vs. cold HPH), and the production temperature. Therefore, three incorporation models have been proposed (45):

1. SLN Type I or homogeneous matrix model,
2. SLN Type II or drug-enriched shell model, and
3. SLN Type III or drug-enriched core model.

The SLN Type I or homogeneous matrix model is derived from a solid solution of lipid and active ingredient. A solid solution can be obtained when SLNs are produced by the cold homogenization method. A lipid blend can be produced containing the active in a molecularly dispersed form. After solidification of this blend, it is ground in its solid state thus avoiding or minimizing the enrichment of active molecules in different parts of the lipid nanoparticle.

The SLN Type II or drug-enriched shell model is achieved when SLNs are produced via the hot HPH technique, and the active ingredient concentration in the melted lipid is low. During the cooling process of the hot o/w nanoemulsion, the lipid will precipitate first, leading to a steadily increasing concentration of active molecules in the remaining lipid melt with increasing fraction of lipid solidified. An active-free lipid core is formed; when the active reaches its saturation solubility in the remaining melt, an outer shell will solidify containing both active

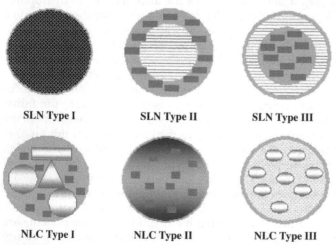

FIGURE 1   (*See color insert.*) Basic types of solid lipid nanoparticles and nanostructured lipid carriers. *Abbreviations*: NLC, nanostructured lipid carrier; SLN, solid lipid nanoparticle. *Source*: From Ref. 44.

and lipid. The enrichment in the outer area of the particles causes burst release. The percentage of active ingredient localized in the outer shell can be adjusted in a controlled way by altering the production parameters. A typical example of an active-enriched shell model is the incorporation of coenzyme Q10 (46,47).

The SLN Type III or drug-enriched core model can take place when the active ingredient concentration in the lipid melt is high and at or relatively close to its saturation solubility. Cooling down of the hot oil droplets will in most cases reduce the solubility of the active in the melt; when the saturation solubility is exceeded, active molecules precipitate leading to the formation of a drug-enriched core.

Regarding the models described for NLCs, Figure 1 also shows three different structures:

1. NLC Type I or imperfect crystal model,
2. NLC Type II or amorphous model, and
3. NLC Type III or multiple model.

NLC type I is defined as the imperfect crystal model, because once in its matrix there are many imperfections which are able to accommodate the active molecules. This model is obtained when mixing solid lipids with small amounts of liquid lipids (oils). Owing to the different chain lengths of the fatty acids and the mixture of mono-, di-, and triacylglycerols, the matrix of NLCs is not able to form a highly ordered structure (5).

NLC type II is called the amorphous model because it is created when mixing special lipids which do not recrystallize anymore after homogenization and cooling, such as hydroxyoctacosanylhydroxystearate and isopropylmyristate. These lipids are able to create solid particles of amorphous lipid structure, which can avoid the occurrence of crystallization, minimizing drug expulsion, because the matrix is maintained in the polymorphic α form.

NLC type III is described as the multiple model. This model has been developed to improve the loading capacity of several drugs, such as the ones whose solubility in liquid lipids is higher than in solid lipids (48,49). This type is derived from w/o/w emulsions, which consist of an oil-in-fat-in-water dispersion. Very small oil nanocompartments are created inside the solid lipid matrix of the nanoparticles generated by a phase-separation process (5). This model is obtained when mixing solid lipids with liquid lipids (oils) in such a ratio that the solubility of the oil molecules in the solid lipid is exceeded. The melted lipid and the hot oil are blended; thus, the two lipids must show a miscibility gap at the used concentrations, at approximatel 40°C. A hot o/w nanoemulsion is produced at a higher temperature (approx. 80°C), then the lipid droplets are cooled. When reaching the miscibility gap, the oil precipitates forming tiny oil droplets in the melted solid lipid. Subsequent solidification of the solid lipid as solid nanoparticle matrix leads to fixation of the oily nanocompartments.

DEVELOPMENT OF COSMETIC AND TRANSDERMAL PRODUCTS BASED ON SOLID LIPID NANOPARTICLES AND NANOSTRUCTURED LIPID CARRIERS

The scientific literature reports several approaches for the development of products based on SLNs and NLCs (4,5).

Incorporation of Solid Lipid Nanoparticles and Nanostructured Lipid Carriers into Semisolid Preparations

Similar to liposomes, polymeric nanoparticles, and microsponge systems, aqueous SLN or NLC dispersions can be added to semisolid preparations such as lotions, creams, and hydrogels (50,51). The advantage of this procedure is the association of a well-established topical formulation with several attractive advantages of the lipid nanoparticles in the same final product.

The incorporation of SLNs or NLCs into a cream consists of the addition of the lipid nanoparticles as a highly concentrated dispersion, that is, with 50% solid (particle) content to a freshly prepared o/w cream or during the production of such cream (49,52). In the first case, a part of the water in the cream formulation is replaced by a highly concentrated SLN or NLC dispersion, and after that the production process is run normally. The lipid nanoparticles are sufficiently stabilized to avoid their coalescence with the inner oil droplets of the emulsion. If the production process of the emulsion is performed at a temperature higher than the melting point of the lipid nanoparticles, these latter will melt but will recrystallize during the cooling at the end of the process. The second approach is more elegant, but in this case the cream is produced as usual, however with a reduced water content in order to compensate for the water added with the aqueous SLN or NLC dispersion. After the production of the cream, the concentrated SLN or NLC dispersion is added by stirring at room temperature. This process avoids the melting of the nanoparticles, avoiding therefore undesired changes within the internal particle structure.

If the aim is the addition of SLNs or NLCs to hydrogels, the procedure is even simpler. The hydrogels can be previously prepared, and after that SLN or NLC dispersion is diluted within the semisolid formulation (50). Alternatively, a concentrated SLN or NLC dispersion is added before the gelation process. However, it should be noted that electrolytes frequently used to jellify synthetic polymers can destabilize the lipid nanoparticles. The surface electrical charge (zeta potential) is reduced leading to aggregation of suspended particles. This phenomenon should be considered when, for example, adding electrolytes in the form of sodium hydroxide for the preparation of carbomer gels. The type of neutralizing agent affects the aggregation of SLNs and NLCs, and it can be avoided or minimized when using Tristan® and Neutrol® TE as neutralizing agents (49). As soon as the gel is formed, aggregation will not occur anymore because SLNs and NLCs will be physically stabilized and entrapped in the gel network. In general, SLN and NLC dispersions, which are unstable because of suboptimal surfactant combination, can be further stabilized after their incorporation into hydrogels. This opens the opportunity to use stabilizers, which are not that efficient in providing a long-term stability of the aqueous dispersion, but are regulatory accepted. The SLN and NLC dispersions need to be stable only for the few hours until they are incorporated into the semisolid formulation, where they will be stabilized by the gel network.

Production of Gels Based on Solid Lipid Nanoparticles and Nanostructured Lipid Carriers

The production of gels based on SLNs and NLCs consists of topical formulations having only lipid nanoparticles in their composition. A lipid nanoparticle dispersion is previously prepared, and then the gelling agent is added, preferentially nonelectrolyte agents, such as cellulose derivatives (49) or other natural gums (53). For many gel preparations, an amount of 4% to 10% of lipid nanoparticles is sufficient. To make production more profitable, a concentrated particle suspension (e.g., 40%–50%) can be prepared and then diluted to the desired final concentration. This approach has certain advantages, such as the release of actives being controlled only by the lipid nanoparticle matrix. The desired properties can be adjusted in a very controlled way by attenuating the lipid nanoparticle features.

Production of Creams Based on Solid Lipid Nanoparticles and Nanostructured Lipid Carriers

The production of creams based on SLNs and NLCs consists of the production of aqueous dispersions of lipid nanoparticles in a high concentration, up to 50% or 60%. When applying higher lipid concentrations, ointments with a bicontinuous structure will be formed, that is, the homogenization process leads to well-defined particles and not to an ointment-like system.

It is known that the viscosity of the preparations increases with the lipid concentration (51), that is, at about 40% to 45% the formulations are cream-like, above 50% they become paste-like, and when increased to a solid content of 80% or 90% the formulations are solid and can be cut with a knife. Cream-like and paste-like formulations are suitable for dermal application of actives, whereas the solid-like systems are usually of high interest for oral administration of lipid particles to exploit the absorption-enhancing effect of lipids (54). For the production of such formulations, a highly concentrated stock suspension (50%–60% lipid nanoparticles) is first prepared by HPH. Then, additional melted lipid is added stepwise and dispersed again, building a concentration of up to 80% or 90% of solid content. In the melted state, the obtained product is still liquid and it has a relatively low viscosity. After cooling down, the system becomes cream-like, paste-like, or solid-like.

FEATURES OF SOLID LIPID NANOPARTICLES AND NANOSTRUCTURED LIPID CARRIERS AND SKIN EFFECTS

Physical Stability in Aqueous Dispersions and in Creams

Physical stability of the aqueous SLN and NLC dispersions, that is, the absence of particle aggregation and creaming, is a prerequisite for the formulation of cosmetic and pharmaceutical products based on SLNs and NLCs. Owing to their small size in the nanometer range, lipid nanoparticles are naturally stable, and creaming of aqueous dispersions or nanoparticle sedimentation might not occur. The particles are kept in suspension by the Brownian motion of the water molecules. Owing to their surface electrical charge, the particles are stabilized by electrostatics repulsion, and the physical stability is even further enhanced when sterically stabilizing polymers, such as Tween 80 or poloxamer, are used as surfactants in the formulation. The high lipid nanoparticle stability as aqueous dispersion has been reported for more than three years (55). Furthermore, if necessary SLN and NLC can be incorporated in creams, gels, lotions, or body milks, to increase their physical stability as reported above.

Apart from aggregation and creaming, another type of instability could be questioned, that is, the dissolution of lipid nanoparticles in the liquid oil of the above-mentioned semisolid formulations. In contrast to liposomes, SLNs and NLCs have the advantage that the stability can be proven quantitatively by differential scanning calorimetry (DSC). In the DSC measurements, the melting of the nanoparticles and the melting energy in Joule per gram can be determined. Comparing the melting energy on the day of nanoparticles incorporation into the cream with the melting energy obtained after a certain storage time, will allow the calculation of the total percentage of nanoparticles still present in the formulation. This is not possible to perform with liposomes. It is easy to prove the existence of liposomes in a product after certain storage time by electron microscopy, however the quantification of their number is not possible or it is extremely difficult to perform (in this case using, e.g., quantitative electron microscopy analysis). This is a major obstacle for introducing a liposomal cosmetic formulation into the market in Japan. However, this is not a major problem with SLNs and NLCs because the exact amount after a certain storage time can be easily analyzed quantitatively by DSC (56).

Loading Capacity, Entrapment Efficiency, and Controlled-Release Properties

Important parameters to evaluate the suitability of a carrier system are the loading capacity and the entrapment efficiency for the active ingredients. A full range of model active ingredients has been incorporated into SLNs and NLCs. An updated list has been recently provided by our group (57). Loading capacity of 10% to 20% was obtained for tetracaine and etomidate with physical stability of the particles remaining (58) (please note that the loading capacity is calculated in percent of the lipid mass). Vitamins A and E and their derivatives have been incorporated into SLNs up to 25% (56). In this study, the incorporation was limited by the fact that higher percentages did not lead to any more solid particles. However, if these active ingredients are blended with even higher melting lipids, then the loading capacity can be further increased. In case of full miscibility of the active ingredient with the lipid, loading capacities of 50% and more can be achieved. The loading capacity can be 100% in cases where the active ingredient is lipophilic and solid itself.

The entrapment efficiency is the percentage of active ingredient which is entrapped inside the lipid particles. For lipophilic active ingredients, the entrapment efficiencies are typically between 90% and 98%. The lowest values observed were approximately 80%, for example, tetracaine (59) and clotrimazole (60). For hydrophilic compounds, the loading capacity and the entrapment efficiency are obviously lower. Values of about 50% have been obtained for the extremely hydrophilic model compound Iotrolan, an X-ray contrast agent (61). Iotrolan was used as a model compound because of its extremely high hydrophilicity; two parts of Iotrolan dissolve in only one part of water. Model drugs for peptides and proteins (e.g., lysozyme) have also been incorporated. It could be proven that lysozyme remained chemically intact after incorporation into the SLN and was still active (62). With hydrophilic peptides, loading capacities up to 20% have been achieved for prolonged release from the particles in vivo in the animal model.

The release of incorporated ingredients from the lipid nanoparticles can be modulated according to the needs from very fast to very slow. Figure 2 compares the release of clotrimazole obtained from SLNs and NLCs using Franz diffusion cells (60).

In NLC formulations, lipid nanoparticles have a liquid core, and clotrimazole is incorporated in the oil less tightly in comparison to the solid lipid matrix of SLN formulations. In the latter, drug molecules are incorporated into the crystalline matrix and their diffusional mobility is decreased (60).

In general, diffusion through the carrier is the main mechanism of controlled release as described by Fick's law of diffusion (5). However, drug diffusion

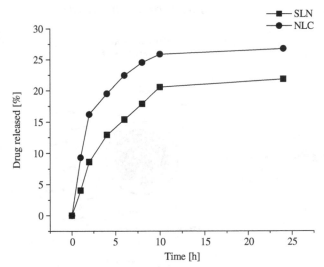

FIGURE 2 Clotrimazole release profiles from tripalmitin-based solid lipid nanoparticles and nano structured lipid carrier. *Abbreviations*: NLC, nanostructured lipid carrier; SLN, solid lipid nanoparticle. *Source*: From Ref. 60.

coefficient cannot be considered constant, but it is dependent upon drug concentration. Owing to a large drug loading, the degree of diffusion can be decreased. There are too many molecules trying to diffuse and they limit their own permeation (hindering effects). Also, the previously described incorporation models for SLNs (drug-enriched core or shell) underline these findings. Drug loading is very important with regard to release characteristics (6). Generally, the increase of drug loading leads to an acceleration of the drug release. However, in particular cases, increasing the drug loading may slow down the release, which can be explained by possible drug crystallization inside the nanoparticles.

Figure 3 shows the redistribution effect occurring during the SLN production by the hot HPH technique (6). According to characteristics, such as drug solubility and its partitioning coefficient, dispersing the drug-containing lipid melt in a hot aqueous surfactant solution will lead to distribution of drug into the aqueous phase. If the aqueous phase contains a higher surfactant concentration, in most cases this leads to a better solubility of the lipophilic drug in the water phase (e.g., by solubilization) and thus more pronounced distribution of drug to the water phase.

The solubility of the active ingredient in the water phase can be further increased by choosing higher production temperatures, that is, in this case more active will partition to the water phase (6). The opposite effect will occur when the obtained hot nanoemulsion is in the cooling process, that is, the solubility of the active in the aqueous phase decreases. Lipid starts to precipitate forming a lipid core with a lower active concentration than in the original drug-containing lipid melt. Further cooling leads to further reduction of the active solubility in the water phase and redistribution back to the lipid phase, however due to the formation of the solid lipid core, only the outer shell is accessible for the active. In this case, most of the active will be released in the form of a burst. The extent of the burst release can be, therefore, modified by controlling the amount of active in the outer shell of the obtained particles. This phenomenon has been observed as a

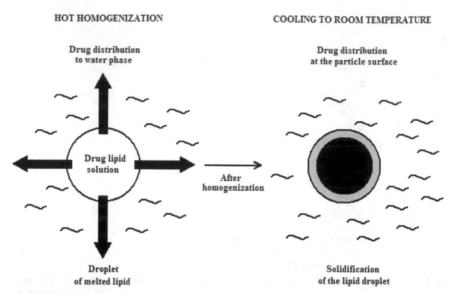

HOT HOMOGENIZATION   COOLING TO ROOM TEMPERATURE

Drug distribution   Drug distribution
to water phase   at the particle surface

Drug lipid
solution

After
homogenization

Droplet   Solidification
of melted lipid   of the lipid droplet

FIGURE 3 Partitioning effect of drug during production of lipid nanoparticles by high-pressure homogenization technique. *Source*: From Ref. 6.

function of production temperature and surfactant concentration. Burst release can also be avoided applying the cold HPH process (63,64).

Chemical Protection of Incorporated Substances
It is known that stabilization of chemically labile actives against degradation (e.g., hydrolysis and oxidation) can be achieved using a solid matrix such as the one of polymeric particles (65). This is also valid for the lipid nanoparticles. The stability of retinol and coenzyme Q10 could be enhanced when incorporated into lipid nanoparticles made from a mixture of Compritol®888 ATO and Miglyol®812 (66,67). Ketoconazole could also be protected to a relative extent using the same lipid (68).

Owing to the fluid character of carriers such as liposomes and emulsions, the active ingredients will partition between the liquid oil and water phases (56). Permanent exchange of molecules between these two phases will decompose the active molecules in the water phase, and simultaneously nondegraded compound will partition from the oil to the water phase (based on partitioning coefficient after Nernst). The partitioning ratio between nondegraded and degraded active will be maintained (Fig. 4, upper). In comparison to a solid matrix (SLN or NLC), the active will be in this case fixed inside the lipid particles. Exchange between the inner and outer phases will not happen or it will occur very slowly (Fig. 4, lower). These observations emphasize the protection and chemical stabilization effects of incorporated actives into SLNs and NLCs (69).

Occlusive Effects and Skin Hydration
Owing to the small particle size of SLNs and NLCs, these carriers show adhesive properties (52,70), properties that have also been observed when using liposomes. When in contact with the skin, lipid nanoparticles create a thin film with very narrow

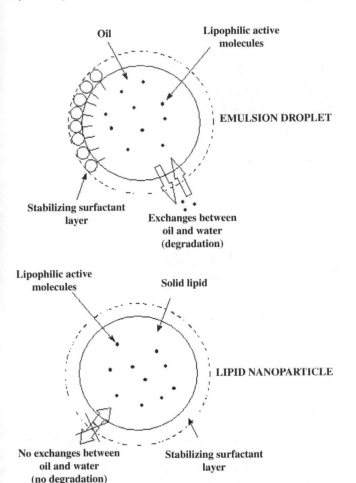

FIGURE 4 Chemical protection of labile actives in emulsion droplets versus lipid nanoparticles. Free partitioning of nondegraded and degraded active molecules in the emulsion system (*upper*), but hindered by the solid state of the lipid nanoparticles (*lower*). *Source*: From Ref. 66.

interspaces between the particles. The formation of this film can be sensed when applying an SLN or NLC formulation onto the skin. Even relatively small amounts of lipid nanoparticles in a cream (e.g., 5%) can create this film (56).

Figure 5 shows that the relatively high occlusivity is a special feature of lipid nanoparticles (Fig. 5, lower), when compared with lipid microparticles (Fig. 5, upper) of identical lipid content. The rather low occlusivity of microparticles is attributed to the large spaces between the micrometer carriers still allowing the evaporation of water. The small spaces (capillaries) between the nanoparticles are hydrodynamically unfavorable and limit water loss (small diameter of pores, higher resistance to water vapor flow). This film hinders water evaporation, which means that an occlusive effect leads to increased skin hydration.

This property might be very interesting for skin protection during the day, when applying placebo SLNs or NLCs. The skin constantly comes into contact with

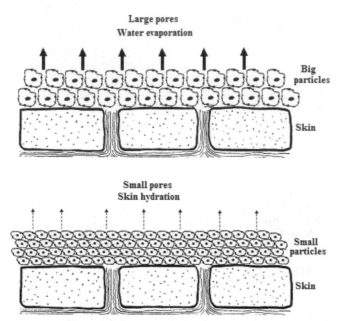

FIGURE 5 Mechanism of the occlusion effect depending on the particle size. A solid lipid micro-particle dispersion (diameter 1 μm, upper) in comparison to an aqueous solid lipid nanoparticles or nanostructured lipid carrier dispersion (diameter 230 nm, lower). *Source*: From Ref. 66.

a wide variety of chemicals which are normally present in the atmosphere. These include water and dissolved mineral salts present as free electrolytes together with the atmospheric gases. Skin's permeability to these different substances varies widely. Occlusion of the skin leads to increased hydration and subsequently to the smoothing of wrinkles—an effect utilized in many cosmetic products. On the basis of this property, SLN- and NLC-containing products are expected to have also anti-aging effects, especially when preparing them with skin-caring active ingredients, such as several vitamins and ceramides. Ceramides can be blended with higher melting lipids leading to solid nanoparticles, and when applied they will promote restoration of the damaged protective lipid layer of the skin (4).

Penetration Enhancement of Incorporated Substances

Owing to occlusion properties of lipid nanoparticles and subsequent increased skin hydration, these carriers can improve the penetration of the incorporated actives into the skin. The penetration-enhancement effect of lipid nanoparticles has been tested with tocopherol and tocopherol acetate. Lipid nanoparticles loaded with those actives have been applied to the skin and the penetration compared to alcoholic solution of the same compounds by applying a stripping test (cumulative penetration as a function of the number of strips). Penetration observed with lipid nanoparticle formulations was twice as high as obtained with the referenced alcoholic solution. In addition, these data also have shown that active ingredients incorporated into lipid nanoparticles were obviously released from the carriers when applied to the skin (66).

SOLID LIPID NANOPARTICLES AND NANOSTRUCTURED LIPID CARRIERS AS VEHICLES FOR COSMETIC, DERMAL, AND TRANSDERMAL ACTIVES

The introduction of lipid particles into pharmaceutical technology is reported to be very old, and recently attempts have been made to introduce lipid nanoparticles into the market by cosmetic and pharmaceutical companies. The first product is already on the market and it has been introduced by the company Yamanouchi (e.g., Nanobase®) in Poland, covered by the Yamanouchi patent (71). This product contains active-free lipid nanoparticles and it is intended for cosmetic purposes.

Even though cosmetic formulations do not necessarily have any physiological function, they resemble topical applications for dermatological use in many aspects. For example, the purpose of a lipstick is essentially decorative, but its formulation embodies a number of excipients commonly used in pharmaceutical products. Having considered the ways in which therapeutic applications are formulated, it is only necessary to examine the modifications of these techniques employed in the cosmetic field, with special reference to fragrance, feel, freshness, appearance, and skin persistence. Factors such as personal taste and fashion also have a strong influence when people purchase the product. Thus, in order to develop a successful product, the formulation must exhibit both functional attributes and esthetic appeal.

Besides lipsticks, facial makeup products can also be developed that have lipid nanoparticles. They serve to improve the uniformity of coloring, add new color, disguise blemishes, and impart a smooth matt finish. The face exposes the greatest single area of the body surface to climatic influence and in view of the major esthetic significance of its appearance, there is a real need for protection. The relative thinness of the facial epidermis adds further importance to such protection. Also cleansing creams, which are oil-miscible preparations useful to remove makeup residues without the energetic degreasing that may result from using soap and water, can be formulated with SLNs and NLCs. The aqueous phase of the dispersion has surfactant properties to remove the makeup while the lipid nanoparticles adhere to the skin protecting it. Other examples are face powders (lipid nanoparticles can be spray-dried) for a basis coloring or masking to cover minor defects, lipsticks, hair dressings, nail preparations, depilatories, and shaving aids.

According to market studies, an important factor for a cosmetic to be purchased is not only that the packaging must have an esthetic appeal, but so must the appearance of the formulation itself. White products are preferred by the consumer, lipid nanoparticles can be used to weaken, for example, yellowish actives (coenzyme Q10, vitamin C). This whitening effect is of special interest for actives which are degraded with degradation products possessing a color, even if they do not influence the product quality (4). Whitening and lightening properties of lipid nanoparticles are currently being explored (71–74).

Deodorants and antiperspirants can also have lipid nanoparticles particularly if formulated with antiseptics, for example, hexachlorophene or trichlorophane, which appear to increase the permeability of the sweat duct and thus reduce the amount of the secretion reaching the surface of the skin.

Aging of the skin has been attributed to a change in the circulating sex hormones, but alterations of the collagen and elastic tissues, which are accelerated by chronic UV exposition, is probably more significant. It is, therefore, likely that UV-absorbing cosmetics should have a truly protective role in this context. Molecular UV blockers have been incorporated into lipid nanoparticles (75–80).

A side effect of these sunscreens is penetration into the skin leading to skin irritation or even allergic reactions (81). Particulate UV blockers frequently used are titanium dioxide particles which have also been loaded into NLCs (82). There is also an ongoing controversial discussion whether and to what extent titanium dioxide particles penetrate into the skin (83,84) where they can potentially interact with the immune system (85). After incorporation of molecular UV blockers into lipid nanoparticles, a synergistic effect of the UV scattering caused by the SLN themselves and the UV absorbance of the molecular sunscreen was observed (86). This opens the question of reducing the concentration of the molecular sunscreen, and simultaneously its potential side effects, while also maintaining the UV-protective level. Apart from reduction of side effects, this result is of commercial interest for expensive UV blockers. In addition, it was found that penetration of molecular sunscreens into the skin was reduced when comparing SLNs to a traditional o/w emulsion system of similar composition (78).

The only element common to nearly all cosmetic products is the employment of a perfume to impart a pleasing fragrance. Lipid nanoparticles can also be used for prolonged release of perfumes, fragrances, and insect repellents, in comparison to o/w emulsions and Eau de Toilettes (84). The release can be slowed down by incorporating the perfume in a solid matrix instead in a liquid lipid particle (oil droplet) (75). This is very interesting if the aim is to create a once a day application with continuing scent. Fundamentally, perfumes are derived from the essential oils of botanical origin and most formulae still rely to a considerable extent in the use of natural oils. Thus, NLCs are suitable to deliver oily fragrances due to the presence of an inner liquid core in their structure. Although oily fragrances are quite expensive, using a prolonged release system such as NLC, lower amounts of oil will be needed; in addition, they can be used in soaps and less expensive products. Prolonged release was also observed for insect repellents, such as lemon oil (75,88–90).

Dermal and transdermal formulations may also be compounded as free-flowing solids (powders), semisolids, or liquids. The decision to employ a particular dosage form is mainly dependent on considerations of functional suitability. The effectiveness of both topical and transdermal systems is related to the extent of percutaneous absorption of the drug. Thus, there is a tendency to view these systems as being closely related in terms of functionality. However, when systems such as SLNs and NLCs are placed on the skin to deliver the incorporated drugs, these can act: (*i*) in the local tissues immediately beneath the application site, (*ii*) in the deep regions in the vicinity of the application site, and (*iii*) in the systemic circulation. Of course, when moving down this progression, the drug-delivery challenge becomes increasingly difficult. To achieve systemic circulation, drug release over long periods must be provided. The main feature of lipid nanoparticles intended for dermal and transdermal delivery of drugs is their controlled-release properties (10,91). The release profile accomplished by lipid nanoparticles is dependent on their structure (60). As discussed previously, depending on the production method (hot vs. cold homogenization), the composition of the formulation (i.e., surfactant, lipids), the solubilizing properties of the matrix for the drug nanoparticles with a different structure will be obtained (5,63,64). Depending on the matrix structure, the release profiles will vary from very fast, medium, or extremely prolonged release (60). The degree of the initial burst release, for example, desired for topical applications, could be explained by the dissolution properties of the drugs during the production process being a function of lipid, surfactant, and production temperature. The understanding of this mechanism allows the controlled production of lipid nanoparticles with a defined initial dose.

To reach pharmacologically adequate systemic levels in transdermal therapy, a sufficient amount of drug needs to cross the skin from the application site to the circulation. Conventional transdermal systems are ointments and adhesive systems of precisely defined size, for which ideally there would be no local accumulation. However, in those cases the drug molecules are forced to cross through a small diffusional window defined by the contact area of the transdermal system. Consequently, irritation and/or sensitizing effects underlying this system might be observed. To overcome such inconvenience, the use of lipid nanoparticles might be beneficial particularly due to the fact that they are composed of physiological and well-accepted lipids. Furthermore, skin lipids (fatty acids, ceramides) can also figure in the lipid nanoparticle composition. In addition to chemical stabilization of incorporated drugs (68), drug penetration can be improved by occlusion and further hydration effects.

CONCLUDING REMARKS

There is no doubt that lipid nanoparticles combine advantages of other carrier systems, such as emulsions, liposomes, and polymeric nanoparticles. Considering their special properties, SLNs and NLCs will find applications in cosmetic products but also in pharmaceutical formulations, that is, for dermal and transdermal delivery.

Over the last decade, dermal and transdermal delivery of drugs has become one of the most promising areas of pharmaceutical research and due to intensive efforts, thousand of patents have been filed dealing with new concepts and new technologies. Apart from their special features, major advantages of SLNs and NLCs are definitely the possibility for large-scale production, the cost-effective production method, and the relatively low cost of excipients and other components. Owing to the worldwide patent protection, the product exclusivity can be guaranteed giving no advantage to competitors. Registered trade names worldwide offer the possibility for sale using a product name optimized considering marketing aspects.

Pharmaceutical and cosmetic preparations are made in a wide range of batch sizes and the scale of operations strongly influences the final quality of the obtained product. Wherever those formulations are prepared, raw materials have to be stored, the ingredients and the final product have to be transferred from one point to another. They have to be transported and processed in contact with various constructional materials and finally stored in bulk before transfer to final containers. When dealing with aqueous SLN and NLC dispersions, these need to be physicochemically stable to avoid failure of the scale of production. Large-scale production is possible for SLNs and NLCs, which means that not only the equipment is available, but also the obtained batches are physicochemically stable (82,92).

REFERENCES

1. Hadgraft J. Passive enhancement strategies in topical and transdermal drug delivery. Int J Pharm 1999; 184:1–6.
2. Müller RH, Lucks J-S. Azneistoffträger aus festen Lipidteilchen–feste Lipid Nanosphären (SLN), Germany. European Patent 0605497, 1996.
3. Müller RH, Mäder K, Lippacher A, Jenning V. Fest-flüssig (halbfeste) Lipidpartikel und Verfahren zur Herstellung hochkonzentrierter Lipidpartikeldispersionen. PCT application PCT/EP00/04565, 1998.
4. Müller RH, Mehnert W, Souto EB. Solid lipid nanoparticles (SLN) and nanostructured lipid carriers (NLC) for dermal delivery. In: Bronaugh L, ed. Percutaneous Absorption. New York: Marcel Dekker, 2005:719–738.

5. Müller RH, Radtke M, Wissing SA. Solid lipid nanoparticles (SLN) and nanostructured lipid carriers (NLC) in cosmetic and dermatological preparations. Adv Drug Deliv Rev 2002; 54:S131–S155.

6. Müller RH, Mäder K, Gohla S. Solid lipid nanoparticles (SLN) for controlled drug delivery—a review of the state of art. Eur J Pharm Biopharm 2000; 50:161–177.

7. Siekmann B, Westesen K. Submicron lipid suspensions (solid lipid nanoparticles) versus lipid nanoemulsions: similarities and differences. In: Benita S, ed. Submicron Emulsions in Drug Targeting and Delivery. Amsterdam: Harwood Academic Publishers, 1998:205–218.

8. Müller RH, Radtke M, Wissing SA. Nanostructured lipid matrices for improved microencapsulation of drugs. Int J Pharm 2002; 242:121–128.

9. Müller RH, Radtke M, Wissing SA. Solid lipid nanoparticles and nanostructured lipid carriers. In: Nalwa HS, ed. Encyclopedia of Nanoscience and Nanotechnology. Los Angeles, California: American Scientific Publishers, 2004:43–56.

10. Müller RH, Wissing SA. Lipopearls for topical delivery of active compounds and controlled release. In: Rathbone MJ, Hadgraft J, Roberts MS, eds. Modified-Release Drug Delivery Systems. New York: Marcel Dekker, 2003:571–587.

11. Mehnert W, Mäder K. Solid lipid nanoparticles—production, characterization and applications. Adv Drug Deliv Rev 2001; 47:165–196.

12. Bunjes H, Westesen K, Koch MHJ. Crystallization tendency and polymorphic transitions in triglyceride nanoparticles. Int J Pharm 1996; 129:159–173.

13. Hunter RJ. Foundations of Colloidal Science. Oxford: Oxford University Press, 1986.

14. Westesen K, Bunjes H. Do nanoparticles prepared from lipids solid at room temperature always possess a solid lipid matrix? Int J Pharm 1995; 115:129–131.

15. Hagemann JW. Thermal behaviour and polymorphism of acylglycerides. In: Garti N, Sato K, eds. Crystallization and Polymorphism of Fats and Fatty Acids. New York: Marcel Dekker, 1988:9–96.

16. Hernqvist L. Crystal structures of fats and fatty acids. In: Garti N, Sato K, eds. Crystallization and Polymorphism of Fats and Fatty Acids. New York: Marcel Dekker, 1988:97–137.

17. Müller BW. Suppositorien. Stuttgart: Wissenschaftliche Verlagsgesellschaft mbH, 1986.

18. Krischner H. Einführung in die Röntgenfeinstrukturanalyse. Vol. 4. Auflage: Vieweg Verlag Braunschweig, 1990.

19. Westesen K, Bunjes H, Koch MHJ. Physicochemical characterization of lipid nanoparticles and evaluation of their drug loading capacity and sustained release potential. J Control Release 1997; 48:223–236.

20. Speiser P. Lipidnanopellets als Trägersystem für Arzneimittel zur peroralen Anwendung. European Patent EP 0167825, 1990.

21. Domb AJ. Lipospheres for controlled delivery of substances. USP Patent USS 188837, 1993.

22. Müller RH, Lucks JS. Arzneistoffträger aus festen Lipidteilchen, Feste Lipidnanosphären (SLN), 1991.

23. Gasco MR. Method for producing solid lipid microspheres having a narrow size distribution. US Patent 5,250,236, 1993.

24. Hallberg D, Holm I, Obel AL, Schuberth O, Wretlind A. Fat emulsion for complete intravenous nutrition. Postgrad Med 1967; 42:A149–A152.

25. Wretlind A. Development of fat emulsions. J Parenter Enteral Nutr 1981; 5:230–235.

26. Wretlind A. Recollections of pioneers in nutrition: landmarks in the development of parenteral nutrition. J Am Coll Nutr 1992; 11:366–373.

27. Cavalli R, Caputo O, Marengo E, Pattarino F, Gasco MR. The effect of the components of microemulsions on both size and crystalline structure of solid lipid nanoparticles (SLN) containing a series of model molecules. Die Pharmazie 1998; 53:392–396.

28. Cavalli R, Marengo E, Rodriguez L, Gasco MR. Effects of some experimental factors on the production process of solid lipid nanoparticles. Eur J Pharm Biopharm 1996; 43:110–115.

29. Sjöström B, Bergenståhl B. Preparation of submicron drug particles in lecithin-stabilized o/w emulsions. I. Model studies of the precipitation of cholesteryl acetate. Int J Pharm 1992; 88:53–62.

30. Fessi C, Devissaguet J-P, Puisieux F, Thies C. Process for the preparation of dispersible colloidal systems of a substance in the form of nanoparticles. US Patent 5,118,528, 1992.
31. Quintanar-Guerrero D, Fessi H, Alléman E, Doelker E. Pseudolatex preparation using a novel emulsion-diffusion process involving direct displacement of partially-water-miscible solvents by distillation. Int J Pharm 1999; 188:155–164.
32. Heurtault B, Saulnier P, Pech B, Proust J-E, Richard J, Benoit J-P. Nanocapsules lipidiques, procédé de préparation et utilisation comme médicament, France, 2000.
33. Heurtault B, Saulnier P, Pech B, Proust J-E, Benoit J-P. A novel phase inversion-based process for the preparation of lipid nanocarriers. Pharm Res 2002; 19:875–880.
34. Siekmann B, Westesen K. Investigations on solid lipid nanoparticles prepared by precipitation in o/w emulsions. Eur J Pharm Biopharm 1996; 43:104–109.
35. Reithmeier H, Herrmann J, Göpferich A. Development and characterization of lipid microparticles as a drug carrier for somatostatin. Int J Pharm 2001; 218:133–143.
36. García-Fuentes M, Torres D, Alonso MJ. Design of lipid nanoparticles for the oral delivery of hydrophilic macromolecules. Colloid Surf B 2002; 27:159–168.
37. Schubert MA, Müller-Goymann CC. Solvent injection as a new approach for manufacturing lipid nanoparticles—evaluation of the method and process parameters. Eur J Pharm Biopharm 2003; 55:125–131.
38. Dubes A, Parrot-Lopez H, Abdelwahed W, et al. Scanning electron microscopy and atomic force microscopy imaging of solid lipid nanoparticles derived from amphiphilic cyclodextrins. Eur J Pharm Biopharm 2003; 55:279–282.
39. Hu FQ, Yuan H, Zhang HH, Fang M. Preparation of solid lipid nanoparticles with clobetasol propionate by a novel solvent diffusion method in aqueous system and physicochemical characterization. Int J Pharm 2002; 239:121–128.
40. Hu FQ, Hong Y, Yuan H. Preparation and characterization of solid lipid nanoparticles containing peptide. Int J Pharm 2004; 273:29–35.
41. Trotta M, Debernardi F, Caputo O. Preparation of solid lipid nanoparticles by a solvent emulsification-diffusion technique. Int J Pharm 2003; 257:153–160.
42. Shahgaldian P, Gualbert J, Aïssa K, Coleman AW. A study of the freeze-drying conditions of calixarene based solid lipid nanoparticles. Eur J Pharm Biopharm 2003; 55:181–184.
43. Heurtault B, Saulnier P, Pech B, et al. The influence of lipid nanocapsule composition on their size distribution. Eur J Pharm Sci 2003; 18:55–61.
44. Souto EB. SLN and NLC for topical delivery of antifungals. Ph.D. Thesis. Berlin: Free University of Berlin, 2005.
45. Mehnert W, zur Mühlen A, Dingler A, Weyhers H, Müller RH. Solid lipid nanoparticles (SLN)—ein neuartiger Wirkstoff-Carrier für Kosmetika und Pharmazeutika. II. Wirkstoff-Inkorporation, Freisetzung und Sterilizierbarkeit. Pharm Ind 1997; 59:511–514.
46. zur Mühlen A. Feste Lipid–Nanopartikel mit prolongierter Wirkstoffliberation: Herstellung, Langzeitsabilität, Charakterisierung, Freisetzungsverhalten und Mechanismen. Ph.D. Thesis. Berlin: Freie Universität Berlin, 1996.
47. Lukowski G, Werner U. Investigation of surface and drug release of solid lipid nanoparticles loaded with acyclovir. Int Symp Control Release Bioact Mater 1998; 25:425–428.
48. Jenning V. Feste Lipid-Nanopartikel (SLN) als Trägersystem für die dermale Applilkation von Retinol. Ph.D. Thesis. Berlin: Freie Universität Berlin, 1999.
49. Jenning V, Schäfer-Korting M, Gohla S. Vitamin A-loaded solid lipid nanoparticles for topical use: drug release properties. J Control Release 2000; 66:115–126.
50. Souto EB, Wissing SA, Barbosa CM, Müller RH. Evaluation of the physical stability of SLN and NLC before and after incorporation into hydrogel formulations. Eur J Pharm Biopharm 2004; 58:83–90.
51. Souto EB, Müller RH. Rheological and in vitro release behaviour of clotrimazole-containing aqueous SLN dispersions and commercial creams. Die Pharmazie.
52. Wissing SA, Lippacher A, Müller RH. Investigations on the occlusive properties of solid lipid nanoparticles (SLN). J Cosmet Sci 2001; 52:313–324.
53. Souto EB. SLN and NLC as drug carriers of clotrimazole for topical formulations. Master Thesis. Oporto: Oporto University, 2003.
54. Müller RH, Keck CM. Challenges and solutions for the delivery of biotech drugs—a review of drug nanocrystal technology and lipid nanoparticles. J Biotechnol 2004; 113:151–170.

55. Müller RH, Dingler A, Weyhers H, zur Mühlen A, Mehnert W. Solid lipid nanoparticles–ein neuartiger Wirkstoff-Carrier für Kosmetika und Pharmazeutika. 3. Mitteilung: Langzeitstabilität, Gefrier- und Sprühtrocknung, Toxizität, Anwendung in Kosmetika und Pharmazeutika. Pharm Ind 1997; 59:614–619.

56. Dingler A, Hildebrand G, Niehus H, Müller RH. Cosmetic anti-aging formulation based on vitamin E-loaded solid lipid nanoparticles. Proc Int Symp Control Release Bioact Mater 1998; 25:433–434.

57. Souto EB, Müller RH. Lipid nanoparticles (SLN and NLC) for drug delivery. In: Domb AJ, Tabata Y, Ravi Kumar MNV, Farber S, eds. Nanoparticles for Pharmaceutical Applications. Los Angeles, California: American Scientific Publishers, 2007:103–122.

58. Müller RH, Mehnert W, Lucks J-S, et al. Solid lipid nanoparticles (SLN)—an alternative colloidal carrier system for controlled drug delivery. Eur J Pharm Biopharm 1995; 41:62–69.

59. Schwarz C, Mehnert W. Solid lipid nanoparticles (SLN) for controlled drug delivery. II. Drug incorporation and physicochemical characterization. J Microencapsul 1999; 16:205–213.

60. Souto EB, Wissing SA, Barbosa CM, Müller RH. Development of a controlled release formulation based on SLN and NLC for topical clotrimazole delivery. Int J Pharm 2004; 278:71–77.

61. Weyhers H. Feste Lipid Nanopartikel (SLN) für die gewebsspezifische Arzneistoffapplikation, Herstellung, Charakterisierung oberflächenmodifizierter Formulierungen. Ph.D. Thesis. Berlin: Freie Universität Berlin, 1995.

62. Almeida AJ, Runge S, Müller RH. Peptide-loaded solid lipid nanoparticles (SLN): influence of production parameters. Int J Pharm 1997; 149:255–265.

63. zur Mühlen A, Mehnert W. Drug release and release mechanism of prednisolone loaded solid lipid nanoparticles. Die Pharmazie 1998; 53:552–555.

64. zur Mühlen A, Schwarz C, Mehnert W. Solid lipid nanoparticles (SLN) for controlled drug delivery—drug release and release mechanism. Eur J Pharm Biopharm 1998; 45:149–155.

65. Sakuma S, Suzuki N, Sudo R, Hiwatari K, Kishida A, Akashi M. Optimized chemical structure of nanoparticles as carriers for oral delivery of salmon calcitonin. Int J Pharm 2002; 239:185–195.

66. Dingler A. Feste Lipid-Nanopartickel als kolloidale Wirkstoffträgersysteme zur dermalen Applikation. Ph.D. Thesis. Berlin: Freie Universität Berlin, 1998.

67. Müller RH, Dingler A. Feste Lipid-Nanopartikel (Lipopearls™) als neuartiger Carrier für kosmetische und dermatologische Wirkstoffe. Pharm Zeit Dermo 1998; 49:11–15.

68. Souto EB, Müller RH. SLN and NLC for topical delivery of ketoconazole. J Microencapsul 2005; 22:501–510.

69. Dingler A, Lukowski G, Pflegel P, Müller RH, Gohla S. Production and characterization of Lipopearls for cosmetics. Proc Int Symp Control Release Bioact Mater 1997; 25:935–936.

70. Wissing SA, Müller RH. The influence of the crystallinity of lipid nanoparticles on their occlusive properties. Int J Pharm 2002; 242:377–379.

71. de Vringer T. Topical preparation containing a suspension of solid lipid particles. European Patent 91200664, 1992.

72. Teeranachaideekul V, Souto EB, Müller RH, Junyaprasert VB. Effect of surfactant on the physical and chemical stability of ascorbyl palmitate-loaded NLC system. In: AAPS annual meeting and exposition, Nashville, U.S.A., November 2005:6–10.

73. Teeranachaideekul V, Souto EB, Junyaprasert VB, Müller RH. Long-term physical stability of Q10-loaded NLC at different storage conditions. In: AAPS annual meeting and exposition, Nashville, U.S.A., November 2005:6–10.

74. Souto EB, Teeranachaideekul V, Junyaprasert VB, Müller RH. Encapsulation of nicotinamide into nanostructured lipid carriers. In: 15th international symposium on microencapsulation, Parma, Italy, September 2005:18–21.

75. Wissing SA. SLN als innovatives Formulierungskonzept für pflegende und protective dermale Zubereitungen. Ph.D. Thesis. Berlin: Freie Universität Berlin, 2002.

76. Wissing SA, Müller RH. The development of an improved carrier system for sunscreens formulations based on crystalline lipid nanoparticles. Int J Pharm 2002; 242:373–375.

77. Wissing SA, Müller RH. Solid lipid nanoparticles as carrier for sunscreens: in vitro release and in vivo skin penetration. J Control Release 2002; 81:225–233.
78. Wissing SA, Müller RH. In vitro and in vivo skin permeation of sunscreens from solid lipid nanoparticles (SLN™), supercooled melts and emulsions. In: Proceedings of the fourth world meeting APGI/APV, Florence, 2002:1135–1136.
79. Wissing SA, Müller RH. A novel sunscreen system based on tocopherol acetate incorporated into solid lipid nanoparticles. Int J Cosmet Sci 2001; 23:233–243.
80. Wissing SA, Müller RH. Solid lipid nanoparticles (SLN) as sunscreens: advantages over conventional emulsion based systems. Proc Int Symp Control Release Bioact Mater 2001; 28:522–523.
81. Mariani E, Neuhoff C, Bargagna A, et al. Synthesis, in vitro percutaneous absorption and phototoxicity of new benzylidene derivatives of 1,3,3-trimethyl-2-oxabicyclo(2.2.2)octan-6-one as potential UV sunscreens. Int J Pharm 1998; 161:65–73.
82. Saupe A. Pharmazeutisch-kosmetische Anwendungen Nanostrukturierter Lipidcarrier (NLC): Lichtschutz und Pflege. Ph.D. Thesis. Berlin: Freie Universität Berlin, 2004.
83. Bennat C. Lichtschutz mit Mikropigmenten–Beitrag zur physikochemischen Charakterisierung, galenischen Stabilisierung und Untersuchung des Penetrationsverhaltens von mikrofeinen Titandioxid und Zinkdioxid. Ph.D. Thesis. Braunschweig: TU Braunschweig, 1999.
84. Bennat C, Müller-Gowmann CC. Skin penetration and stabilization of formulations containing microfine titanium dioxide as physical UV filter. Int J Cosmet Sci 2000; 22:271–283.
85. Hagedorn-Leweke U, Lippold BC. Accumulation of sunscreens and other compounds in keratinous substrates. Eur J Pharm Biopharm 1998; 46:215–221.
86. Müller RH, Wissing SA, Mäder K. Sunscreens containing UV radiation reflecting of absorbing agents, protecting against harmful UV radiation and reinforcing the natural skin barrier. PCT Int Appl WO 01/03652, 2001.
87. Hommoss A, Souto EB, Müller RH. Assessment of the release profiles of a perfume incorporated into NLC dispersions in comparison to reference nanoemulsions. In: AAPS annual meeting and exposition, Nashville, U.S.A., November 2005:6–10.
88. Yaziksiz-Iscan Y, Wissing SA, Müller RH, Hekimoglu S. Different production methods for solid lipid nanoparticles (SLN) containing the insect repellent DEET. In: Proceedings of the fourth world meeting APGI/APV, Florence, 2002:789–790.
89. Yaziksiz-Iscan Y, Hekimoglu S, Sargon MF, Kas S, Hincal AA. In vitro release and skin permeation of DEET incorporated solid lipid nanoparticles in various vehicles. In: Proceedings of the fourth world meeting APGI/APV, Florence, 2002:1183–1184.
90. Yaziksiz-Iscan Y, Wissing SA, Hekimoglu S, Müller RH. Development of a novel carrier system for vitamin K using solid lipid nanoparticles (SLN™). In: Proceedings of the fourth world meeting APGI/APV, Florence, 2002:787–788.
91. Müller RH, Lippacher A, Gohla S. Solid lipid nanoparticles (SLN) as carrier system for the controlled release of drugs. In: Wise D, ed. Handbook of Pharmaceutical Controlled Release Technology. New York: Marcel Dekker, 2000:377–391.
92. Schneppe T. Entwicklung und Qualifizierung einer Pilotanlage zur GMP- und QM-gerechten Herstellung von festen Lipid-Nanopartickeln. Ph.D. Thesis. Berlin: Freie Universität Berlin, 1998.

15 Nano-Carriers of Drugs and Genes for the Treatment of Restenosis

Einat Cohen-Sela[†], Victoria Elazar[†], Hila Epstein-Barash[†], and Gershon Golomb
Department of Pharmaceutics, School of Pharmacy, The Hebrew University of Jerusalem, Jerusalem, Israel

INTRODUCTION

Restenosis

Percutaneous coronary interventions (PCIs) are widely employed for the revascularization of arteries obstructed by an atherosclerotic plaque in patients with symptomatic coronary artery disease, which usually presents as angina or myocardial infarction (1). The PCI procedures include balloon dilation, endoluminal stenting, excisional atherectomy, intravascular brachytherapy, and laser ablation. The successful treatment of stenotic coronary arteries by PCI is limited by the occurrences of restenosis, which continues to be a serious complication (2–6). Restenosis is characterized by three stages of response to the vessel wall injury: (*i*) acute elastic recoil, (*ii*) negative remodeling, and (*iii*) neointimal proliferation (7). Coronary artery stenting following balloon angioplasty significantly decreased restenosis rate by solving the problems of elastic recoil and vessel negative remodeling (5,8–10), however, in-stent restenosis, due to neointimal proliferation, remains the major limiting factor of PCI. An inflammatory healing response is triggered by the mechanical damage to the arterial wall (11–14). At first, platelets are activated and attached around the site of injury, followed by adhesion of inflammatory cells. Cytokines and growth factors are secreted by adjacent platelets, macrophages, and/or endothelial cells, including platelet-derived growth factor (PDGF), fibroblast growth factor (FGF), and interleukin-1β (IL-1β) (15), leading to proliferation and migration of smooth muscle cells (SMCs) towards the arterial lumen, with subsequent secretion of abundant extracellular matrix forming neointima and narrowing the artery.

The multifactorial pathogenesis of restenosis allows several options where pharmacological agents might be applied to prevent the disease process (16,17). A large number of clinical trials have investigated various systemic drug therapies in an attempt to reduce restenosis. Pharmacological therapies can be divided into categories based on mechanisms of action: prevention of thrombus formation, prevention of vascular recoil and remodeling, and prevention of inflammation and cell proliferation (16). None of the human trials demonstrated any beneficial effect on the incidence of restenosis. Systemic pharmacological approaches have failed in humans due to inability to achieve the required dose at the site of injury without causing systemic side effects (18). As a response to the failure of the systemic administration, the concept of local drug delivery emerged, offering the advantage of high local concentration and minimizing systemic side effects due to the relatively lower systemic concentrations. Until recently, locally delivered drugs have been unsuccessful in humans due to rapid washout of the drug (19), indicating the need

[†]Equal contribution to this work.

for a controlled administration of the drug for an adequate period of time. The most successful approach to date is drug-eluting stents, delivering medication directly to the site of vascular injury from polymeric coated stents (20–24). The first approved and commercially available drug-eluting stent was the Cypher (Cordis, a Johnson & Johnson Company; New Brunswick, New Jersey, U.S.A.), containing Rapamycin (Sirolimus), a naturally occurring macrolide antibiotic and a potent immunosuppressive agent (25,26). Taxus (Boston Scientific Corporation; Natick, Massachusetts, U.S.A.) was the second approved drug-eluting stent containing Paclitaxel (PXL), a microtubule-stabilizing agent with potent antiproliferative activity (27,28). However, despite their clinical success, the long-term efficacy and safety of these two drug-eluting stents are yet to be confirmed.

Nano-Carriers

Nano-carrier systems, such as liposomes, oil-in-water emulsions, and polymeric nanoparticles (NP), have been extensively investigated over the last few decades as a way to modify the biodistribution of drugs (29–36). An encapsulated drug follows the distribution of the carrier, rather than depending on the drug's physicochemical properties and molecular structure. The therapeutic efficacy of pharmacological agents is dependent on their biodistribution, as well as their elimination route and kinetics; thus, nano-carriers can be used to improve the therapeutic index of drugs. Nano-carriers have attractive biological properties, since carrier-incorporated pharmaceuticals are protected from the inactivation effect of external conditions, yet do not cause undesirable side reactions (37–39). In addition, nano-carriers may be utilized to achieve targeted therapies; targeting to a desirable site may lead to a more effective therapeutic drug action and prevent side effects (40).

Liposomes

Liposomes are microscopic phospholipid vesicles with a bilayered membrane structure and have received a lot of attention during the past 30 years as pharmaceutical carriers of great potential (41,42). Liposomes are formed by the self-assembly of phospholipid molecules in an aqueous environment. Liposomes are used as biocompatible carriers of drugs, peptides, proteins, plasmid DNA, and antisense oligonucleotides or ribozymes for pharmaceutical, cosmetic, and biochemical purposes (42). The enormous versatility in particle size (43,44) and in the physical parameters of the lipids affords an attractive potential for constructing tailor-made vehicles for a wide range of applications (45–63). Liposomes can be divided into three subgroups: classical (conventional) liposomes that are short circulating (64); long circulating liposomes, typically membrane-modified with polyethyleneglycol (PEG) (37,39,65–68); and immunoliposomes, liposomes with surface-attached ligands capable of recognizing and binding to cells of interest (69,70).

Nanoparticles

NP are solid colloidal particles in the nano-size range and, when formulated from biocompatible polymers, they can be used as drug carriers for therapeutic applications. Depending on their design, NP can be divided into two major subgroups: nanospheres (NS) and nanocapsules (NC). The NS are composed of a matrix structure, and NC are characterized by a polymeric rate-limiting membrane (71). The drug may be chemically bound to the particle-forming polymer, adsorbed on the NP surface, or entrapped in the NP (72,73).

The NP can be prepared by methods involving either polymerization of dispersed monomers or dispersion of preformed polymers. The use of preformed polymers is preferable, since they are well characterized and contain no residual monomers or polymerization reagents (74). The choice of the polymer depends upon the therapeutic application of the system, desired drug release, and bio-compatibility. The NP may be fabricated using biopolymers (gelatin, albumin, casein, polysaccharides, lectins, etc.) and synthetic polymers (polycianoacrylates, polyesters, polyanhydride, etc.). The biopolymers are not capable of providing protracted release kinetics for small drug molecules, thus limiting possible applications to delivery of biological macromolecules or drugs for which immediate action is desirable. The polymers most commonly used in this field of research are the synthetic aliphatic biodegradable polyesters, polylactide (PLA), polyglycolide (PLG), and their co-polymer (PLGA). The PLGA polymers have been used widely as biomaterials for medical applications over the last 30 years and are regarded as biocompatible and nontoxic (33).

Nano-Carriers in the Treatment of Restenosis
In designing a delivery system, it is important to consider the route of administration (local or systemic) and medication dose, as well as mechanism and duration of the desired drug action. Liposomes and NP as drug carriers can be utilized for the treatment of restenosis. The nanocarriers can be designed to have varying degradation and drug release profiles according to specific requirements (73), as well as tissue and cell localization properties, allowing control of their pharmacological action selectivity. Optimal drug delivery requires preferential localization to the site of injury, while maintaining a reservoir of drug sufficient for desired activity duration, in order to avoid uptake into noninjured segments of the artery and nonspecific cells (75,76). Several modifications of liposomes were proposed to cause selective cell targeting for the cardiovascular system (77). Modifications promoting targeting to the injured artery can be divided according to the specific ligands and receptors on cells involved: (*i*) GPIIb-IIIa receptor on activated platelets (78), (*ii*) tissue factor (TP) on vascular endothelial cells, (*iii*) upregulated PDGF receptor for SMCs migration/proliferation, and (*iv*) E- and/or P-selectine both on endothelial cells and platelets (79,80). Specific targeting for activated cells causes reduction of side effects in the nonactivated noninjured site due to lower or no expression on resting vascular cells (81).

LOCAL DRUG DELIVERY IN RESTENOSIS
It is accepted that the ultimate antirestenotic therapy will utilize the concept of local drug delivery, considering the regional nature of the restenotic process. This hypothesis is strongly supported by the virtual failure of systemically administered pharmacological agents to control restenosis (17,82), on one hand, and the success of drug-eluting stents (27,28), on the other. Local delivery of drugs directed against particular steps in the pathogenesis of restenosis enhances efficacy by increasing drug concentration to therapeutic levels in the immediate vicinity of vascular injury with minimal or the absence of systemic side effects (83–90). In addition, therapeutic agents with short half-life or chemically unstable agents are delivered directly to their site of target with minimal loss of therapeutic activity prior to their uptake. Furthermore, the incorporation of the drug into a carrier system allows controlling its release, thus fitting the drug release to the pathology demands (73).

Liposomes for local drug delivery offer the advantages of extensive uptake by a variety of cells and specific localization in the cells (43,44). By controlling liposome size, one can control the delivery (48,91–94). Small vesicles (<150 nm diameter) bind to cell surface receptors and are transported by receptor-mediated endocytosis. After internalization, the vesicle fuses with lysosomes, which induce the breakdown of the lipids and release of their contents (95–105). Large particles (>150 nm diameter), on the other hand, are taken up principally by phagocytosis, which is usually limited to phagocytic cells but can be induced in many other cell types with appropriate ligands (106). In both cases, the liposome could either be degraded in the low pH environment, or it could fuse directly with the endosomal or lysosomal membrane. Furthermore, the incorporation of drug within liposomal vector allows combination of rapid burst release and, at the same time, sustained release by simple controlling of the liposomal formulation.

In local drug delivery, the ultrasmall size of NP is an important advantage, since it enables higher arterial uptake because of the apparent ease of access to the arterial wall (107). Fishbein et al. (108) have shown that rhodamine B containing polymeric NP was traced in rat carotid arteries 24 hours after intraluminal delivery, whereas no fluorescent dye was present in the arterial segments treated with an equal amount of rhodamine B in solution (Fig. 1), indicating that the NP were able to prevent the rapid elimination of the free drug. Furthermore, NP offer the possibility of intra-arterial delivery via porous catheters that could be included as a final step in interventional cardiac catheterization (109–111).

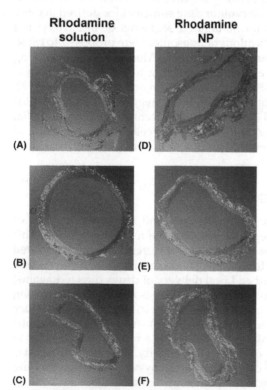

Rhodamine solution   **Rhodamine NP**

(A)   (D)

(B)   (E)

(C)   (F)

FIGURE 1 (*See color insert.*) Confocal images of balloon-injured rat carotid arteries after intaluminal delivery of rhodamine solution and rhodamine-containing nanoparticles. The arteries were harvested 90 minutes (**A** and **D**), eight hours (**B** and **E**), and one day (**C** and **F**) after delivery. *Abbreviation*: NP, nanoparticles. *Source*: From Ref. 108.

Gene Therapy for the Treatment of Restenosis

The local nature of the restenosis phenomenon makes it an attractive target for gene therapy, given that the tissue reaction that develops is directly accessible by the intervention itself (112). The success of gene therapy in the prevention of restenosis depends on the identification of appropriate molecular targets, a suitable vector system chosen for efficient vessel wall targeting, and methods for vascular gene delivery without producing undue damage or distal tissue ischemia (113). The appropriate genetic modification, performed locally at the time of angioplasty, could induce a long-term benefit in potency by fundamentally redirecting the healing response at its roots (114).

Several molecular species have been implicated in the stimulation of vascular smooth muscle cells (VSMCs) to initiate the intimal hyperplasic process (115,116): PDGF, basic fibroblast growth factor (bFGF), transforming growth factor beta (TGF- β), angiotensin II, and activator protein-1 (AP-1) (117–120).

Another strategy is focused on the cell cycle machinery of cells involved in proliferation and neointima formation (121,122). The VSMC proliferation depends on the increased expression of certain cell cycle regulatory proteins at critical points along the cell cycle, including proliferating cell nuclear antigen (PCNA), transcription factor E2F, nuclear factor-κB, cell division cycle 2 (cdc2) kinase, the cyclins, cyclin-dependent kinase (cdk), and nuclear protooncogenes (c-myc and c-myb), molecules that appear to be critical in the mitogenic signaling events (123–128). It has been hypothesized that by blocking the gene expression or function of one or more of these proteins, one could prevent the progression of VSMC through the cell cycle and inhibit neointimal growth. Thus, different regulatory molecules can be specific targets for gene therapy (2,129).

Gene therapy can be defined as a transfer of nucleic acids to the somatic cells of an individual with a resulting therapeutic effect, such as synthesis of missing or defective proteins (introduction of intact gene sequences) or expression blockade of disease-related genes (antisense technology, decoy oligonucleotides, and ribozymes) (130–133). Somatic gene therapy has emerged as a promising approach for the prevention of restenosis (134). The aim of antisense-short double-stranded DNA or RNA oligonucleotides strategy is to inhibit protein synthesis by selectively blocking the initiation of translation or increasing the mRNA degradation by RNase H (131,132,135). Natural phosphodiester antisense oligomers are susceptible to rapid degradation by nucleases. To overcome this problem, a number of chemically modified nuclease resistant analogs, such as phosphorotioated oligodeoxynucleotides (PT-ODNs) and chimeric oligomers (morpholino and peptide nucleic acids) have been designed (136–138). Some success in altering intimal hyperplasia in restenosis has been achieved using antisense oligonucleotides in *cell culture* and in animal models (139,140). Treatment with PT-ODNs against c-myc, using a polymer-based delivery system, resulted in only partial inhibition of VSMC growth in vitro and failed to reduce overall intimal hyperplasia in rat arterial injury model (141). Introduction of c-myb PT-ODNs, incorporated in the same carrier system, using the same animal model, was found to be effective in vivo (142). However, in further studies, the results were not confirmed.

Transfection of cis-element double-stranded oligodeoxynucleotides (decoy) has been reported as a powerful tool in a new class of antigene strategies for gene therapy. Synthetic double-stranded DNA with high affinity for a target transcription factor may be introduced into target cells as a "decoy" cis element to bind the transcriptional factor. Transfection of such "decoy" oligonucleotides results in attenuation of authentic cis–trans interaction, leading to the removal of the trans-factors from the endogenous cis-element with subsequent modulation of gene expression (143). Several studies have provided evidence of the in vivo application of this molecular approach as a therapeutic strategy against cardiovascular disease (133).

A major problem encountered with gene therapy and, particularly, the therapeutic use of oligonucleotides, is the low cellular permeability due to their large molecular size and high charge density and lysosomal degradation. The uptake of foreign genetic material (naked DNA, RNA, or oligonucleotide) by mammalian cells is an inefficient process (118,144). To improve their cellular delivery, several vector systems were developed (145,146). Viruses are among the most precise and stable gene vectors. Retroviral, adenoviral, and adeno-associated vectors have the advantage of exploiting the natural mechanisms of the body's cell receptors, thus increasing their efficacy and leading to a stable and long-term expression of the genetic material in the cells where they have been inserted (147,148). However, endogenous virus recombination, oncogenic effects, immunogenicity, and unknown long-term effects lead to serious limitations regarding their use in gene therapy (145,149–153). Moreover, the recent severe toxicity and side effects of acute T-cell leukemia in some patients that emerged in a recent clinical trial of retroviral vector in X-linked severe combined immunodeficiency highlights the importance of nonviral gene delivery (149,154).

Liposomal Gene Delivery

Nonviral transfection systems, such as cationic liposomes, hemagglutinating virus of Japan (HVJ)-liposomes, and biodegradable polymeric NP, are generally preferred over viruses because they are nonimmunogenic, relatively easy to assemble, form stable complexes with plasmid DNA, provide protection of the plasmid DNA from degradative nucleases, and are amenable to scale-up for industrial production (155,156). Their drawback is that they are less efficient than the viral vectors (113,157).

Cationic Liposomes

Complexing recombinant DNA with cationic liposomes consisting of cationic and neutral lipids, also known as cationic lipoplexes, are relatively efficient in delivering DNA into cells (158), however, the complex can be inactivated in the presence of serum, and there have been reports of instability upon storage (159). In addition, cytotoxicity of cationic liposomes remains a concern (160,161). The degree of successful gene transfer is highly dependent on the cationic lipid type, liposomal formulation, and cell type (162–165). Cationic vectors bind to negatively charged DNA, resulting in a condensation reaction and the formation of stable complexes in the nano range. Fusion with the cell membrane or endocytosis allows incorporation of DNA into the cell (166). Recent reports suggest that new liposomal formulations, individually optimized for the targeted tissue, with better protocols and/or continuously administered (poly-)-cationic liposomes may substantially increase transfection efficiencies (167–169). Transfection results have been different in various cell types and cell lines; thus, each reagent apparently has celltype-specific and additional species-specific characteristics (170). Newer lipids are being developed in order to enhance vascular gene transfer while minimizing toxicity. New compounds, such as (±)-N-(3-aminopropyl)-N,N-dimethyl-2,3-bis(dodecyloxy)-1-propanaminium bromide (GAP-DLRIE), and dioleoylphosphatidylethanolamine (DOPE), have been shown to increase the vascular delivery of plasmid DNA by 15-fold compared with previous cationic liposomes (171), screened nonviral formulations transfecting primary VSMCs in vitro with different concentrations and combinations of nonviral vectors as well as varying DNA/vector ratios and adjuvants. Uptake efficiencies ranged from 0.1% to 20% of transfected VSMC by changing liposomal parameters.

Use of cationic liposomes (Lipofectamine) for introduction of PT-ODNs, targeting human PCNA mRNA, in vitro influenced the oligonucleotide uptake in human VSMC and human atherosclerotic plaque, did not enhance antisense effect, but increased the magnitude of specific VSMC inhibition compared to the naked sequences (172). Nuclear factor-κB (NF-κB) decoy oligonucleotides transfected by cationic liposome method (Lipofectamine and TfX50) inhibited tumor necrosis factor-α (TNF-α)-induced expression of interleukin-6 (IL-6) and intracellular adhesion molecule-1 (ICAM-1) in mouse endothelial cells (173) and proliferation of rabbit VSMC (174) in vitro. 1,3-Dioleoyloxy-2-(N-[5]-carbamoyl-spermine)-propane (DOCSPER), a recently developed polycationic spermin with no addition of neutral lipid, has shown the best efficiency with less toxicity. In vivo studies, comparing 1,3-dioleoyloxy-2-(6-carboxy-spermyl)-propylamide (DOSPER) and Lipofectamine (DOSPA/DOPE 3:1 W/W) conducted in the pig balloon angioplasty model using plasmids coding for the antibacterial peptide cecropin A, showed greater reduction in neointima formation using DOSPER cationic liposomes in comparison to Lipofectamine as nonviral vector (175). The mechanism of enhancement of gene transfection rate using DOCSPER is not well understood. Nonviral vectors facilitate gene transfer in different ways, even in the same cell type, due to complex extracellular and intracellular events involved during the transfection process (176,177). Membrane binding, internalization, endosomal release, uncoating, and nuclear translocation constitute basic cellular events during nonviral gene transfer and may be involved in different degrees depending on the vector used. Combination of anionic liposomes/DNA and calcium ions has been suggested by Patil et al. (178) to enable efficient transfection with safer profile. Increased transfection of nonviral vector can be achieved in vitro as well as in vivo by controlling liposomal formulation and transfer conditions (175,177,179).

Fusigenic Liposome Hemagglutinating Virus of Japan-Liposomes (Virosom)

The HVJ or Sendai virus is a member of the murine paramyxovirus family, containing a single-stranded RNA virus genome with an envelope (165,180). The HVJ-envelope contains two glycoproteins: HN (hemagglutinating neuraminidase) and F (fusion protein). These HVJ-envelope proteins are involved in cell fusion. The HVJ virus is an enveloped large particle ranging from 300 to 600 nm in diameter. The viral particle, which is negatively charged and attached to sialic acid (the HVJ receptor), fuses with cell membrane, and releases its genome into cytoplasm directly, rather via the endocytosis (181).

The HVJ-liposome gene transfer technology was developed in late 1980s (e.g., Ref. 182) and early 1990s (e.g., Refs. 183 and 192) to introduce nucleic acids, oligodeoxynucleotide (ODN), and protein with high efficiency. The molecules included in HVJ-liposomes are delivered directly into various types of mammalian cells by means of the virus cell fusigenic character of HVJ. The HVJ-liposomes are constructed by a combination of inactivated viral particles and cationic liposomes to produce a nonviral gene transfer system (165,182,183). The HVJ-liposome nucleic acids or ODN are more efficient and safer than other nonviral vectors (184,185). Moreover, ODN delivered by HVJ-liposomes showed rapid accumulation in the nucleus, which persisted up to two weeks. In the second generation, HVJ-liposomes were modified from cationic to anionic. Anionic HVJ-liposomes showed a 5- to 10-fold higher gene expression in several cell types (186). The HVJ-liposomes have low immunogenic and low pathogenic profile (safety experiments were conducted in monkeys that demonstrated the safety, feasibility, and therapeutic potential of the HVJ-liposome vector for humans) (123,187). The HVJ-liposomes' versatility offered a wide range of different molecules and high transfection efficiency into a variety of cells both in vitro and in vivo (117,133,144,186–194).

Intact gene sequences were transferred using HVJ-liposomes for prevention of experimental restenosis. Plasmids, containing cDNA of endogenous neointimal growth inhibitors, such as nitric oxide synthase (NOS), prostacyclin synthase (PGIS), tissue factor pathway inhibitor (TFPI), were delivered to the vessel wall in vivo by means of HVJ-liposomes (186,188,189). Transfection of NOS inhibited neointima formation by 70%, 14 days after balloon injury of rat carotid artery (188). Introduction of cDNA encoding human PGIS into endothelium-denuded rat carotid arteries resulted in strong PGIS expression in neointimal cells at day 7 and significant inhibition of vascular lesion formation generated at day 14 after balloon injury (neointimal/medial area: 1.2 ± 0.4), in comparison to vehicle control group (1.7 ± 0.5; $P < 0.01$) (189). One week after angioplasty and TFPI gene delivery to rabbit iliac artery, TFPI protein was detected in neointima and media of the vessel wall. At four weeks, the minimal luminal diameter was significantly greater ($P < 0.01$) and the mean percentage of stenosis was significantly lower (37 ± 18 vs. $83 \pm 18\%$, $P < 0.01$) in the TFPI-transfected group than in the other three control groups (186).

The HVJ-liposomes were utilized to enhance the efficiency of cellular uptake and the stability of most commonly used phosphorothioated antisense oligonucleotides, while minimizing their nonspecific toxicity in several in vitro and in vivo studies (123,190–192). Cyclin B1 and cdc2 kinase antisense oligonucleotides, transferred into injured rat carotid arteries by HVJ-liposomes, were localized primarily in cell nuclei and caused partial, but specific and significant reduction of intimal hyperplasia up to eight weeks after transfection, whereas cyclin B1/cdc2 antisense combination completely abolished neointima formation (123). Transfection of antisense angiotensin-converting enzyme (ACE) oligonucleotides resulted in inhibition of neointimal growth by 50% without effect on blood pressure, heart rate, and serum ACE activity (193). Sustained inhibition of neointima growth was produced by a single administration of HVJ-liposomes containing antisense cdk2 kinase (65% neointima inhibition) or combinations of cdk2/cdc2 (85%) and cdc2/PCNA (50–60%) oligonucleotides (191,192). Transfection of decoy ODNs targeting transcription factor E2F using HVJ-liposomes inhibited the induction of c-myc, cdc2, and PCNA expression, as well as VSMC proliferation in vitro and markedly suppressed neointima formation compared with control-treated vessels in the model of rat carotid injury (neointima/media ratio for E2F-transfected segments: 0.291 ± 0.061 vs. untransfected ones: 1.117 ± 0.138) (194). HVJ-liposomal transfer of AP-1 decoy ODN resulted in significantly decreased VSMC growth ($P < 0.05$) and migration ($P < 0.01$) in cell culture and attenuation of intimal hyperplasia in rat vessel wall in vivo. Pretreatment of rat carotid artery with AP-1 decoy ODN before balloon injury was more effective than post-treatment ($P < 0.01$) in inhibiting neointimal formation (117,193,194).

Polymeric NP for Gene Delivery

Biodegradable NP also present a potentially advantageous drug delivery system to transfer genes for restenosis prevention, due to their nonviral nature and their ability to produce local activity of derived gene products (195). Antisense ODNs utilized to inhibit the function of growth regulatory or cell-cycle genes (c-myb, c-myc, PCNA, cdc2, and cdk2) of SMCs have been shown to decrease intimal thickening in experimental restenosis (139,140,142,191,196,197). Nevertheless, fully phosphorothioated antisense ODNs analogs were tested, which demonstrate high affinity for various cellular proteins, resulting in nonspecific effects. In addition, high concentrations of phosphorothioated ODNs inhibit DNA-polymerases and RNase H, which impairs their effectiveness as antisense agents (131). Cohen et al. (198) synthesized a novel partially phosphorothioated antisense ODN sequence for the purpose of minimizing the nonspecific effects of the fully phosphorothioated ODNs. The ODN was designed to downregulate PDGFR-β, which plays a pivotal role in the enhancement of SMCs migration after balloon angioplasty (199). The antisense was incorporated into a PLGA-based nanopaticulate system, and the antirestenotic efficacy was examined in the rat carotid artery model (Fig. 2A). The purpose of the encapsulation in NP was to enable the intracellular delivery of the ODN, which exhibit low cellular permeability due to its large molecular weight and high charge density.

The double emulsion–solvent evaporation method (200) was employed for the preparation of the PLGA-antisense NP, yielding NP with a spherical shape, homogeneous size distribution (~300 nm), high encapsulation efficiency (81%), and sustained release of PDGFR-β antisense for over a month. In order to achieve high encapsulation, calcium ions were added to the formulation, that minimized the escape of the negatively charged ODNs to the exterior phase (Fig. 2B), similar to plasmid DNA encapsulation as was previously reported by the same group (Fig. 2C) (201).

Partially phosphorothioated antisense sequences were found to be more specific than the fully phosphorothioated analogs in vitro. The in vivo efficiency was examined by locally administrating treatment and controls to rat carotid arteries, immediately after balloon injury. The rats were sacrificed after 14 days. Scrambled ODN sequence (naked and encapsulated) did not show any effect, which indicates that the antirestenotic effect was sequence-specific. A significant antirestenotic effect of the naked antisense sequence and the antisense-loaded NP was observed in comparison to blank NP that had no deleterious effect on the arteries, while the naked antisense showed a strong trend towards a greater effect than the nanoparticulate antisense, although this trend did not reach statistical significance. It was suggested that the dose of the ODN delivered from the NP was markedly lower in comparison to the naked antisense, since the release of the antisense from the NP was very slow. It was also proposed that the uptake into the artery was in favor of the dissolved material rather than the suspended NP. It can be concluded that while a more specific and effective antisense sequence was designed, the formulation should be further improved to meet the specific requirements of the disease. The failures of human clinical studies (130,202–204) suggest that the promise of gene therapy in restenosis was not fulfilled.

Local Drug Delivery of Drugs
Tyrphostins
Tyrphostins are a family of structurally related drugs that possess inhibitory activity against receptor-bound and cytoplasmic protein tyrosine kinases (PTK) (205,206). Derivatization of the basic structure of these compounds gives rise to inhibitors

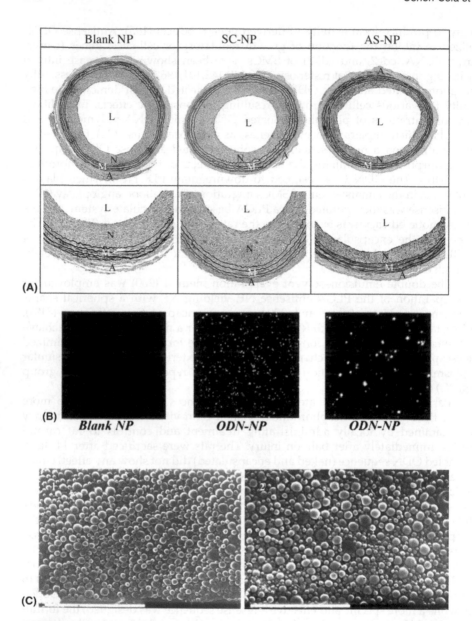

FIGURE 2 (**A**) (*See color insert.*) Inhibition of neointimal formation 14 days after balloon injury to rat carotid artery and intraluminal instillations with 20 µM (1 nmole) antisense or scrambled partially phosphorothioated oligodeoxynucleotides (PT-ODNs) encapsulated in PLGA nanoparticles (total of 50 µL suspension). Photomicrographs of representative histological sections. Verchoeff's elastin stain, magnification ×12.5. (**B**) (*See color insert.*) Fluorescence micrographs of blank and PT-ODN-loaded PLGA nanoparticles. The PT-ODNs were covalently labeled with FITC prior encapsulation. Note fluorescence signal in over 90% of the particles. (**C**) Scanning electron micrographs of blank (1) and plasmid DNA loaded (2) PLGA nanoparticles, prepared by double emulsion–solvent evaporation method. Gold coating (200 seconds), magnification ×5K, 30 kV, bar = 10 µM. *Abbreviations*: A, adventitia; L, lwnen; M, media; N, neointima; NP, nanoparticles; SC-NP, scrambled NP; AS-NP, antisense NP. *Source*: From Refs. 198 and 201.

exhibiting a high degree of specificity to PTK of a given type, such as PDGFR-β (207,208). The antirestenotic efficacy of locally delivered inhibitors AG-1295 and AGL-2043, formulated in PLA-based NP, has recently been evaluated (108,110,209). These two tyrphostins are low MW, aromatic compounds, whereas AGL-2043 has some solubility in water due to the presence of a polar moiety in its structure and AG-1295 is practically insoluble in water. Tyrphostin AG-1295 demonstrated SMC-specific inhibitory effect on cell growth in vitro and ex vivo (111,210) via inhibition of PDGFR-β-autophosphorilation, which supports the suggested mechanism of action. The AGL-2043 is a novel tyrphostin characterized by a higher affinity to the receptor and increased inhibitory potency (207). The tyrphostins were successfully entrapped in the PLA-based NP by the nanoprecipitation method (211), which involves a spontaneous gradient-driven diffusion of water miscible organic solvents into continuous aqueous phase (110,212,213). The release of both tyrphostins was studied using the external sink method. The AGL-2043 exhibited a more rapid release in comparison to AG-1295, apparently due to partial adsorption of the former on the NP (110,214). Rapid drug release associated with substantial drug distribution onto NP surface has previously been reported for other semi-polar compounds formulated in NP by nanoprecipitation (215).

Selected NP formulations of AG-1295 and AGL-2043 were evaluated in animal models of restenosis (108,110). Neointimal formation was significantly reduced by locally delivered 90 nm NP of both AG-1295 and AGL-2043 in comparison to control animals, but not by 160 nm NP at the same drug doses (108,110). The insignificant effect of the 160 nm particles might be associated with the less efficient ingress in the arterial tissue (108) and possibly with reduced uptake by SMCs (216). The small NP were characterized by a rapid elimination in the first 90 minutes followed by a slower late elimination (108). The early faster elimination of the smaller particles was probably caused by the easier migration to the adventitia, facilitating their elimination through the vasa vasorum. Their reduced late washout was probably due to their better penetration into deep arterial structures and creation of a drug depot that is relatively inaccessible to leaching by blood flow. The inferior antirestenotic effect of the large particles is in good accord with their low tissue drug level at advanced time points. The NP of AGL-2043 exhibited higher antirestenotic efficacy compared to AG-1295 loaded NP of comparable size and molar drug loading, which may be attributed to the lower potency of the second molecule. The pig model is considered to be more relevant for the pathophysiology of human restenosis (217). Further examination of the antirestenotic effect of NP formulations of the two tyrphostins was performed in the pig model, and a significant antirestenotic effect was observed in comparison with unloaded NP of the same size (110).

Dexamethasone

Dexamethasone (DXM) is a glucocorticosteroid drug that was found to significantly reduce neointimal proliferation in the rat carotid artery model, following periadventitial delivery (218). There are several possible mechanisms for the antirestenotic effect of glucocorticosteroids, including inhibition of PDGF production (219), IL-1β transcription (220) (a cytokine that stimulates SMCs proliferation), and reduction of the inflammatory response (221). In light of these results, Guzman et al. have decided to examine the antirestenotic efficacy of locally delivered DXM PLGA-based NP (109).

The result of the in vivo efficacy study in the rat carotid artery model demonstrated a significant decrease in the intima/media ratio with DXM NP, in comparison to blank NP and DXM NP injected intraperitoneally (IP) (109,222). The DXM levels in the arterial wall were detectable up to two weeks following intra-arterial administration of DXM NP, while no detectable DXM levels were observed beyond three hours after IP administration, indicating the successful localized delivery of the NP (109,222). The antirestenotic effect of DXM delivered in NP was compared to silicone perivasular delivery. The efficacy of the silicone implant was found to be higher by more than two-fold, in spite of the higher drug dose delivered into the artery by the NP (109,218,222). It was hypothesized that the inferior effect of the NP was due to their less efficient arterial uptake and shorter residence time in the artery, indicating the need for formulation improvement.

2-Aminochromone U-86893 (U86)

The U-86 is an antiproliferative cytostatic drug that was found to have an antichemotactic and antimutagenic activity on SMCs in vitro (223). A significant antirestenotic effect in balloon-injured rat carotid arteries was achieved by systemically injected U-86. However, due to rapid plasma clearance and poor oral availability, the IV doses required to achieve the therapeutic effect were very high and prolonged (223). Humphrey et al. (224) examined the inhibitory effect of PLGA-based U-86 NP on neointimal proliferation in porcine coronary arteries subjected to balloon injury. The emulsification solvent evaporation method was employed to formulate NP of 110 ± 40 nm. The release was biphasic and relatively prolonged; over 40% of the loaded drug was released over the first 24 hours, followed by a slow phase with exponentially decreasing release rate over the next two weeks. It was found that 9 mg of U-86 encapsulated within 60 mg of PLGA NP, locally administered by direct intramural infusion via the Dispatch® catheter, significantly reduces neointimal hyperplasia development in severely balloon-injured porcine coronary arteries. The antiproliferative effect of locally delivered nanoparticulate U-86 was limited primarily to those arteries that had extensive IEL/medial ruptures. No effect was observed in moderately injured vessels, which was probably due to insufficient retention of active drug in these vascular sites.

The Effect of Formulation Characteristics and Delivery Conditions on Arterial Uptake

In order to optimize the intra-arterial localization of therapeutic agents using the NP nano-carrier system, several groups examined the performance of NP as a function of formulation characteristics as well as delivery conditions.

Particle size was found to be an important determinant of the arterial uptake. Song et al. (225) reported on a three-fold lower arterial uptake of large PLGA-based NP (266 nm) in comparison to small-sized NP (100 nm) in the ex vivo dog femoral model. Westedt (226) demonstrated a size-dependent NP penetration into an intact rabbit vessel wall: while smaller NP (100–200 nm) were deposited in the inner regions of the vessel, larger NP (514 nm) accumulated primarily at the luminal surface of the aorta. It was demonstrated by the authors that the residence properties of tyrphostins-loaded NP in rat carotid arteries were influenced by their size. The smaller NP (90 nm) showed better ingress into the arterial tissue than the large NP (160 nm), as indicated by a 3.4-fold higher initial drug concentration in the tissue, more than eight-fold higher amount of NP remaining associated with the artery following the rapid NP washout phase and higher local drug levels maintained over 14 days following administration (108). Furthermore, the 90 nm NP, but not the 160 nm NP, significantly reduced neointimal hyperplasia in the rat carotid model, establishing for the first time a correlation between NP size and antirestenotic efficacy (108,110).

Drug loading in the NP carrier was also found to be a significant factor in the arterial uptake of NP. It was demonstrated that higher U-86 loading reduced the arterial U-86 levels in both ex vivo and in vivo studies (76), which can be attributed to faster release kinetics of the drug from the formulation containing the higher drug loading. An increase in the NP concentration in the infusion solution increased the arterial U-86 levels up to a certain NP concentration beyond which the arterial uptake of the NP was limited, probably due to charge neutralization (76). The same group also investigated the influence of surface modifications of PLGA-based NP containing U-86 on their arterial uptake (76,227). In general, cationic surface modifying agents demonstrated increased arterial drug levels. The NP surface, modified with a cationic compound didodecyldimethylammonium bromide (DMAB), demonstrated 7- to 10-fold greater U-86 arterial levels in comparison to unmodified NP in different ex vivo and in vivo studies. The mechanism responsible for the enhanced arterial uptake was assumed to involve an alteration in the NP surface charge (76).

The aforementioned data confirm that NP properties, such as size and surface chemistry, play a critical role in their arterial uptake and deposition; however, their successful application also depends on the delivery conditions, as well as on possible encountered anatomic barriers. In particular, for NP delivered to the artery by infusion through a balloon catheter delivery system, it was reported that the infusion duration and pressure influence the NP arterial localization. Repeated short infusions of NP suspension were found to be two-fold more effective in terms of drug arterial levels than a single prolonged infusion, which was not significantly different in efficacy from a short single infusion (227). In a different study, an enhancement of particle deposition at the delivery site was observed as a consequence of an infusion pressure increased from 2 to 4 atm. Recently, it was also reported that the localization of the NP in a coronary artery of a pig was influenced by the catheter type (228). The efficiency of arterial localization of NP was evaluated in the porcine coronary model using two catheters differing in their work principle. In the Dispach® catheter, the drug is infused into small closed chambers formed when the balloon is inflated and can diffuse into the arterial wall under pressure. The infusion using this catheter can be prolonged, since the blood continues to flow. The second catheter was the Infiltrator® in which the micro-injector-ports on the surface of the balloon penetrate the arterial wall upon inflation of the balloon and allow intramural delivery. This catheter cannot be used for prolonged infusion since it blocks the blood flow completely. The Dispach® was found to be more efficient than the Infiltrator®; it was suggested that that the micro-injector-ports may have failed to penetrate the intimal layer. Possible anatomic barriers to any particle transportation through the wall tissue are the intact internal and external elastic lamina. Moreover, the presence of an atherosclerotic plaque on the inner luminal surface strongly influences the particle penetration into the arterial wall (226). This observation points to at an additional aspect of local NP delivery strategies in restenosis that should be taken under consideration.

In summary, while NP present a promising drug carrier system for arterial local drug delivery, NP formulation properties, as well as their delivery protocol, should be carefully optimized to achieve the antirestenotic effect. The lack of clinical trials suggests that the promise from the studies was not fulfilled.

SYSTEMIC DRUG DELIVERY

The failure of the numerous systemic treatment attempts to prevent arterial restenosis in humans raises doubts regarding the feasibility of the systemic approach. However, an efficient systemic treatment could potentially address problems inherent in the local treatment strategy, regardless of its initial success rate. As opposed to local therapy, a systemic drug delivery system may allow the treatment of multiple lesions with a single injection and provide an option for convenient administration of repeat doses for the treatment optimization, as well as flexibility in choosing the type and number of stents to be deployed for varying lesion lengths, artery sizes, and anatomic locations.

Numerous studies established the potential of systemic treatment with liposomal and nanoparticulate formulations (95–97). By controlling their formulation characteristics and composition, these nano-carriers can present a highly efficient drug device with specific release profile and definite target sites (38,39,64,91,92,94, 229–232). In addition, due to their small size and biocompatible components, liposomes and NP are safe for parenteral administration. Furthermore, liposomes and NP can be surface-modified with tissue-specific ligand to achieve arterial localization, following systemic administration; however, to date, no significant developments have been reported for targeted delivery systems in vivo.

Systemic nano-carriers therapy for restenosis includes systemic administration intended for arterial localization, attained either passively (by controlling the formulation properties) or actively (by attaching the ligand on the nano-carrier surface), and systemic administration aimed at a systemic target.

Systemic Delivery for Arterial Localization
Doxorubicin
Doxorubicin is a drug clinically used for the treatment of cancer; it is often administered as a liposomal formulation pegylated or in ultrasmall nanosize in order to reduce its uptake by the mononuclear phagocyte system (mps) and reduce the drug toxicity (233). Doxorubicin damages DNA by intercalation of the anthracycline portion, metal ion chelation, or by generation of free radicals. It has also been shown to inhibit DNA topoisomerase II, which is critical to DNA function. The cytotoxic activity of the drug is not cell-cycle specific. NK911 are core-shell NP formed by PEG-based block copolymer encapsulating doxorubicin (234). When NK911 components are dissolved in the aqueous phase, they form stable NP (polymeric micelles) with an average diameter of 40 nm. NK911 NP were found to selectively penetrate through tumor vessel walls, having enhanced permeability (234). Enhanced vascular permeability that was first recognized in tumor tissues (235) was later on also observed in inflammatory and infected tissues (236–238). Uwatoku et al. (239) hypothesized that balloon-injured coronary arteries also have enhanced permeability and suggested that they could be a good target for NK911. They confirmed that balloon injury causes a marked and sustained increase in the vascular permeability for at least seven days using Evans Blue staining. The NK911 accumulated in the vascular lesion, where permeability was increased; the tissue concentrations of doxorubicin were up to four-fold higher three hours following IV injection of NK911 in comparison to free doxorubicin. Low drug levels were observed in the uninjured contralateral arteries used as a control. The accumulation was attributed to two factors: the size of the NP, which was adequate for enhanced accumulation, and the NP negative surface charge, which created an attraction of the formulation to

the positively charged luminal surface of the injured blood vessel. The IV injected NK911 immediately and three and six days after the balloon injury, but not doxorubicin alone, significantly inhibited restenosis in the rat carotid artery four weeks after the injury in both single- and double-injury models. It was demonstrated by immunostaining that the antirestenotic efficacy of doxorubicin NP was achieved by the inhibition of SMCs proliferation, rather than due to enhancement of apoptosis or inhibition of inflammatory cell recruitment. The RNA protection assay demonstrated that the expression of several cytokines was inhibited by NK911, but not that of apoptosis-related molecules. However, even in light of the encouraging results using the NK911 particles, the clinical potential of this formulation is limited due to the high toxicity of doxorubicin.

Paclitaxel
The PXL is a potent antiproliferative drug clinically used to treat cancer. The PXL promotes polymerization of the α- and β-units of tubulin and causes abnormal stabilization of microtubules required for G2 transition into M-phase (240,241). In low doses, the structural changes in the cytoskeleton result in a nearly complete inhibition of growth and proliferation and migration of SMCs for a long period. The most common delivery of PXL for the prevention of restenosis is local via drug-eluting stents (28). Kolodgie et al. (242) chose to examine the feasibility of systemic administration of nanopariculate PXL for the treatment of restenosis. The rationale was that systemic delivery of PXL would provide a more uniform stented arterial segment exposure to the drug, treatment of multiple lesions, and readily adjusted target dose. Nevertheless, it should be noted that the NP were administrated locally to the iliac bifurcation. A systemic IV infusion was only employed for the repeat dose at 28 days. The NP used was a novel albumin-stabilized 130 nm NP formulation of PXL (nPXL) (243). Using albumin as the stabilizer solved the hypersensitivity reactions (despite prophylaxis) and long infusion rates of 3 to 24 hours associated with the former nPXL containing Cremophor EL as the surfactant (244). Doses of nPXL were administrated as a 10-minute intra-arterial infusion through a balloon catheter at the iliac bifurcation to NZ white rabbits, immediately after bilateral iliac artery stent implantation. The nPXL reduced neointimal growth at 28 days produced in a dose–response manner, accompanied by incomplete healing. The efficacy was not sustained after 90 days following a single dose of nPXL of the highest dose tested (5 mg/kg). However, a second 3.5 mg/kg dose administrated intravenously 28 days after stenting led to persistent reduction of neointimal formation at 90 days with almost complete healing. It was suggested that the novel PXL formulation may offer an antirestenotic therapy with reduced toxicity that may overcome some of the limitations of the drug-coated stents. However, there are no proven advantages over the clinically used, highly successful, Taxus, drug-eluting stent.

Systemic Delivery for a Systemic Target
Better insights and understanding of the involvement of innate immunity as a vital factor in the progression of restenosis allowed the evolution of a new systemic therapy, directed against the immune cells. Innate immunity triggers the healing response that leads to neointimal formation (245–247). Monocytes/macrophages play a key role in the inflammation cascade, resulting in restenosis of blood vessels (248,249). Emerging experimental and clinical data indicate that the inflammatory cell number within the vessel wall is a powerful predictor of the extent of cellular

proliferation and intimal thickening (250,251). Monocytes/macrophages comprise up to 60% of neointimal cells after stent-induced arterial injury in rabbit, porcine, and nonhuman primate models and in human autopsy specimens (251). It was recently shown by Fukuda et al. (252) that the circulating monocytes count in human patients increased and reached its peak two days after stent implantation, and that the maximum monocytes count after stent implantation showed significant positive correlation with in-stent neointimal volume at six months follow-up in patients after stent implantations.

Macrophages belong to the MPS. They originate from pluripotent stem cells of bone marrow that are precursors for all hematopoietic cells, that is, lymphocytes, erythrocytes, osteoclasts, neutrophils, and mononuclear phagocytes (253). After certain differentiation steps in the bone marrow, the committed stem cells give rise to monocytes, which move to the circulation, migrate to distinct tissue compartments, and differentiate into macrophages. Macrophages are an essential part of the immune system; in normal steady state in the body, they form a constant population with a balance between renewal and cell death. In inflammation, the distribution and development of macrophages changes significantly (254–256). Following a stimulus such as inflammation, the amount of circulating monocytes and their migration to the site of inflammation increases significantly. It was hypothesized by the authors that systemic inactivation of monocytes and macrophages may lead to attenuation of neointimal formation. In order to target therapeutic agents to monocytes and macrophages, the authors used liposomes. Liposomes are readily taken up by cells of the MPS (formerly known as RES), macrophages, in particular, and to some extent, neutrophils, by the process of phagocytosis. Cell-specific delivery system for monocytes and macrophages depletion could be beneficial for the attenuation of the restenotic processes, while causing minimal toxicity to non-phagocytic cells (245).

Monocyte depletion was previously achieved by administration of other particulates, silica, asbestors (257), and carrageenan (258). These methods resulted in partial depletion as well as unwanted effects on non-phagocytic cells. Rooijen (259) was the first to use a liposomal formulation containing a bisphosphonate (BP) in order to deplete systemic monocytes. Liposomes for the treatment of restenosis via monocytes/macrophages depletion should possess optimal size distribution, since liposomes size control circulation time. The general trend for liposomes of similar composition is that increasing size translates into more rapid uptake by MPs (91,94), in particular by circulation monocytes.

Liposomes surface charge is also an important factor; charged liposomes are cleared more rapidly than neutral, and negatively charged liposomes are eliminated faster than positively charged liposomes (63,229,260). The effect of lipids composition, choosing lipids with specific transition phase, is an additional important factor that is intricately interrelated with the effect of charge. Circulation time is dependent on membrane packing and permeability considerations, as the inclusion of high-phase transition lipids will increase circulation lifetime. The presence of cholesterol in liposomes probably has one of the most important roles in the maintenance of membrane bilayer stability and, consequently, long circulation time in vivo (261). In the absence of cholesterol, liposomes are destabilized by high-density lipoprotein (HDL) particles and, upon release, their components can be readily eliminated from the circulation (262,263). Liposomes with cholesterol display negative correlation between clearance and stability in plasma (262). Designing an optimal liposomal formulation for the treatment of restenosis requires consideration of all these factors together. Negatively charged liposomes at the range of 200 nm are preferable due to the compromise between high phagocytic capacity by monocytes and lower systemic toxicity. In order to achieve optimal release profile and plasma stability, incorporation of cholesterol is essential. Conventional liposomes, negatively charged with an average size of 20 nm containing cholesterol, were utilized to achieve better and improved phagocytosis capacity and, at the same time, suitable release pattern and plasma stability. Thus, the MPS cells, mainly monocytes, are the target site for the systemic treatment of restenosis.

Bisphosphonates

The BPs, bone-seeking agents, are a family of drugs that inhibit bone resorption via osteoclast inactivation and are used clinically in several calcium-related disorders, such as tumor osteolysis and osteoporosis. The BPs are hydrophilic-charged molecules that do not penetrate cells (264,265). After administration to patients or animals, they accumulate mainly in bone tissue, and are cleared rapidly from the circulation into the urine (264–266). The in vivo effect on bone by BPs is mediated by the phagocytosis of the bone-adsorbed BP by osteoclasts. Osteoclasts and macrophages share a common hematopoietic progenitor cell in the bone marrow. Liposomes, a particulate dosage form, can be used to enhance the intracellular delivery of BPs into phagocytic cells, such as, monocytes/macrophages, in cell culture and in animals (259,267).

Negatively charged liposomes were prepared by thin lipid film hydration. The liposomes were composed of distearoylphosphatidylcholine (DSPC), phosphatidylglycerol (DSPG), and cholesterol (CHOL) at a ratio of 3:2:1, respectively (Fig. 3A). Anionic liposomes are nontoxic, and, after phagocytosis by monocytes/macrophages, the lipid bilayers of the liposomes are disrupted under the influence of the lysosomal phospholipases in the macrophage. The drug, which is dissolved in the aqueous compartments, is released into the cell. Furthermore, a free BP, released by leakage from liposomes or released from dead macrophages, will not enter cells in amounts that are able to disturb their metabolism. This approach, named the liposome-mediated macrophage "suicide" technique, was intensively used to eliminate macrophages from different compartments of the body in animals to study the role of macrophages in pathological and immunological conditions (268).

In macrophages, cell line (RAW264) and human monocytes (primary culture), highly endocytotic cells, it was found that encapsulation of BPs in liposomes enhances their inhibitory activity 20- to 1000-fold compared with free drug (Fig. 3B) (269–272). The SMCs and endothelial cells (ECs) are insensitive to the liposomal drug delivery (245). Enhanced phagocytosis into cells may be achieved by negative and positive charge of the liposomes (45,59,63,229,267). Positively charged lipids are not approved by the FDA for clinical use. The surface charge density of the liposomal bisphosphonates (LBPs) has been optimized for minimal leakage and effective intracellular delivery of encapsulated drugs (260,271).

Activated macrophages secrete cytokines and growth factors, leading to enhanced inflammation, and induce SMC proliferation and migration towards the arterial lumen, forming neointima and narrowing the artery (273–280). The BPs have numerous biochemical effects on cellular metabolism, ranging from the inhibition of general cell metabolism to modulation of cytokine secretion (281). Nonamino BPs as clodronate and etidronate have anti-inflammatory properties (282–284). They reduce cytokine secretion upon stimuli. In contrast to the non-amino-BPs, clodronate and etidronate, the amino-containing BPs, alendronate and pamidronate at a dose that does not kill the cells, showed proinflammatory properties on macrophage

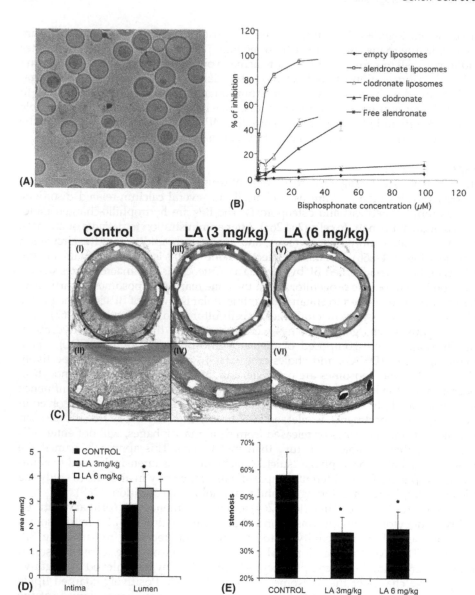

FIGURE 3 (**A**) Cryo-TEM microscopy of DSPC:DSPG:CHOL liposomes obtained by thin film hydration method, and extruded through 0.2 μm polycarbonate membranes. (**B**) Effect of liposomal formulations: bisphosphonates (BPs) (alendronate and clodronate), empty and free drugs on RAW 264 cell survival. Curves represent percent of cell inhibition with different BP concentrations. Cell count in buffer only was determined to be 100% (*n* = 3). (**C**) (*See color insert.*) Low- and high-power photomicrographs of hypercholesterolemic rabbit iliac artery stents at 28 days (Verhoeff staining) of control (I and II) and of animals treated with LA 3mg/kg (III and IV) and 6mg/kg (V and VI). (**D**) Bar graph showing reduction in intimal area and increased luminal area in treated animals. (**E**) Bar graph showing reduction in stenosis (%) in LA-treated animals (*n* = 16 arteries/group, **P* < 0.05). *Abbreviation*: LA, liposomal alendronate. *Source*: From Refs. 269 and 292.

functions by inducing the secretion of cytokines from macrophages (285). It has been shown that BPs also diminish secretion of reactive oxygen species by human neutrophils, polymorphonuclear leukocytes, and macrophages in vitro (286–288).

Encapsulation of BPs in liposomal formulations enhanced their potency. Liposomal clodronate (LC) was more than ten times more potent an inhibitor of cytokine secretion from RAW 264 than the free drug (289).

The PDGF-BB is a strong chemoattractant for vascular SMCs involved in neointima formation secondary to vascular injury (290,291). In vivo studies conducted in the authors' laboratory revealed that PDGFβR activation (i.e., tyrosine phosphorylation) is markedly increased to 135% of baseline levels in balloon-injured arteries of untreated rats, whereas it was barely detectable in LC-treated rats (i.e., below baseline activity) (269). Macrophages are a rich source of growth factors and cytokines, which facilitates SMCs migration to the injured vessel (248). Suppression of these mediators activation in treated animals (rat and rabbit) corresponds to a substantial reduction of PDGF-BB protein levels in the lesion, which can explain the reduced SMC migration and neointimal formation in treated animals. The authors' data are in conjunction with reduction in arterial and blood cytokines, IL-1β, TNFα, NFκB and MMP-2 activity, following injury (245). The systemic inactivation results in reduced expression of local inflammatory mediators, leading to reduced activation and proliferation of SMC and decreased neointimal formation.

It was reported by the authors that LBPs deplete blood monocytes (FACS), tissue macrophages, and total WBC (Coulter) count in the rabbit balloon angioplasty model (with or without stenting) (245,269). Systemic administration of LBP reduced circulating monocytes as well as tissue infiltration and accumulation of macrophages. The WBC count increased slightly 48 hours after surgery, with no significant difference between controls and the LBP groups (269). Monocyte number at 24 and 48 hours after balloon injury and stenting was significantly lower in LBPs-treated animals. Blood monocytes depletion and elevating WBC was partial and transient, lasting six days after IV injection of LBPs. Site-specific reduction of macrophages numbers was observed at the injured arterial site in LBPs-treated rabbits, three and six days after injury (245). Furthermore, the number of tissue macrophages in liver and spleen were reduced by LBPs at 6 days after treatment.

Liposomes loaded with the fluorescent marker, Rhodamine, with or without a BP were utilized to support the notion that LBPs exert their effects systemically (245,269). Depletion of systemic monocytes that carry the liposomes to the injured site should result in reduced arterial uptake of liposomes. Indeed, fluorescent-labeled LBPs significantly reduced the fluorescent signal in the injured arterial wall, whereas massive fluorescent was detected without the BP (245).

The LBPs were injected at different dosage regimens to rats and hypercholesterolemic rabbits to examine the therapeutic effect.

The rat carotid artery injured by a balloon catheter has been widely used as a model of angioplasty. The rat model is a "proliferation" model without foam cells. This form of injury causes immediate coagulation and thrombosis cascade in which platelets adhere, spread, and degranulate on the denuded surface of the artery, and, approximately 24 hours later, SMC begin to proliferate. The LBPs, clodronate and alendronate, were injected to male sabra rats, 15 mg/kg and 3 mg/kg, respectively. Marked neointimal formation and decreased luminal area were observed in control animals. The LC and liposomal alendronate (LA) suppressed intimal growth when administered IV on day −1 and +6. The N/M ratios were reduced by 60% and 69% for LC and LA, respectively (245,269,292).

The hypercholesterolemic rabbit model simulates the human model, since foam cells are involved. Liposomal clodronate and alendronate were injected one day before balloon angioplasty and six days after (15 mg/kg and 1.5 mg/kg, respectively), resulting in significant attenuation of intimal hyperplasia and luminal stenosis 28 days after surgery (245,269). Stenosis was reduced from $75 \pm 8\%$ in the control: empty liposomes, saline and free BP, to $41 \pm 8\%$ with LC treatment and $68 \pm 5\%$ with LA (3 mg/kg) treatment. Stenting procedure in the Iliac artery resulted in abundant concentric neointimal formation composed of SMC and foam cells, with both intraluminal and outward neointimal growth. Luminal stenosis 28 days after stenting was $58 \pm 11\%$. The LA (3 mg/kg) significantly reduced neointimal formation compared with control groups. No significant difference was observed between animals treated with 3 or 6 mg/kg LA or 15 mg/kg LC (Fig. 3C).

Different dosage regiments were examined; multiple doses of LC (15 mg/kg) or LA (1.5 mg/kg) one day before balloon angioplasty and six days after were found to have the same effect as one dose at day −1. Changing the time of injection from −1 to one injection six days after surgery had no effect. Treatment of LA, a single dose, at the time of injury required dose adjustment, elevation of dose from 1.5 to 3 mg/kg (269). A drug potency effect relationship of reducing restenosis was established by the authors, alendronate > pamidronate > ISA-13-1 > clodronate (266,293). Nonamino BPs as clodronate are several orders of magnitude less potent than the amino BP, alendronate, in inhibiting osteoclasts and consequently bone-related disorders, such as tumor osteolysis and osteoporosis (265). Consistent effect was established with monocytes/macrophage inhibition (245).

Having established the antirestenotic effect of BPs encapsulated in liposomes, the authors further investigated the use of polymeric NP for the same purpose, in order to examine whether a polymeric nanoparticulate formulation containing BPs could exert a comparable effect on LBPs. Similar to liposomes, a successful targeting to monocytes/macrophages requires knowledge of the particle characteristics that promote their phagocytosis. The physicochemical properties of NP, such as size and surface chemistry, also play an important role in opsonin adsorption and the elimination of NP from the circulation (294,295). Phagocytosis may be increased with increasing surface charge of the particle, particularly when the charge is negative (296). In addition, larger-sized particles are more inclined to be phagocytosed than smaller ones (297). Encapsulation of hydrophilic agents, such as BPs, in a nano-carrier based on a lipophilic polymer is challenging due to the agents' affinity for the external aqueous phase (40,225,298,299). The encapsulation efficiency of hydrophilic BPs in NP may be optimized by the in situ formation of their salts with low solubility in water, such as poorly water soluble complex with calcium. The double emulsion–solvent evaporation method (200) was used for the NP preparation, and their antirestenotic effect was examined in animal models. Unlike other NP formulations examined for restenosis therapy releasing the therapeutic agent in a slow release manner, the release rate of the BPs was designed to be rapid inside the phagocytic cell, protecting the drug in circulation for a sufficient period till phagocytosis. The NP of an aminobisphosphonate (ISA) were found to release 88% of the drug within 20 minutes and the release was completed within two hours. The ISA NP with encapsulation yield of 69% and average size of 392 nm, both subcutaneously and intravenously injected one day before balloon angioplasty (15 mg/kg), resulted in significant attenuation of intimal hyperplasia and stenosis at 14 days in the rat carotid injury model compared with control animals treated with free ISA, carrier solution or blank NP. Alendronate NP with encapsulation yield of 55.1% and average size of 223 nm, subcutaneously administered (1.5 mg/kg) one day before and six days after balloon angioplasty, resulted in a reduction of intimal hyperplasia and stenosis at 28 days in the rabbit model.

The effect of BPs encapsulated in nano-carriers on SMCs proliferation is indirectly mediated by the inhibitory effect on monocytes/macrophages. By systemic administration of BPs encapsulated in nano-carriers, systemic monocytes and tissue macrophages depletion is achieved, reducing the number of monocytes/macrophages available, and thereby reducing their accumulation in the arterial wall and the subsequent contribution to SMCs migration and proliferation. This approach, biologic targeting, is fundamentally different than any other treatment modality in restenosis. While other nano-carrier formulations, even if administrated systemically, are aimed to effect locally inhibiting local events related with the restenotic course of action, the encapsulated BPs present a systemic therapy to a systemic process, regardless of the procedure and the devices used. If effective in a clinical setting, it may be an easily administered, cost-effective modality that allows flexibility in choosing the type and number of stents to be deployed and may serve as an adjunct therapy in high-risk patients.

SUMMARY

To date, local drug delivery is considered to be the most favorable treatment for restenosis, with drug-eluting stents being the leading approach in clinical practice; however, their long-term efficacy and toxicity should be further examined. In addition, the antirestenotic effectiveness in high-risk groups, as well as in cases of small vessels, long lesions, and ostial or bifurcation lesions is yet to be established.

Another strategy for the prevention of restenosis by the local route investigated over the last few decades is nano-carriers, including liposomes and NP. These carriers offer a potentially improved delivery system, since they incorporate the advantages of local drug delivery and, in addition, enable targeting to specific cells. Liposomes and polymeric NP were found to be highly efficient in the local delivery of both pharmaceutical agents and gene products. In the field of gene therapy for restenosis, numerous liposomal formulations were examined. The formulations were modified by either surface charge or nonimmunogenic viral vectors for the enhancement of their penetration through the arterial wall as well as their incorporation into specific cells and specific intracellular localization. However, thus far, all the approaches in gene therapy for the prevention of restenosis failed to produce satisfactory results in clinical trails. The use of NP for gene therapy in restenosis is in its early stages. The systemic approach for restenosis prevention (with a free drug in solution) failed to produce satisfactory results in clinical trials. This is because therapeutic drug levels in the injured artery were not achieved following systemic administration.

The strategy of most systemic experimental therapies for restenosis is to achieve arterial localization following the systemic delivery of a pharmaceutical agent. The single unique approach of systemic administration aimed at a systemic target, termed "biological targeting," is the BPs-encapsulated nano-carriers. This latter approach was developed in view of the paradigm change that restenosis is a systemic disease manifested in local hyperplasia, which calls for a systemic intervention. Encapsulated BPs are targeted to deplete circulating monocytes, which are converted into macrophages at the site of injury, and play an important role in the course of restenosis. Such targeting requires specific formulation properties, including relatively larger particle size and high surface charge. Both liposomes and NP were found to be effective carriers for targeting of BP to monocytes, showing highly promising results as an antirestenosic therapy in rat and rabbit restenosis models.

Nano-carriers with their diverse size, high drug entrapment capacity, the ability to control their characteristics, and drug release profile present an advantageous delivery system for therapeutic agents in restenosis, suitable for both local and systemic administration. The systemic approach, if addressed properly, could provide significant advantages over local drug delivery.

REFERENCES

1. Garas SM, Huber P, Scott NA. Overview of therapies for prevention of restenosis after coronary interventions. Pharmacol Ther 2001; 92(2–3):165–178.
2. Bennett MR, O'Sullivan M. Mechanisms of angioplasty and stent restenosis: implications for design of rational therapy, Pharmacol Ther 2001; 91(2):149–166.
3. Bittl JA. Advances in coronary angioplasty. N Engl J Med 1996; 335(17):1290–1302.
4. Chorny M, Fishbein I, Golomb G, Drug delivery systems for the treatment of restenosis, Crit Rev Ther Drug 2000; 17(3):249–284.
5. Fischman DL, Leon MB, Baim DS, et al. A randomized comparison of coronary-stent placement and balloon angioplasty in the treatment of coronary-artery disease. N Engl J Med 1994; 331(8):496–501.
6. Libby P, Ganz P. Restenosis revisited—new targets, new therapies. N Engl J Med 1997; 337(6):418–419.
7. Mintz GS, Popma JJ, Pichard AD, et al. Arterial remodeling after coronary angioplasty–A serial intravascular ultrasound study. Circulation 1996; 94(1):35–43.
8. Hoffmann R, Mintz GS, Dussaillant GR, et al. Patterns and mechanisms of in-stent restenosis—a serial intravascular ultrasound study. Circulation 1996; 94(6):1247–1254.
9. Lowe HC, Oesterle SN, Khachigian LM. Coronary in-stent restenosis: current status and future strategies. J Am Coll Cardiol 2002; 39(2):183–193.
10. Mudra H, Regar E, Klauss V, et al. Serial follow-up after optimized ultrasound-guided deployment of Palmaz-Schatz stents—in-stent neointimal proliferation without significant reference segment response. Circulation 1997; 95(2):363–370.
11. Brasen JH, Kivela A, Roser K, et al. Angiogenesis, vascular endothelial growth factor and platelet-derived growth factor-BB expression, iron deposition, and oxidation-specific epitopes in stented human coronary arteries. Arterioscl Throm Vas 2001; 21(11):1720–1726.
12. Farb A, Sangiorgi G, Carter AJ, et al. Pathology of acute and chronic coronary stenting in humans. Circulation 1999; 99(1):44–52.
13. Grewe PH, Deneke T, Machraoui A, Barmeyer J, Muller KM. Acute and chronic tissue response to coronary stent implantation:pathologic findings in human specimen. J Am Coll Cardiol 2000; 35(1):157–163.
14. Kornowski R, Hong MK, Tio FO, Bramwell O, Wu HS, Leon MB. Instent restenosis: contributions of inflammatory responses and arterial injury to neointimal hyperplasia. J Am Coll Cardiol 1998; 31(1):224–230.
15. Bayes-Genis A, Campbell JH, Carlson PJ, Holmes DR, Schwartz, RS. Macrophages, myofibroblasts and neointimal hyperplasia after coronary artery injury and repair. Atherosclerosis 2002; 163(1):89–98.
16. Herrman JPR, Hermans WRM, Vos J, Serruys PW. Pharmacological approaches to the prevention of restenosis following angioplasty—the search for the holy-grail.1. Drugs 1993; 46(1):18–52.
17. Landzberg BR, Frishman WH, Lerrick K. Pathophysiology and pharmacological approaches for prevention of coronary artery restenosis following coronary artery balloon angioplasty and related procedures. Prog Cardiovasc Dis 1997; 39(4):361–398.
18. Faxon DP. Systemic drug therapy for restenosis—"Deja vu all over again," Circulation 2002; 106(18):2296–2298.

19. Versaci F, Gaspardone A, Tomai F, et al. Immunosuppressive therapy for the prevention of restenosis after coronary artery stent implantation (IMPRESS study). J Am Coll Cardiol 2002; 39(5):15a–15a.
20. Colombo A, Drzewiecki J, Banning A, et al. Randomized study to assess the effectiveness of slow- and moderate-release polymer-based paclitaxel-eluting stents for coronary artery lesions. Circulation 2003; 108(7):788–794.
21. Grube E, Silber S, Hauptmann KE, et al. Six- and twelve-month results from a randomized, double-blind trial on a slow-release paclitaxel-eluting stent for de novo coronary lesions. Circulation 2003; 107(1):38–42.
22. Morice M, Serruys PW, Sousa JE, et al. A randomized comparison of a sirolimus-eluting stent with a standard stent for coronary revascularization. New Engl J Med 2002; 346(23):1773–1780.
23. Moses JW, Leon MB, Popma JJ, et al. Sirolimus-eluting stents versus standard stents in patients with stenosis in a native coronary artery. New Engl J Med 2003; 349(14):1315–1323.
24. Schofer J, Schluter M, Gershlick AH, et al. Sirolimus-eluting stents for treatment of patients with long atherosclerotic lesions in small coronary arteries: double-blind, randomised controlled trial (E-SIRIUS). Lancet 2003; 362(9390):1093–1099.
25. Marx SO, Jayaraman T, Go LO, Marks AR. Rapamycin-FKBP inhibits cell cycle regulators of proliferation in vascular smooth muscle cells. Circ Res 1995; 76(3):412–417.
26. Poon M, Marx SO, Gallo R, Badimon JJ, Taubman MB, Marks AR. Rapamycin inhibits vascular smooth muscle cell migration. J Clin Invest 1996; 98(10):2277–2283.
27. Park SJ, Shim WH, Ho DS, et al. A paclitaxel-eluting stent for the prevention of coronary restenosis. N Engl J Med 2003; 348(16):1537–1545.
28. Stone GW, Ellis SG, Cox DA, et al. A polymer-based, paclitaxel-eluting stent in patients with coronary artery disease. N Engl J Med 2004; 350(3):221–231.
29. Ahsan FL, Rivas IP, Khan MA, Suarez AIT. Targeting to macrophages: role of physicochemical properties of particulate carriers-liposomes and microspheres—on the phagocytosis by macrophages. J Control Release 2002; 79(1–3):29–40.
30. Allen TM, Moase EH. Therapeutic opportunities for targeted liposomal drug delivery. Adv Drug Deliv Rev 1996; 21:117–133.
31. Kreuter J. Drug Targeting with nanoparticles. Eur J Drug Metab Ph 1994; 19(3):253–256.
32. Leroux JC, Cozens R, Roesel JL, et al. Pharmacokinetics of a novel HIV-1 protease inhibitor incorporated into biodegradable or enteric nanoparticles following intravenous and oral administration to mice. J Pharm Sci 1995; 84(12):1387–1391.
33. Moghimi SM, Hunter AC, Murray JC, Long-circulating and target-specific nanoparticles: theory to practice. Pharmacol Rev 2001; 53(2):283–318.
34. Nishioka Y, Yoshino H. Lymphatic targeting with nanoparticulate system. Adv Drug Deliv Rev 2001; 47(1):55–64.
35. Torchilin VP. Drug targeting. Eur J Pharm Sci 2000; 11(suppl 2):S81–S91.
36. Yokoyama M, Okano T. Targetable drug carriers: present status and a future perspective. Adv Drug Deliver Rev 1996; 21:77–80.
37. Gabizon A, Chemla M, Tzemach D, Horowitz AT, Goren D. Liposome longevity and stability in circulation: effects on the in vivo delivery to tumors and therapeutic efficacy of encapsulated anthracyclines. J Drug Target 1996; 3(5):391–398.
38. Gabizon A, Chisin R, Amselem S, et al. Pharmacokinetic and imaging studies in patients receiving a formulation of liposome-associated adriamycin. Br J Cancer 1991; 64(6):1125–1132.
39. Gabizon A, Papahadjopoulos D. Liposome formulations with prolonged circulation time in blood and enhanced uptake by tumors. Proc Natl Acad Sci USA 1988; 85(18):6949–6953.
40. Govender T, Stolnik S, Garnett MC, Illum L, Davis SS. PLGA nanoparticles prepared by nanoprecipitation: drug loading and release studies of a water soluble drug. J Control Release 1999; 57(2):171–185.
41. Torchilin VP. Liposomes as targetable drug carriers. Crit Rev Ther Drug Carrier Syst 1985; 2(1):65–115.
42. Torchilin VP. Recent advances with liposomes as pharmaceutical carriers. Nat Rev Drug Discov 2005; 4(2):145–160.

43. Szoka F, Olson F, Heath T, Vail W, Mayhew E, Papahadjopoulos D. Preparation of unilamellar liposomes of intermediate size (0.1–0.2 mumol) by a combination of reverse phase evaporation and extrusion through polycarbonate membranes. Biochim Biophys Acta 1980; 601(3):559–571.

44. Olson F, Hunt CA, Szoka FC, Vail WJ, Papahadjopoulos D. Preparation of liposomes of defined size distribution by extrusion through polycarbonate membranes. Biochim Biophys Acta 1979; 557(1):9–23.

45. Kosobe T, Moriyama E, Tokuoka Y, Kawashima N. Size and surface charge effect of 5-aminolevulinic acid-containing liposomes on photodynamic therapy for cultivated cancer cells. Drug Dev Ind Pharm 2005; 31(7):623–629.

46. Zhu J, Yan F, Guo Z, Marchant RE. Surface modification of liposomes by saccharides: vesicle size and stability of lactosyl liposomes studied by photon correlation spectroscopy. J Colloid Interface Sci 2005; 289(2):542–550.

47. Nomura SM, Mizutani Y, Kurita K, Watanabe A, Akiyoshi K, Changes in the morphology of cell-size liposomes in the presence of cholesterol: formation of neuron-like tubes and liposome networks. Biochim Biophys Acta 2005; 1669(2):164–169.

48. Nagayasu A, Uchiyama K, Kiwada H. The size of liposomes: a factor which affects their targeting efficiency to tumors and therapeutic activity of liposomal antitumor drugs. Adv Drug Deliv Rev 1999; 40(1–2):75–87.

49. Ishida O, Maruyama K, Sasaki K, Iwatsuru M. Size-dependent extravasation and interstitial localization of polyethyleneglycol liposomes in solid tumor-bearing mice. Int J Pharm 1999; 190(1):49–56.

50. Bajoria R, Contractor SF. Effect of the size of liposomes on the transfer and uptake of carboxyfluorescein by the perfused human term placenta. J Pharm Pharmacol 1997; 49(7):675–681.

51. Nagayasu A, Shimooka T, Kiwada H. Effect of vesicle size on in vivo release of daunorubicin from hydrogenated egg phosphatidylcholine-based liposomes into blood circulation. Biol Pharm Bull 1995; 18(7):1020–1023.

52. Nagayasu A, Shimooka T, Kinouchi Y, Uchiyama K, Takeichi Y, Kiwada H. Effects of fluidity and vesicle size on antitumor activity and myelosuppressive activity of liposomes loaded with daunorubicin. Biol Pharm Bull 1994; 17(7):935–939.

53. Liu D, Mori A, Huang L. Role of liposome size and RES blockade in controlling biodistribution and tumor uptake of GM1-containing liposomes. Biochim Biophys Acta 1992; 1104(1):95–101.

54. Jones MN, Nicholas AR. The effect of blood serum on the size and stability of phospholipid liposomes. Biochim Biophys Acta 1991; 1065(2):145–152.

55. Barza M, Stuart M, Szoka F, Jr. Effect of size and lipid composition on the pharmacokinetics of intravitreal liposomes. Invest Ophthalmol Vis Sci 1987; 28(5):893–900.

56. Sato Y, Kiwada H, Kato Y. Effects of dose and vesicle size on the pharmacokinetics of liposomes. Chem Pharm Bull (Tokyo) 1986; 34(10):4244–4252.

57. Richards RL, Habbersett RC, Scher I, et al. Influence of vesicle size on complement-dependent immune damage to liposomes. Biochim Biophys Acta 1986; 855(2):223–230.

58. Magin RL, Hunter JM, Niesman MR, Bark GA. Effect of vesicle size on the clearance, distribution, and tumor uptake of temperature-sensitive liposomes. Cancer Drug Deliv 1986; 3(4):223–237.

59. Schwendener RA, Lagocki PA, Rahman YE. The effects of charge and size on the interaction of unilamellar liposomes with macrophages. Biochim Biophys Acta 1984; 772(1):93–101.

60. Margolis LB, Neyfakh AA, Jr. The distribution of solid liposomes of different size on the surface of epithelial cells. Eur J Cell Biol 1983; 31(2):256–262.

61. Yager P, Sheridan JP, Peticolas WL, Changes in size and shape of liposomes undergoing chain melting transitions as studied by optical microscopy. Biochim Biophys Acta 1982; 693(2):485–491.

62. Rahman YE, Cerny EA, Patel KR, Lau EH, Wright BJ. Differential uptake of liposomes varying in size and lipid composition by parenchymal and kupffer cells of mouse liver. Life Sci 1982; 31(19):2061–2071.

63. Juliano RL, Stamp D. The effect of particle size and charge on the clearance rates of liposomes and liposome encapsulated drugs. Biochem Biophys Res Commun 1975; 63(3):651–658.

64. Lasic DD. Novel applications of liposomes. Trends Biotechnol 1998; 16(7):307–321.
65. Lasic DD, Martin FJ, Gabizon A, Huang SK, Papahadjopoulos D. Sterically stabilized liposomes: a hypothesis on the molecular origin of the extended circulation times. Biochim Biophys Acta 1991; 1070(1):187–192.
66. Lasic DD, Vallner JJ, Working PK. Sterically stabilized liposomes in cancer therapy and gene delivery. Curr Opin Mol Ther 1999; 1(2):177–185.
67. Papahadjopoulos D, Allen TM, Gabizon A, et al. Sterically stabilized liposomes: improvements in pharmacokinetics and antitumor therapeutic efficacy. Proc Natl Acad Sci USA 1991; 88(24):11,460–11,464.
68. Woodle MC, Lasic DD. Sterically stabilized liposomes. Biochim Biophys Acta 1992; 1113(2):171–199.
69. Hosokawa S, Tagawa T, Niki H, Hirakawa Y, Nohga K, Nagaike K. Efficacy of immunoliposomes on cancer models in a cell-surface-antigen-density-dependent manner. Br J Cancer 2003; 89(8):1545–1551.
70. Huang A, Kennel SJ, Huang L. Interactions of immunoliposomes with target cells. J Biol Chem 1983; 258(22):14,034–14,040.
71. Allemann E, Gurny R, Doelker E. Drug-loaded nanoparticles—preparation methods and drug targeting issues. Eur J Pharm Biopharm 1993; 39(5):173–191.
72. Kreuter J. Nanoparticle-based drug delivery systems. J Control Release 1991; 16(1–2):169–176.
73. Labhasetwar V, Song CX, Levy RJ. Nanoparticle drug delivery system for restenosis. Adv Drug Deliver Rev 1997; 24(1):63–85.
74. Soppimath KS, Aminabhavi TM, Kulkarni AR, Rudzinski WE. Biodegradable polymeric nanoparticles as drug delivery devices. J Control Release 2001; 70(1–2):1–20.
75. Labhasetwar V. Levy RJ. Implants for site-specific drug delivery. J Appl Biomater 1991; 2(3):211–212.
76. Labhasetwar V, Song C, Humphrey W, Shebuski R, Levy RJ. Arterial uptake of biodegradable nanoparticles: effect of surface modifications. J Pharm Sci 1998; 87(10):1229–1234.
77. Lestini BJ, Sagnella SM, Xu Z, et al. Surface modification of liposomes for selective cell targeting in cardiovascular drug delivery. J Control Release 2002; 78(1–3):235–247.
78. Ghaffari S, Kereiakes DJ, Lincoff AM, et al. Platelet glycoprotein IIb/IIIa receptor blockade with abciximab reduces ischemic complications in patients undergoing directional coronary atherectomy. EPILOG Investigators. Evaluation of PTCA to improve long-term outcome by c7E3 GP IIb/IIIa receptor blockade. Am J Cardiol 1998; 82(1):7–12.
79. Everts M, Koning GA, Kok RJ, et al. In vitro cellular handling and in vivo targeting of E-selectindirected immunoconjugates and immunoliposomes used for drug delivery to inflamed endothelium. Pharm Res 2003; 20(1):64–72.
80. Huwyler J, Cerletti A, Fricker G, Eberle AN, Drewe J. By-passing of Pglycoprotein using immunoliposomes. J Drug Target 2002; 10(1):73–79.
81. Edelman ER, Karnovsky MJ. Contrasting effects of the intermittent and continuous administration of heparin in experimental restenosis. Circulation 1994; 89(2):770–776.
82. Lefkovits J, Topol EJ. Pharmacological approaches for the prevention of restenosis after percutaneous coronary intervention. Prog Cardiovasc Dis 1997; 40(2):141–158.
83. Itoh T, Nonogi H, Miyazaki S, et al. Local delivery of argatroban for the prevention of restenosis after coronary balloon angioplasty: a prospective randomized pilot study. Circ J 2004; 68(7):615–22.
84. Kavanagh CA, Rochev YA, Gallagher WM, Dawson KA, Keenan AK. Local drug delivery in restenosis injury: thermoresponsive co-polymers as potential drug delivery systems. Pharmacol Ther 2004; 102(1):1–15.
85. Tepe G, Duda SH, Kalinowski M, et al. Local intra-arterial drug delivery for prevention of restenosis: comparison of the efficiency of delivery of different radiopharmaceuticals through a porous catheter. Invest Radiol 2001; 36(5):245–249.
86. Ettenson DS, Edelman ER. Local drug delivery: an emerging approach in the treatment of restenosis. Vasc Med 2000; 5(2):97–102.
87. Bonan R. Local drug delivery for the treatment of thrombus and restenosis. J Invasive Cardiol 1996; 8(8):399–402.

88. Brieger D. Topol E. Local drug delivery systems and prevention of restenosis. Cardiovasc Res 1997; 35(3):405–413.

89. Gradus-Pizlo I, Wilensky RL, March KL, et al. Local delivery of biodegradable microparticles containing colchicine or a colchicine analogue: effects on restenosis and implications for catheter-based drug delivery. J Am Coll Cardiol 1995; 26(6):1549–1557.

90. Lincoff AM, Topol EJ, Ellis SG. Local drug delivery for the prevention of restenosis. Fact, fancy, and future. Circulation 1994; 90(4):2070–2084.

91. Allen TM, Austin GA, Chonn A, Lin L, Lee KC. Uptake of liposomes by cultured mouse bone marrow macrophages: influence of liposome composition and size. Biochim Biophys Acta 1991; 1061(1):56–64.

92. Allen TM, Hansen C, Rutledge J. Liposomes with prolonged circulation times: factors affecting uptake by reticuloendothelial and other tissues. Biochim Biophys Acta 1989; 981(1):27–35.

93. Allen TM, Mehra T. Recent advances in sustained release of antineoplastic drugs using liposomes which avoid uptake into the reticuloendothelial system. Proc West Pharmacol Soc 1989; 32:111–114.

94. Allen TM, Chonn A. Large unilamellar liposomes with low uptake into the reticuloendothelial system. FEBS Lett 1987; 223(1):42–46.

95. Michaelis M, Zimmer A, Handjou N, Cinatl J, Cinatl J, Jr. Increased systemic efficacy of aphidicolin encapsulated in liposomes. Oncol Rep 2005; 13(1):157–160.

96. Asrani S, D'Anna S, Alkan-Onyuksel H, Wang W, Goodman D, Zeimer R. Systemic toxicology and laser safety of laser targeted angiography with heat sensitive liposomes. J Ocul Pharmacol Ther 1995; 11(4):575–584.

97. Qi XR, Maitani Y, Nagai T. Rates of systemic degradation and reticuloendothelial system uptake of calcein in the dipalmitoylphosphatidylcholine liposomes with soybean-derived sterols in mice. Pharm Res 1995; 12(1):49–52.

98. Zuwala-Jagiello J. Endocytosis mediated by receptors—function and participation in oral drug delivery. Postepy Hig Med Dosw 2003; 57(3):275–291.

99. Muro S, Koval M, Muzykantov V. Endothelial endocytic pathways: gates for vascular drug delivery. Curr Vasc Pharmacol 2004; 2(3):281–299.

100. Bathori G, Cervenak L, Karadi I. Caveolae—an alternative endocytotic pathway for targeted drug delivery. Crit Rev Ther Drug Carrier Syst 2004; 21(2):67–95.

101. Rejman J, Oberle V, Zuhorn IS, Hoekstra D. Size-dependent internalization of particles via the pathways of clathrin- and caveolae-mediated endocytosis, Biochem J 2004; 377(Pt 1):159–169.

102. Ruckert P, Bates SR, Fisher AB. Role of clathrin- and actin-dependent endocytotic pathways in lung phospholipid uptake. Am J Physiol Lung Cell Mol Physiol 2003; 284(6): L981–L989.

103. Takei K, Slepnev VI, Haucke V, De Camilli P. Functional partnership between amphiphysin and dynamin in clathrin-mediated endocytosis. Nat Cell Biol 1999; 1(1):33–39.

104. Perry DG, Daugherty GL, Martin WJ, II. Clathrin-coated pit-associated proteins are required for alveolar macrophage phagocytosis. J Immunol 1999; 162(1):380–386.

105. Beck KA, Chang M, Brodsky FM, Keen JH. Clathrin assembly protein AP-2 induces aggregation of membrane vesicles: a possible role for AP-2 in endosome formation. J Cell Biol 1992; 119(4):787–796.

106. Yamashita C, Sone S, Ogura T, Kiwada H, Potential value of cetylmannosidemodified liposomes as carriers of macrophage activators to human blood monocytes. Jpn J Cancer Res 1991; 82(5):569–576.

107. Eccleston DS, Lincoff AM. Catheter-based drug delivery for restenosis. Adv Drug Deliver Rev 1997; 24(1):31–43.

108. Fishbein I, Chorny M, Banai S, et al. Formulation and delivery mode affect disposition and activity of tyrphostin-loaded nanoparticles in the rat carotid model. Arterioscler Thromb Vasc Biol 2001; 21(9):1434–1439.

109. Guzman LA, Labhasetwar V, Song CX, et al. Local intraluminal infusion of biodegradable polymeric nanoparticles—A novel approach for prolonged drug delivery after balloon angioplasty. Circulation 1996; 94(6):1441–1448.

110. Banai S, Chorny M, Gertz SD, et al. Locally delivered nanoencapsulated tyrphostin (AGL-2043) reduces neointima formation in balloon-injured rat carotid and stented porcine coronary arteries, Biomaterials 2005; 26(4):451–461.
111. Banai S, Wolf Y, Golomb G, et al. PDGF-receptor tyrosine kinase blocker AG1295 selectively attenuates smooth muscle cell growth in vitro and reduces neointimal formation after balloon angioplasty in swine. Circulation 1998; 97(19):1960–1969.
112. Caplice N, Simari R. Gene transfer for coronary restenosis. Curr Interv Cardiol Rep 1999; 1(2):157–164.
113. Ehsan A, Mann MJ. Antisense and gene therapy to prevent restenosis. Vasc Med 2000; 5(2):103–114.
114. Dedieu JF, Mahfoudi A, Le Roux A, Branellec D. Vectors for gene therapy of cardiovascular disease. Curr Cardiol Rep 2000; 2(1):39–47.
115. Pauletto P, Sartore S, Pessina AC. Smooth-muscle-cell proliferation and differentiation in neointima formation and vascular restenosis. Clin Sci (Lond) 1994; 87(5):467–479.
116. Finkel T. Epstein E. Gene therapy for vascular disease. FASEB J 1995; 9:843–851.
117. Ahn JD, Morishita R, Kaneda Y, et al. Inhibitory effects of novel AP-1 decoy oligodeoxynucleotides on vascular smooth muscle cell proliferation in vitro and neointimal formation in vivo. Circ Res 2002; 90(12):1325–1332.
118. Kaiser S, Toborek M. Liposome-mediated high-efficiency transfection of human endothelial cells. J Vasc Res 2001; 38(2):133–143.
119. Tomita N, Azuma H, Kaneda Y, Ogihara T, Morishita R. Gene therapy with transcription factor decoy oligonucleotides as a potential treatment for cardiovascular diseases. Curr Drug Targets 2003; 4(4):339–346.
120. Kume M, Komori K, Matsumoto T, et al. Administration of a decoy against the activator protein-1 binding site suppresses neointimal thickening in rabbit balloon-injured arteries. Circulation 2002; 105(10):1226–1232.
121. Kullo IJ, Simari RD, Schwartz RS, Vascular gene transfer: from bench to bedside. Arterioscler Thromb Vasc Biol 1999; 19(2):196–207.
122. Li JM, Brooks G. Cell cycle regulatory molecules (cyclins, cyclin-dependent kinases and cyclin-dependent kinase inhibitors) and the cardiovascular system; potential targets for therapy? Eur Heart J 1999; 20(6):406–420.
123. Morishita R, Gibbons GH, Kaneda Y, Ogihara T, Dzau VJ. Pharmacokinetics of antisense oligodeoxyribonucleotides (cyclin-B-1 and Cdc-2 kinase) in the vessel wall in vivo—enhanced therapeutic utility for restenosis by Hvj-liposome delivery. Gene 1994; 149(1):13–19.
124. Clowes AW, Schwartz SM. Significance of quiescent smooth muscle migration in the injured rat carotid artery. Circ Res 1985; 56(1):139–145.
125. Fingerle J, Johnson R, Clowes AW, Majesky MW, Reidy MA. Role of platelets in smooth muscle cell proliferation and migration after vascular injury in rat carotid artery. Proc Natl Acad Sci USA 1989; 86(21):8412–8416.
126. Clowes AW, Clowes MM, Au YP, Reidy MA, Belin D. Smooth muscle cells express urokinase during mitogenesis and tissue-type plasminogen activator during migration in injured rat carotid artery. Circ Res 1990; 67(1):61–67.
127. Chan AK, Kalmes A, Hawkins S, Daum G, Clowes AW. Blockade of the epidermal growth factor receptor decreases intimal hyperplasia in balloon-injured rat carotid artery. J Vasc Surg 2003; 37(3):644–649.
128. Shi Y, Hutchinson HG, Hall DJ, Zalewski A. Down-regulation of c-myc expression by antisense oligonucleotides inhibits proliferation of human smooth-muscle cells. Circulation 1993; 88(3):1190–1195.
129. Isobe M, Morishita R, Suzuki J. New approaches to treat cardiovascular diseases targeting NFkB. J Mol Cell Cardio 2004; 37(1):316–316.
130. Cavazzana-Calvo M, Thrasher A, Mavilio F. The future of gene therapy, Nature 2004; 427(6977):779–781.
131. Stein CA. The experimental use of antisense oligonucleotides: a guide for the perplexed. J Clin Invest 2001; 108(5):641–644.
132. Lambert G, Fattal E, Couvreur P. Nanoparticulate systems for the delivery of antisense oligonucleotides. Adv Drug Deliv Rev 2001; 47(1):99–112.

133. Morishita R, Aoki M, Kaneda Y. Decoy oligodeoxynucleotides as novel cardiovascular drugs for cardiovascular disease. Ann NY Acad Sci 2001; 947, 294–301; discussion 301–302.

134. Gottschalk U, Chan S. Somatic gene therapy: present situation and future perspective. Drug Res 1998; 48:1111–1120.

135. Deshpande D, Rojanasakul Y. Antisense oligonucleotide therapeutics: a class of its own. Pharmaceutical News 1996; 3:15–18.

136. Santiago FS, Khachigian LM. Nucleic acid based strategies as potential therapeutic tools: mechanistic considerations and implications to restenosis. J Mol Med 2001; 79(12):695–706.

137. Taylor MF. Emerging antisense technologies for gene functionalization and drug delivery. DDT 2001; 6:S97–S101.

138. Scanlon KJ, Ohta Y, Ishida H, et al. Oligonucleotide-mediated modulation of mammalian gene expression. FASEB J 1995; 9(13):1288–1296.

139. Sirois MG, Simons M, Edelman ER. Antisense oligonucleotide inhibition of PDGFR-beta receptor subunit expression directs suppression of intimal thickening. Circulation 1997; 95(3):669–676.

140. Villa AE, Guzman LA, Poptic EJ, et al. Effects of antisense c-myb oligonucleotides on vascular smooth muscle cell proliferation and response to vessel wall injury. Circ Res 1995; 76(4):505–513.

141. Edelman ER, Simons M, Sirois MG, Rosenberg RD. C-myc in vasculoproliferative disease. Circ Res 1995; 76(2):176–182.

142. Simons M, Edelman ER, DeKeyser JL, Langer R, Rosenberg RD. Antisense c-myb oligonucleotides inhibit intimal arterial smooth muscle cell accumulation in vivo. Nature 1992; 359(6390):67–70.

143. Morishita R, Higaki J, Tomita N, Ogihara T. Application of transcription factor "decoy" strategy as means of gene therapy and study of gene expression in cardiovascular disease. Circ Res 1998; 82(10):1023–1028.

144. McKay MJ. Gaballa MA. Gene transfer therapy in vascular diseases. Cardiovasc Drug Rev 2001; 19(3):245–262.

145. Mahato RI, Takakura Y, Hashida M, Development of targeted delivery systems for nucleic acid drugs. J Drug Target 1997; 4(6):337–357.

146. Tomita N, Morishita R. Antisense oligonucleotides as a powerful molecular strategy for gene therapy in cardiovascular diseases. Curr Pharm Des 2004; 10(7):797–803.

147. Nabel E, Plautz GE, Nabel G, Site-specific gene expression in vivo by direct gene transfer into the arterial wall. Science 1990; 249:1285–1288.

148. Wilson J, Biriny L, Salomon R. Implantation of vascular graft lined with genetically modified endothelial cells. Science 1989; 244:1344–1346.

149. Twombly R. For gene therapy, now-quantified risks are deemed troubling. J Natl Cancer Inst 2003; 95(14):1032–1033.

150. Smith AE. Viral vectors in gene therapy. Annu Rev Microbiol 1995; 49:807–838.

151. Miller DP, Adam M, Miller A. Gene transfer by retrovirus vectors occurs only in cells that are actively replicating at the time of infection. Mol Cell Biol 1990; 10:4239–4242.

152. Yang Y, Nunes F, Berencsi K, Cellular immunity to viral anti-gene limits E1 deleted adenoviruses for gene therapy. Proc Natl Acad Sci USA 1994; 91(10):4407–4411.

153. Newman K, Dunn P, Owens J. Adenovirus-mediated gene transfer into normal rabbit arteries results in prolong vascular cell activation, inflammation, and neointimal hyperplasia. J Clin Invest 1995; 96:2955–2965.

154. Marwick C, FDA halts gene therapy trials after leukaemia case in France. BMJ 2003; 326(7382):181.

155. Brown MD, Schatzlein AG, Uchegbu IF. Gene delivery with synthetic (non viral) carriers. Int J Pharm 2001; 229(1–2):1–21.

156. Zhdanov RI, Podobed OV, Vlassov VV. Cationic lipid-DNA complexeslipoplexes-for gene transfer and therapy. Bioelectrochemistry 2002; 58(1):53–64.

157. Khurana R, Martin JF, Zachary I. Gene therapy for cardiovascular disease: a case for cautious optimism, Hypertension 2001; 38(5):1210–1216.

158. Clark P, Hersh E. Cationic lipid mediated gene transfer: current concepts. Curr Opin Mol Ther 1999; 1:158–176.

159. Marshall J, Nietupski JB, Lee ER, et al. Cationic lipid structure and formulation considerations for optimal gene transfection of the lung, J Drug Target 2000; 7(6):453–469.
160. Filion MC, Phillips NC. Toxicity and immunomodulatory activity of liposomal vectors formulated with cationic lipids toward immune effector cells. Biochim Biophys Acta 1997; 1329(2):345–356.
161. Dokka S, Toledo D, Shi X, Castranova V, Rojanasakul Y. Oxygen radicalmediated pulmonary toxicity induced by some cationic liposomes. Pharm Res 2000; 17(5):521–525.
162. Filion MC, Phillips NC. Anti-inflammatory activity of cationic lipids. Br J Pharmacol 1997; 122(3):551–557.
163. Duzgunes N, Goldstein JA, Friend DS, Felgner PL. Fusion of liposomes containing a novel cationic lipid, N-[2,3-(dioleyloxy)propyl]-N,N,N-trimethylammonium: induction by multivalent anions and asymmetric fusion with acidic phospholipid vesicles. Biochemistry 1989; 28(23):9179–9184.
164. Campbell RB, Fukumura D, Brown EB, et al. Cationic charge determines the distribution of liposomes between the vascular and extravascular compartments of tumors. Cancer Res 2002; 62(23):6831–6836.
165. Dzau VJ, Mann MJ, Morishita R, Kaneda Y. Fusigenic viral liposome for gene therapy in cardiovascular diseases. Proc Natl Acad Sci USA 1996; 93(21):11421–11425.
166. Felgner JH, Kumar R, Sridhar CN, et al. Enhanced gene delivery and mechanism studies with a novel series of cationic lipid formulations. J Biol Chem 1994; 269(4):2550–2561.
167. Felgner PL, Gadek TR, Holm M, et al. Lipofection: a highly efficient, lipid-mediated DNA-transfection procedure. Proc Natl Acad Sci USA 1987; 84(21):7413–7417.
168. Felgner PL, Tsai YJ, Sukhu L, et al. Improved cationic lipid formulations for in vivo gene therapy. Ann NY Acad Sci 1995; 772; 126–139.
169. Kichler A, Zauner W, Ogris M, Wagner E. Influence of the DNA complexation medium on the trasfection efficiency of lipospermine/DNA particles. Gene Ther 1998; 5:855–860.
170. Groth D, Keilb O, Lehmana C, Schneider M, Rudo M. Preparation and characterisation of a new liposperamine for gene delivery into various cells. Int J Pharm 1998; 162, 143–157.
171. Armeanu S, Pelisek J, Krausz E, et al. Optimization of nonviral gene transfer of vascular smooth muscle cells in vitro and in vivo. Mol Ther 2000; 1(4):366–375.
172. Pickering JG, Isner JM, Ford CM, et al. Processing of chimeric antisense oligonucleotides by human vascular smooth muscle cells and human atherosclerotic plaque. Implications for antisense therapy of restenosis after angioplasty. Circulation 1996; 93(4):772–780.
173. Tomita N, Morishita R, Tomita S, et al. Transcription factor decoy for nuclear factor-kappaB inhibits tumor necrosis factor-alpha-induced expression of interleukin-6 and intracellular adhesion molecule-1 in endothelial cells. J Hypertens 1998; 16(7):993–1000.
174. Kalinowski M, Viehofer K, Hamann C, et al. Local administration of NF-kappa B decoy oligonucleotides to prevent restenosis after balloon angioplasty: an experimental study in New Zealand white rabbits. Cardiovasc Intervent Radiol 2005; 28(3):331–337.
175. Nikol S, Pelisek J, Engelmann MG, Rolland PH, Armeanu S. Prevention of restenosis using the gene for cecropin complexed with DOCSPER liposomes under optimized conditions. Int J Angiol 2000; 9(2):87–94.
176. Liu Y, Fong S, Debs RJ. Cationic liposome-mediated gene delivery in vivo. Methods Enzymol 2003; 373:536–550.
177. Liu Y, Liggitt D, Zhong W, Tu G, Gaensler K, Debs R. Cationic liposomemediated intravenous gene delivery. J Biol Chem 1995; 270(42):24,864–24,870.
178. Patil SD, Rhodes DG, Burgess DJ. Anionic liposomal delivery system for DNA transfection. AAPS J 2004; 6(4):e29.
179. Miller AD. The problem with cationic liposome/micelle-based non-viral vector systems for gene therapy. Curr Med Chem 2003; 10(14):1195–1211.
180. Bitzer M, Armeanu S, Lauer UM, Neubert WJ. Sendai virus vectors as an emerging negative-strand RNA viral vector system. J Gene Med 2003; 5(7):543–553.

181. Nakanishi M, Uchida T, Sugawa H, Ishiura M, Okada Y, Efficient introduction of contents of liposomes into cells using HVJ. Exp Cell Res 1985; 159:399–409.

182. Keneda Y, Iwai K, Uchida T. Introduction and expression of the human insulin gene in adult rat liver. J Biol Chem 1989; 186:129–134.

183. Tomita N, Higaki J, Morishita R, Kato H, Mikami H, Keneda Y. Direct in vivo gene introduction into rat kidney. Biochem Biophys Res Commun 1992; 186:129–134.

184. Keneda Y, Iwai K, Uchida T. Increased expression of DNA cointroduced with nucear protein in adult rat liver. Science 1989; 243, 375–378.

185. Keneda Y, Saeki Y, Morishita R. Gene therapy using HVJ-liposomes: best of both worlds? Mol Med Today 1999; 5, 298–303.

186. Yin X, Yutani C, Ikeda Y, et al. Tissue factor pathway inhibitor gene delivery using HVJ-AVE liposomes markedly reduces restenosis in atherosclerotic arteries. Cardiovasc Res 2002; 56(3):454–463.

187. Morishita R, Gibbons GH, Kaneda Y, Ogihara T, Dzau VJ. Noval and effective gene transfer technique for study of vascular renin angiotensin system. J Clin Invest 1993a; 91:2580–2585.

188. VD Leyen HE, Gibbons GH, Morishita R, et al. Gene theraphy inhibiting neointimal vascular lesion: in vivo transfer of endothelial cell nitric oxide synthase gene. Proc Natl Acad USA 1995; 92, 1137–1141.

189. Todaka T, Yokoyama C, Yanamoto H, et al. Gene transfer of human prostacyclin synthase prevents neointimal formation after carotid balloon injury in rats. Stroke 1999; 30(2):419–426.

190. Aoki M, Morishita R, Matsushita H, et al. Inhibition of the p53 tumor suppressor gene results in growth of human aortic vascular smooth muscle cells. Potential role of p53 in regulation of vascular smooth muscle cell growth. Hypertension 1999; 34(2):192–200.

191. Morishita R, Gibbons GH, Ellison KE, et al. Intimal hyperplasia after vascular injury is inhibited by antisense cdk 2 kinase oligonucleotides. J Clin Invest 1994; 93(4):1458–1464.

192. Morishita R, Gibbons GH, Ellison KE, et al. Single intraluminal delivery of antisense cdc2 kinase and proliferating-cell nuclear antigen oligonucleotides results in chronic inhibition of neointimal hyperplasia. Proc Natl Acad Sci USA 1993; 90(18):8474–8478.

193. Morishita R, Gibbons GH, Tomita N, et al. Antisense oligodeoxynucleotide inhibition of vascular angiotensin-converting enzyme expression attenuates neointimal formation: evidence for tissue angiotensin-converting enzyme function. Arterioscler Thromb Vasc Biol 2000; 20(4):915–922.

194. Morishita R, Gibbons GH, Horiuchi KE, et al. A gene therapy strategy using a transcription factor decoy of the E2F binging site inhibits smooth muscle proliferation in vivo. Proc Natl Acad USA 1995; 92:5855–5859.

195. Labhasetwar V, Chen BR, Muller DWM, et al. Gene-based therapies for restenosis. Adv Drug Deliver Rev 1997; 24(1):109–120.

196. Iaccarino G, Smithwick LA, Lefkowitz RJ, Koch WJ. Targeting G(beta gamma) signaling in arterial vascular smooth muscle proliferation: a novel strategy to limit restenosis, Proc Nat Acad Sci USA 1999; 96(7):3945–3950.

197. Indolfi C, Avvedimento EV, Rapacciuolo A, et al. Inhibition of cellular ras prevents smooth-muscle cell-proliferation after vascular injury in-vivo. Nat Med 1995; 1(6):541–545.

198. Cohen-Sacks H, Najajreh Y, Tchaikovski V, et al. Novel PDGF beta R antisense encapsulated in polymeric nanospheres for the treatment of restenosis. Gene Ther 2002; 9(23):1607–1616.

199. Hughes AD, Clunn GF, Refson J, Demoliou-Mason C. Platelet-derived growth factor (PDGF): actions and mechanisms in vascular smooth muscle, Gen Pharmacol 1996; 27(7):1079–1089.

200. Zambaux MF, Bonneaux F, Gref R, et al. Influence of experimental parameters on the characteristics of poly(lactic acid) nanoparticles prepared by a double emulsion method. J Control Release 1998; 50(1–3):31–40.

201. Cohen H, Levy RJ, Gao J, et al. Sustained delivery and expression of DNA encapsulated in polymeric nanoparticles. Gene Ther 2000; 7(22):1896–1905.

202. Morishita R. Recent progress in cardiovascular gene therapy; Emerging to real drug? Preface. Curr Gene Ther 2004; 4(2):i–i(1).

203. Morishita R, Perspective in progress of cardiovascular gene therapy. J Pharmacol Sci 2004; 95(1):1–8.
204. Morishita R, Recent progress in gene therapy for cardiovascular disease. Circ J 2002; 66(12):1077–1086.
205. Levitzki A, Tyrphostins: tyrosine kinase blockers as novel antiproliferative agents and dissectors of signal transduction. FASEB J 1992; 6(14):3275–3282.
206. Levitzki A, Gazit A. Tyrosine kinase inhibition: an approach to drug development. Science 1995; 267(5205):1782–1788.
207. Gazit A, Yee K, Uecker A, et al. Tricyclic quinoxalines as potent kinase inhibitors of PDGFR kinase, Flt3 and Kit. Bioorg Med Chem 2003; 11(9):2007–2018.
208. Kovalenko M, Ronnstrand L, Heldin CH, et al. Phosphorylation site-specific inhibition of platelet-derived growth factor beta-receptor autophosphorylation by the receptor-blocking tyrphostin AG1296. Biochemistry 1997; 36(21):6260–6269.
209. Fishbein I, Chorny M, Rabinovich L, Banai S, Gati I, Golomb G. Nanoparticulate delivery system of a tyrphostin for the treatment of restenosis. J Control Release 2000; 65(1–2):221–229.
210. Fishbein I, Waltenberger J, Banai S, et al. Local delivery of platelet-derived growth factor receptor-specific tyrphostin inhibits neointimal formation in rats. Arterioscler Thromb Vasc Biol 2000; 20(3):667–676.
211. Fessi H, Puisieux F, Devissaguet JP, Ammoury N, Benita S. Nanocapsule formation by interfacial polymer deposition following solvent displacement. Int J Pharm 1989; 55(1), R1–R4.
212. Quintanar-Guerrero D, Allemann E, Fessi H, Doelker E. Preparation techniques and mechanisms of formation of biodegradable nanoparticles from preformed polymers. Drug Dev Ind Pharm 1998; 24(12):1113–1128.
213. Chorny M, Fishbein I, Danenberg HD, Golomb G. Lipophilic drug loaded nanospheres prepared by nanoprecipitation: effect of formulation variables on size, drug recovery and release kinetics. J Control Release 2002; 83(3):389–400.
214. Chorny M, Fishbein I, Danenberg HD, Golomb G. Study of the drug release mechanism from tyrphostin AG-1295-loaded nanospheres by in situ and external sink methods. J Control Release 2002; 83(3):401–414.
215. Brigger I, Chaminade P, Marsaud V, et al. Tamoxifen encapsulation within polyethylene glycol-coated nanospheres. A new antiestrogen formulation. Int J Pharm 2001; 214(1–2):37–42.
216. Prabha S, Zhou WZ, Panyam J, Labhasetwar V. Size-dependency of nanoparticle-mediated gene transfection: studies with fractionated nanoparticles. Int J Pharm 2002; 244(1–2):105–115.
217. Schwartz RS. Neointima and arterial injury: dogs, rats, pigs, and more. Lab Invest 1994; 71(6):789–791.
218. Villa AE, Guzman LA, Chen W, Golomb G, Levy RJ, Topol EJ. Local delivery of dexamethasone for prevention of neointimal proliferation in a rat model of balloon angioplasty. J Clin Invest 1994; 93(3):1243–1249.
219. Berk BC, Rao GN. Angiotensin II-induced vascular smooth muscle cell hypertrophy: PDGF A-chain mediates the increase in cell size. J Cell Physiol 1993; 154(2):368–380.
220. Lee SW, Tsou AP, Chan H, et al. Glucocorticoids selectively inhibit the transcription of the inter-leukin 1 beta gene and decrease the stability of interleukin 1 beta mRNA. Proc Natl Acad Sci USA 1988; 85(4):1204–1208.
221. Kling D, Fingerle J, Harlan JM. Inhibition of leukocyte extravasation with a monoclonal antibody to CD18 during formation of experimental intimal thickening in rabbit carotid arteries. Arterioscler Thromb 1992; 12(9):997–1007.
222. Guzman LA, Labhasetwar V, Song C, Jang Y, Lincoff AM, Levy R. Single intraluminal infusion of biodegradable polymeric nanoparticles matrixed with dexamethasone decreases neointimal formation after vascular injury. Circulation 1995; 92(8): 1394–1394.
223. Erickson LA, Bonin PD, Wishka DG, et al. In vitro and in vivo inhibition of rat vascular smooth muscle cell migration and proliferation by a 2-aminochromone U-86983. J Pharmacol Exp Ther 1994; 271(1):415–421.
224. Humphrey WR, Erickson LA, Simmons CA, et al. The effect of intramural delivery of polymeric nanoparticles loaded with the antiproliferative 2-aminochromone U-86983

on neointimal hyperplasia development in balloon-injured porcine coronary arteries. Adv Drug Deliver Rev 1997; 24(1):87–108.

225. Song CX, Labhasetwar V, Murphy H, et al. Formulation and characterization of biodegradable nanoparticles for intravascular local drug delivery, J Control Release 1997; 43(2–3):197–212.

226. Westedt U, Barbu-Tudoran L, Schaper AK, Kalinowski M, Alfke H, Kissel T. Deposition of nanoparticles in the arterial vessel by porous balloon catheters: localization by confocal laser scanning microscopy and transmission electron microscopy. AAPS PharmSci 2002; 4(4):E41.

227. Song C, Labhasetwar V, Cui X, Underwood T, Levy RJ. Arterial uptake of biodegradable nanoparticles for intravascular local drug delivery: results with an acute dog model. J Control Release 1998; 54(2):201–211.

228. Panyam J, Lof J, O'Leary E, Labhasetwar V. Efficiency of dispatch and infiltrator cardiac infusion catheters in arterial localization of nanoparticles in a porcine coronary model of restenosis. J Drug Target 2002; 10(6):515–523.

229. Gabizon A. Papahadjopoulos D. The role of surface charge and hydrophilic groups on liposome clearance in vivo. Biochim Biophys Acta 1992; 1103(1):94–100.

230. Gabizon A, Price DC, Huberty J, Bresalier RS, Papahadjopoulos D. Effect of liposome composition and other factors on the targeting of liposomes to experimental tumors: biodistribution and imaging studies. Cancer Res 1990; 50(19):6371–6378.

231. Lasic DD. Colloid chemistry. Liposomes within liposomes. Nature 1997; 387(6628): 26–27.

232. Lasic DD, Papahadjopoulos D. Liposomes revisited. Science 1995; 267(5202):1275–1276.

233. Gabizon A, Shmeeda H, Barenholz Y. Pharmacokinetics of pegylated liposomal doxorubicin–review of animal and human studies. Clin Pharmacokinet 2003; 42(5):419–436.

234. Nakanishi T, Fukushima S, Okamoto K, et al. Development of the polymer micelle carrier system for doxorubicin. J Control Release 2001; 74(1–3):295–302.

235. Maeda H. The enhanced permeability and retention (EPR) effect in tumor vasculature: the key role of tumor-selective macromolecular drug targeting. Adv Enzyme Regul 2001; 41:189–207.

236. Maeda H. Role of microbial proteases in pathogenesis. Microbiol Immunol 1996; 40(10): 685–699.

237. Maeda H, Wu J, Okamoto T, Maruo K, Akaike T. Kallikrein-kinin in infection and cancer. Immunopharmacology 1999; 43(2–3):115–128.

238. Molla A, Yamamoto T, Akaike T, Miyoshi S, Maeda H. Activation of Hageman-factor and prekallikrein and generation of kinin by various microbial proteinases. J Biol Chem 1989; 264(18):10589–10594.

239. Uwatoku T, Shimokawa H, Abe K, et al. Application of nanoparticle technology for the prevention of restenosis after balloon injury in rats, Circ Res 2003; 92(7):e62–e69.

240. Rowinsky EK, Donehower RC. Drug-therapy–Paclitaxel (Taxol). New Engl J Med 1995; 332(15):1004–1014.

241. Schiff PB, Horwitz SB. Taxol stabilizes microtubules in mouse fibroblast cells. Proc Natl Acad Sci USA. 1980; 77(3):1561–1565.

242. Kolodgie FD, John M, Khurana C, et al. Sustained reduction of in-stent neointimal growth with the use of a novel systemic nanoparticle paclitaxel. Circulation 2002; 106(10):1195–1198.

243. Ibrahim NK, Desai N, Legha S, et al. Phase I and pharmacokinetic study of ABI-007, a cremophor-free, protein-stabilized, nanoparticle formulation of paclitaxel. Clin Cancer Res 2002; 8(5):1038–1044.

244. Weiss RB, Donehower RC, Wiernik PH, et al. Hypersensitivity Reactions from Taxol. J Clin Oncol 1990; 8(7):1263–1268.

245. Danenberg HD, Fishbein I, Gao J, et al. Macrophage depletion by clodronate-containing liposomes reduces neointimal formation after balloon injury in rats and rabbits. Circulation 2002; 106(5):599–605.

246. Feldman LJ, Aguirre L, Ziol M, et al. Interleukin-10 inhibits intimal hyperplasia after angioplasty or stent implantation in hypercholesterolemic rabbits. Circulation 2000; 101(8):908–916.

247. Rogers C, Edelman ER, Simon DI, A mAb to the beta2-leukocyte integrin Mac-1 (CD11b/ CD18) reduces intimal thickening after angioplasty or stent implantation in rabbits. P Natl Acad Sci USA 1998; 95(17):10,134–10,139.

248. Ross R. Mechanisms of disease–atherosclerosis—an inflammatory disease, N Engl J Med 1999; 340(2):115–126.

249. Rogers C, Welt FG, Karnovsky MJ, Edelman ER. Monocyte recruitment and neointimal hyperplasia in rabbits. Coupled inhibitory effects of heparin. Arterioscler Thromb Vasc Biol 1996; 16(10):1312–1318.

250. Tanaka H, Sukhova GK, Swanson SJ, et al. Sustained activation of vascular cells and leukocytes in the rabbit aorta after balloon injury. Circulation 1993; 88(4 Pt 1):1788–1803.

251. Welt F, Tso C, Edelman E, et al. Leukocyte recruitment and expression of chemokines following different forms of vascular injury, Vasc Med 2003; 8:1–7.

252. Fukuda D, Shimada K, Tanaka A, Kawarabayashi T, Yoshiyama M, Yoshikawa J. Circulating monocytes and in-stent neointima after coronary stent implantation. J Am Coll Cardiol 2004; 43(1):18–23.

253. van Furth R. Origin and turnover of monocytes and macrophages. Curr Top Pathol 1989; 79:125–150.

254. Van Furth R, Phagocytic cells: development and distribution of mononuclear phago- cytes in normal steady state and inflammation. In: Inflammation: Basic Principles and Clinical Correlates. Snyder R, ed. New York: Raven Press, Ltd, 1988:281–295.

255. Pakianathan DR, Extracellular-matrix proteins and leukocyte function. J Leukoc Biol 1995; 57(5):699–702.

256. Carlos TM, Harlan JM. Leukocyte-endothelial adhesion molecules. Blood 1994; 84(7):2068–2101.

257. Kagan E, Hartmann DP. Elimination of macrophages with silica and asbestos. Methods Enzymol 1984; 108:325–335.

258. Shek PN, Lukovich S. The role of macrophages in promoting the antibody response mediated by liposome-associated protein antigens. Immunol Lett 1982; 5(6):305–309.

259. van Rooijen N, van Nieuwmegen R. Elimination of phagocytic cells in the spleen after intravenous injection of liposome-encapsulated dichloromethylene diphosphonate. An enzyme-histochemical study. Cell Tissue Res 1984; 238(2):355–358.

260. Caselles T, Villalian J, Frernandez J. Influence of liposome charge and composition on their interaction with human blood serum proteins. Mol Cell Biochem 1993; 120:119–126.

261. Gregoriadis G, Davis C. Stability of liposome in vivo and in vitro is promoted by their cholesterol content and the presence of blood cells. Biochem Biophys Res Commun 1979; 89:1287–1293.

262. Senior J, Gregoriadis G. Stability of small unilamellar liposomes in serum and clearance from the circulation: the effect of the phospholipid and cholesterol components. Life Sci 1982; 30:2123–2136.

263. Damen J, Dijkstra J, Regts J, Scherphof G. Effect of lipoprotein-free plasma on the inter- action of human plasma high density lipoprotein with egg yolk phosphatidylcholin liposomes. Biochem Biophys Acta 1980; 620:90–99.

264. Fleisch H, Bisphosphonates–Pharmacology and use in the treatment of tumor-induced hypercalcemic and metastatic bone-disease. Drugs 1991; 42(6):919–944.

265. Fleisch H. Bisphosphonates: mechanisms of action. Endocr Rev 1998; 19(1):80–100.

266. Rodan, GA. Mechanisms of action of bisphosphonates. Annu Rev Pharmacol Toxicol 1998; 38:375–388.

267. Monkkonen J, Valjakka R, Hakasalo M, Urtti A. The effects of liposome surface-charge and size on the intracellular delivery of clodronate and gallium in-vitro. Int J Pharm 1994; 107(3):189–197.

268. Van Rooijen N. The liposome-mediated macrophage `suicide' technique. J Immunol Methods 1989; 124(1):1–6.

269. Danenberg HD, Fishbein I, Epstein H, et al. Systemic depletion of macrophages by liposomal bisphosphonates reduces neointimal formation following balloon-injury in the rat carotid artery. J Cardiovasc Pharmacol 2003; 42(5):671–679.

270. Monkkonen J, Heath TD. The effects of liposome-encapsulated and free clodronate on the growth of macrophage-like cells in-vitro—the role of calcium and iron. Calcif Tissue Int 1993; 53(2):139–146.
271. Monkkonen J, Liukkonen J, Taskinen M, Heath TD, Urtti A. Studies on liposome formulations for intraarticular delivery of clodronate. J Controlled Rel 1995; 35(2–3):145–154.
272. Selander KS, Monkkonen J, Karhukorpi EK, Harkonen P, Hannuniemi R, Vaananen HK. Characteristics of clodronate-induced apoptosis in osteoclasts and macrophages. Mol Pharmacol 1996; 50(5):1127–1138.
273. Diacovo TG, Roth SJ, Buccola JM, Bainton DF, Springer TA. Neutrophil rolling, arrest, and transmigration across activated, surface-adherent platelets via sequential action of P-selectin and the beta 2-integrin CD11b/CD18. Blood 1996; 88(1):146–157.
274. Larsen E, Celi A, Gilbert GE, et al. PADGEM protein: a receptor that mediates the interaction of activated platelets with neutrophils and monocytes. Cell 1989; 59(2):305–312.
275. Hamburger SA, Mcever RP. Gmp-140 mediates adhesion of stimulated platelets to neutrophils. Blood 1990; 75(3):550–554.
276. McEver RP, Cummings RD. Role of PSGL-1 binding to selectins in leukocyte recruitment. J Clin Invest 1997; 100(11):S97–S103.
277. Simon DI, Chen Z, Xu H, et al. Platelet glycoprotein ibalpha is a counterreceptor for the leukocyte integrin Mac-1 (CD11b/CD18), J Exp Med 2000; 192(2):193–204.
278. Diacovo TG, Defougerolles AR, Bainton DF, Springer TA, A functional integrin ligand on the surface of platelets–Intercellular-adhesion molecule-2. J Clin Invest 1994; 94(3):1243–1251.
279. Weber C, Springer, TA. Neutrophil accumulation on activated, surface-adherent platelets in flow is mediated by interaction of Mac-1 with fibrinogen bound to alpha IIb beta 3 and stimulated by platelet-activating factor. J Clin Invest 1997; 100(8):2085–2093.
280. Libby P, Shcwartz D, Brogi E, Tanaka H, Clinton S. A cascade model for restenosis. A special case of atherosclerosis progression. Circulation 86(6S), III47–III52, 1992.
281. Fast DK, Felix R, Dowse C, Neuman WF, Fleisch H. The effects of diphosphonates on the growth and glycolysis of connective-tissue cells in culture. Biochem J 1978; 172(1):97–107.
282. Felix R, Bettex JD, Fleisch H. Effect of diphosphonates on the synthesis of prostaglandins in cultured calvaria cells. Calcif Tissue Int 1981; 33(5):549–552.
283. Ohya K, Yamada S, Felix R, Fleisch H. Effect of Bisphosphonates on prostaglandin synthesis by rat bone-cells and mouse calvaria in culture. Clin Sci 1985; 69(4):403–411.
284. Giuliani N, Pedrazzoni M, Passeri G, Girasole G. Bisphosphonates inhibit IL-6 production by human osteoblastic-like cells. Scand J Rheumatol 1998; 27(1):38–41.
285. Makkonen N, Salminen A, Rogers MJ, et al. Contrasting effects of alendronate and clodronate on RAW 264 macrophages: the role of a bisphosphonate metabolite. Eur J Pharm Sci 1999; 8(2):109–118.
286. Hyvonen PM, Kowolik MJ, Human neutrophil priming: chemiluminescence modified by hydroxyapatite and three bisphosphonates in vitro. J Clin Lab Immunol 1993; 40(2):69–76.
287. Serretti R, Core P, Muti S, Salaffi F. Influence of dichloromethylene diphosphonate on reactive oxygen species production by human neutrophils. Rheumatol Int 1993; 13(4):135–138.
288. Mian M, Benetti D, Aloisi R, Rosini S, Fantozzi R. Effects of bisphosphonate derivatives on macrophage function. Pharmacology 1994; 49(5):336–342.
289. Monkkonen J, Pennanen N, Lapinjoki S, Urtti A. Clodronate (Dichloromethylene Bisphosphonate) inhibits LPS-stimulated Il-6 and TNF production by Raw-264 cells. Life Sciences 1994; 54(14):Pl229–Pl234.
290. Majesky MW, Reidy MA, Bowen-Pope DF, Hart CE, Wilcox JN, Schwartz SM. PDGF ligand and receptor gene expression during repair of arterial injury. J Cell Biol 1990; 111(5 Pt 1):2149–2158.
291. Waltenberger J. Modulation of growth factor action: Implications for the treatment of cardiovascular diseases. Circulation 1997; 96(11):4083–4094.
292. Danenberg HD, Golomb G, Groothuis A, et al. Liposomal alendronate inhibits systemic innate immunity and reduces in-stent neointimal hyperplasia in rabbits. Circulation 2003; 108(22):2798–2804.

293. Cohen H, Alferiev IS, Monkkonen J, et al. Synthesis and preclinical pharmacology of 2-(2-aminopyrimidinio) ethylidene-1,1-bisphosphonic acid betaine (ISA-13-1)-a novel bisphosphonate. Pharm Res 1999; 16(9):1399–1406.

294. Ogawara K, Yoshida M, Kubo J, et al. Mechanisms of hepatic disposition of polystyrene microspheres in rats: Effects of serum depend on the sizes of microspheres. J Control Release 1999; 61(3):241–250.

295. Ogawara K, Yoshida M, Takakura Y, Hashida M, Higaki K, Kimura T. Interaction of polystyrene microspheres with liver cells: roles of membrane receptors and serum proteins. Bba-Gen Subjects 1999; 1472(1–2):165–172.

296. Roser M, Fischer D, Kissel T. Surface-modified biodegradable albumin nano- and microspheres. II: effect of surface charges on in vitro phagocytosis and biodistribution in rats. Eur J Pharm Biopharm 1998; 46(3):255–263.

297. Tabata Y, Ikada Y. Effect of surface charges on in vitro phagocytosis and biodistribution in rats. Biomaterials 1998; 9(4):356–362.

298. Niwa T, Takeuchi H, Hino T, Kunou N, Kawashima Y. Preparations of biodegradable nanospheres of water-soluble and insoluble drugs with D,L-lactide glycolide copolymer by a novel spontaneous emulsification solvent diffusion method, and the drug release behavior. J Control Release 1993; 25(1–2):89–98.

299. Niwa T, Takeuchi H, Hino T, Kunou N, Kawashima Y. In-vitro drug-release behavior of D,L-lactide/glycolide copolymer (Plga) nanospheres with nafarelin acetate prepared by a novel spontaneous emulsification solvent diffusion method. J Pharm Sci 1994; 83(5):727–732.

Ocular Applications of Nanoparticulate Drug-Delivery Systems

Annick Ludwig
Department of Pharmaceutical Sciences, University of Antwerp, Antwerp, Belgium

INTRODUCTION

The absorption of topically applied ophthalmic drugs is very poor because of efficient mechanisms protecting the eye from harmful materials and agents. These protective mechanisms, such as reflex blinking, lachrymation, tear turnover, and drainage, result in the rapid removal of foreign substances from the eye surface. Moreover, the very tight epithelium of the cornea also compromises the permeation of drug molecules. Consequently, the contact time of conventional eye drops is only about five minutes, and typically less than 5% of the applied dose penetrates passively across the cornea and reaches the intraocular tissues (1).

Thus, frequent instillations of eye drops are necessary to maintain therapeutic drug level in the tear film or at the site of action. However, the frequent use of highly concentrated drug solutions may induce toxic side effects after absorption via the blood vessels in the conjunctival stroma or nasal mucosa into systemic circulation. Moreover, cellular damage at the ocular surface could occur (2–4).

The rationale for the development of various particulate systems for sustained drug delivery is based on possible entrapment of the particles in the ocular mucus layer covering the eye surface, and the interaction of bioadhesive polymer chains with mucins. This will increase the precorneal residence time of the drug, allowing for an extension of the absorption time. Furthermore, by controlling drug release and enhancing drug absorption, this could also improve corneal drug penetration. One attractive feature of utilizing nanoparticles for ocular drug delivery is that it is in a liquid dosage form which can be easily administered by patients (4–8).

Another significant challenge is to deliver therapeutic doses of drugs to treat diseases affecting the posterior segment of the eye. It is difficult to deliver drugs to the posterior segment by topical application because of the diffusional distance and the counter-directional intraocular convection from the ciliary body to Schlemm's canal. The most logical way is to deliver drugs by intraocular injections thus bypassing anatomical and physiological barriers. However, drugs of short half-lives (e.g., antibiotics, antiviral drugs) would require repeated injections, which could increase the risk of retinal detachment or hemorrhage. Therefore, biodegradable nanoparticles were developed for intraocular administration in order to obtain a controlled, sustained drug release and thus reducing the number of injections required (9).

The choice of the polymer for preparing particulate systems will depend on the physicochemical properties of the drug. The goal is to achieve high drug loading in order to minimize the required volume to be instilled into the eye. Corneal uptake and transport of nanoparticles should be facilitated by small particle size (100–200 nm) (8).

Drug-release kinetics are regulated by the composition and preparation procedure of the particles, the molecular weight and degradation of the polymers, and the physicochemical properties of the entrapped drug molecule (4,6–8). As excellent reviews on the use of nanoparticles in ocular drug delivery have been published previously, this chapter will mainly focus on the latest relevant research reported in literature (5–9).

POLYMERS OF NATURAL ORIGIN

As they are biocompatible, polymers of natural origin such as proteins and polysaccharides have been investigated for use in the production of micro- and nanoparticles. A denaturation process induced by either heating or cooling and subsequent chemical cross-linking procedures to create a denser particle matrix prepare protein nanoparticles. Another preparation method is based on desolvation of the macromolecules, which leads to precipitation or the formation of a coacervate phase. A cross-linking agent (e.g., glutaraldehyde) is added to harden the native particles (5,6,10). Owing to the presence of charged groups, protein nanoparticles can be used as a matrix in which the drug molecules may be physically entrapped or covalently linked (11). Some examples of particles for ocular purpose reported in literature are summarized in Table 1.

Various in vivo studies in rabbits reported that a prolonged effect of drugs (pilocarpine, piroxicam) incorporated in albumin particles was observed when compared to commercial preparations or aqueous and viscous solutions (4,5,11).

TABLE 1 Types of Ocular Particulate Dosage Forms Used in Animal Studies Which Were Prepared from Proteins and Polysaccharides

Polymer	Drug	Observations	References
Albumin	Piroxicam	Increased bioavailability compared to commercial eye drops	(12)
Albumin	Ganciclovir	After intravitreal injection in rats, the residence time is prolonged (2 weeks); no inflammation; good tolerance	(13)
Chitosan	Cyclosporin A	Therapeutic concentrations in cornea and conjunctiva during at least 48 hrs	(14)
Chitosan	Fluorescent label	High amounts of nanoparticles into corneal and conjunctival epithelia	(15)
Chitosan PEO insert	Ofloxacin	C_{max} in aqueous humor increased compared to plain PEO inserts	(16)
Pectin	Piroxicam	2.5-fold higher bioavailability in aqueous humor compared to commercial eye drops	(17)
Starch acetate	—	After 3 hrs incubation, 8% of cultured retinal epithelial cells took up microspheres	(18)
Carrageenan gelatin	Timolol	5.6- and 2.5-fold higher bioavailability in aqueous humor compared to commercial eye drops and in situ gelling system, respectively	(19)

Note: Unless as indicated, in vivo tests were performed on rabbits.
Abbreviation: PEO, poly(ethylene oxide).

However, in one study, topical application of hydrocortisone-loaded albumin particles in rabbits resulted in a lower tissue concentration of the drug as compared to the application of a simple drug solution (5). This result is possibly due to the strong binding of the drug to the particles. The retention of nanoparticles was found to be higher in inflamed tissue as compared with the normal tissue (5).

Ganciclovir, the most widely used antiviral drug for the treatment of cytomegalovirus retinitis, was formulated in nanoparticles for intravitreal administration in rats. A prolonged residence in the vitreous cavity (two weeks) showed no evidence of inflammatory reaction in the retinal tissue and also did not affect the vision (13).

The types of polysaccharides which have been investigated for the production of ocular particulates are chitosan, pectin, and carrageenan.

Chitosan, a deacetylated chitin, is biodegradable, biocompatible, and nontoxic (7,8). The polycationic chitosan was investigated as an ophthalmic vehicle because of its probable superior mucoadhesiveness due to its ability to produce molecular attractive forces by electrostatic interactions with the negative charges of the mucus. Numerous studies indicated an increase in the precorneal retention time of chitosan solutions (7). Moreover, chitosan appears to enhance the permeability of the cornea transiently due to the interaction with tight junction structures (7).

For the preparation of chitosan nanoparticles, a number of techniques are employed. These include covalent chemical cross-linking, ionic cross-linking (e.g., ionotropic gelation with tripolyphosphate), or desolvation. Chitosan microspheres have been prepared by water-in-oil evaporation and spray-drying. By adjusting the molecular weight and the deacetylation degree of the polymer used, one could achieve the degradation and release rate required for a specific drug (7).

In one study, the animals treated with cyclosporine A-loaded nanoparticles were found to show significantly higher corneal and conjunctival drug levels than those treated with a suspension of cyclosporin A in a chitosan aqueous solution or in water (2–6-fold increase) (14). In a recent study in rabbits, De Campos and coworkers showed that the amounts of fluorescent nanoparticles in cornea and conjunctiva were significantly higher than those for a control solution. These amounts were fairly constant for up to 24 hours. A higher retention of chitosan nanoparticles in the conjunctiva as compared to that in the cornea was observed. Confocal microscopy studies suggest that nanoparticles penetrate into the corneal and conjunctival epithelia by a paracellular/transcellular pathway which is different from the pathway used by the poly(alkylcyanoacrylate) (PACA) and poly(epsilon-caprolacton) (PECL) nanoparticles (7,15).

To improve the release kinetics of ofloxacin, chitosan microspheres loaded with ofloxacin were also incorporated in poly(ethylene oxide) (PEO) inserts. The in vivo results in rabbits did not demonstrate a biopharmaceutical improvement compared to plain PEO inserts. However, a significant increase in the C_{max} value in the aqueous humor was observed which could partly be due to the permeability-enhancing effect of chitosan across the cornea (16).

Pectin nanoparticles loaded with fluorescein showed an increase in the precorneal retention time from 0.5 to 2.5 hours, when compared with a fluorescein solution. In vivo tests with piroxicam-loaded pectin particles indicated a 2.5-fold increase in the amount of drug concentration in the aqueous humor as compared to a commercial eye drop solution (17).

Tuovinen et al. (18) reported the first study on enzyme-sensitive microparticles made of the natural biodegradable potato starch acetate for retinal targeting.

After a three-hour incubation, about 8% of the cells of a retinal pigment epithelium (RPE) culture took up microparticles. The viability of cultured RPE cells was at least 82% after 24-hour incubation with the microparticles. The degradation of potato starch acetate in RPE cells is catalyzed by esterases and amylases. Considering the low toxicity, it seems that these microparticles are suitable for drug delivery to the posterior segment of the eye (18).

Carrageenans are a group of water-soluble sulfated galactans extracted from brown seaweed. Microspheres containing gelatin, lambda carrageenan, and timolol were prepared by spray-drying. The different ratios of carrageenan and gelatin proved to be useful in modulating the drug-release profiles and mucoadhesive properties. After administration of a microsphere (50/50 mixture) suspension, the bioavailability (AUC values) of timolol in the aqueous humor in rabbits were 5.6 and 2.5 times higher in comparison with commercial eye drops and in situ gelling system, respectively (19).

ACRYLATES
Poly(alkylcyanoacrylates)
In the past, two biodegradable and biocompatible polymers, PACAs and poly(alkylmethacrylates), were quite popular for use in the preparation of drug carriers of particle size range from 200 to 500 nm. The use of these polymers is based on their mucoadhesive or bioadhesive properties. The difference between the two polymers lies mainly in their degradation rate: polymers with a longer side chain are degraded more slowly, resulting in a slower release of the drug incorporated in PACA particles (4–6).

The drug is either incorporated in PACA particles during the polymerization process or adsorbed to the nanoparticle surface after the particle is formed. The ultimate particle size of the particles and the degree of drug loading are dependent on several preparation parameters such as the pH of the preparation medium and the type of stabilizer or surfactant used (4–6,8).

PACA nanospheres were shown to adhere to the eye surface, and were taken up by a transcellular pathway in the outer cell layers of conjunctiva and cornea. This could be explained by either endocytosis or lysis of the cell wall induced by particle degradation products. Although the concentration of the drug in ocular tissues was shown to be higher in inflamed tissues, a condition where the permeability of the cell membrane is increased, no full penetration across the cornea into the anterior chamber was observed (5).

Many studies confirmed that the use of nanoparticles with these polymers can improve the clinical effects of a therapeutic agent (i.e., in glaucoma therapy or antibiotic therapy) and also minimizes its side effects (4–6). Sustained drug release from the polymer matrix and prolonged therapeutic effect were observed, except in the situation where the drug had a high affinity for the polymer. The increased biological response was attributed to improved ocular penetration and bioadhesion. The precorneal residence time of PACA nanoparticles could further be increased by incorporating the particles into a polyethylene glycol (PEG) gel or coating the particles with PEG (20,21). Acyclovir-loaded, PEG-coated polyethyl-2-cyanoacrylate showed a 25-fold increase in the drug level in aqueous humor when compared with an aqueous solution of the free drug. This result is probably due to a longer interaction of the nanoparticles with the corneal epithelium and the penetration-enhancing effect of PEG (21).

Acrylate Derivatives

Polyacrylic acid (PAA) and carbomers are used in the preparation of viscous eye drops, artificial tears, hydrogels, and inserts. The mucoadhesive properties of these polymers are mainly due to hydrogen bonding and interpenetration of the polymer chains and the mucus layer at the eye surface (4).

The hydration state and pH of microspheres in the lacrimal fluid were shown to be a factor affecting the residence time of the microspheres in the eye. In one study, radiolabeled PAA microspheres made with Carbopol® 907 cross-linked with maltose was applied either in dry form or in a prehydrated form. The clearance rate of the microspheres applied in the dry form was found to be higher than the prehydrated form probably due to incomplete hydration in the lachrymal fluid. Furthermore, the clearance of hydrated microspheres at pH 7.4 is higher than at pH 5.0 because the presence of protonated carboxyl groups at pH 5.0 in PAA permits enhanced bioadhesion through hydrogen bond formation with mucins (Table 2) (22).

In a recent study, De et al. (28) demonstrated the biocompatibility and adhesive properties of PAA nanoparticles on human corneal epithelial cells. A controlled release of the partly ionically entrapped brimonidine was obtained due to the cation-exchange properties of the polyanionic PAA matrix of the nanoparticles (28).

A major problem of PACA nanoparticles is the low loading capacity for hydrophilic drugs. To improve drug loading, attempts are made to increase the hydrophilicity of the particle surface by copolymerization of methylmethacrylate (MMA) and sulfopropylmethacrylate (SPM). Bound drug molecules are released from the carrier by competitive replacement by other ions. These copolymer nanoparticles loaded with the muscarinic agonists arecaidine propargyl ester (APE) and (S)-(+)aceclidine were evaluated in rabbits. A twofold increase in drug absorption was obtained when the nanoparticles were instilled together with bioadhesive hyaluronan (23).

Various cationic acrylic copolymers were also examined to prepare nanoparticles with a positive charge in order to facilitate an effective adhesion of the delivery system to the ocular surface (8). Pignatello et al. (24–26) formulated nanoparticles with

TABLE 2 Overview of In Vivo Studies Carried Out in Rabbits Using Nanoparticles Prepared with Acrylate Derivatives

Type of polymer	Drug	Observations	References
Carbopol 907	[111]Indium	Faster elimination of microspheres in dry form than when instilled as a dispersion	(22)
Copolymers MMA–SPM	Propargyl ester (APE) (S)-(+)aceclidine	Combination with mucoadhesive polymers increased bioavailability by twofold	(23)
Eudragit RL100 and RS100	Ibuprofen; Flurbiprofen	Higher drug levels in the aqueous humor compared to aqueous solution due to sustained release and increased precorneal retention	(24–26)
PNIPAAm	Epinephrine	Eightfold longer decrease of IOP after administration of cross-linked particles compared to eye drops	(27)

Abbreviations: APE, arecaidine propargyl ester; IOP, intraocular pressure; MMA, methylmethacrylate; PNIPAAm, poly-*N*-isopropylacrylamide; SPM, sulfopropylmethacrylate.

Eudragit® RL and RS using a modified quasiemulsion solvent diffusion technique and solvent evaporation method. Using these nanoparticles, they demonstrated that sustained release and increased absorption of the incorporated nonsteroidal, antiinflammatory drugs were achieved. Furthermore, no inflammation or discomfort was observed in the rabbit's eye, suggesting that the nanoparticles were well tolerated (24).

Hsiue et al. (27) investigated the use of a thermosensitive polymer, poly-N-isopropylacrylamide (PNIPAAm), in controlled-release delivery systems for glaucoma therapy. Cross-linked PNIPAAm nanoparticles containing epinephrine were administrated to rabbits, and its effect on the intraocular pressure (IOP) was monitored. The results indicated that a decreased pressure response which lasted eight times longer than that of conventional eye drops was observed.

POLY(EPSILON-CAPROLACTON)

Another biocompatible and biodegradable polymer is PECL. It is slightly more hydrophobic when compared with PACA (6,29). PECL nanoparticles and nanocapsules for ophthalmic use can be prepared by solvent extraction or solvent evaporation method (6).

Upon instillation, the PECL particles form aggregates and reside in the cul-de-sac, gradually releasing the drug. This hypothesis was put forward to explain the much more pronounced reduction in IOP in glaucomatous rabbits after administration of PECL nanoparticles when compared to PACA and PLGA microspheres (4–6). PECL nanoparticles also seem to be able to penetrate the outer corneal cell layers, but contrary to PACA, no cellular damage was observed. This suggests that an endocytic mechanism may be involved. The penetration of the particles is found to be size-dependent: nanoparticles but not microspheres were found in the corneal cells (4–6).

Numerous in vivo studies demonstrated that enhanced corneal absorption and prolonged therapeutic effects of drugs are possible when the drugs are incorporated in PECL nanoparticles. The drugs tested were: betaxolol, metipranolol, carteolol, cyclosporin A, and indomethacin. Furthermore, nanocapsules seem to display a better effect than nanospheres, probably because the drug entrapped was in the unionized form in the oily core of the delivery system and could diffuse more easily to the cornea (4–6,8).

A strategy designed to enhance the interaction with the mucus layer in the eye has been investigated by Calvo et al. (30) who coated PECL particles with cationic bioadhesive polymers. Compared with noncoated particles, the corneal and aqueous humor indomethacin concentrations were doubled for chitosan-coated nanocapsules. However, coating with polylysine did not seem to improve the bioavailability of the tested drug. The rise in bioavailability was attributed to the structural similarity between chitosan and mucin, rather than to its positive charge (30). Chitosan-coated PECL particles exhibit an important interaction with the mucus layer, but the penetration in the corneal epithelium is lower when compared with that of the uncoated particles (7).

De Campos et al. (31) compared the effect of coating PECL nanocapsules with PEG versus chitosan on the interaction of PECL nanocapsules with the ocular mucosa. The in vivo study showed that the nanoparticles entered the corneal epithelium by a transcellular pathway. The penetration rate and depth were dependent on the coating composition. PEG coating enhanced the passage of the PECL particles nanocapsules across the whole epithelium, whereas the chitosan coating favored the retention in the superficial layers of the epithelium (31). Consequently, the design of colloidal carriers with different ocular distribution seems to be possible.

POLY(D,L-LACTIC ACID) AND POLY(D,L-LACTIDE-CO-GLYCOLIDE)

As poly(D,L-lactic acid) (PLA) and poly(D,L-lactide-co-glycolide) (PLGA) are FDA-approved products (additives) for parenteral use, microspheres and nanoparticles made of these polymers were investigated primarily for the controlled release of drugs after intravitreal or subconjunctival injection rather than for topical application (4,5,9,29).

PLA is a synthetic, biocompatible, and biodegradable polymer and PLGA a copolymer of poly(lactic acid) and poly(glycolic acid). The degradation rate depends on the molecular weight, conformation, and polymer composition (9,29,32). The drug is released out of the spheres by diffusion and by hydrolysis of the PLA/PLGA matrix. In an attempt to optimize the mucoadhesive properties, PLA can be copolymerized with other polymers (e.g., PECL or PEG), so that more appropriate "tailor-made" polymers can be developed (33).

Several methods have been proposed for the preparation of the PLA/PLGA particles. However, the most popular technique is the emulsification solvent evaporation method (9,32). The uptake of PLGA nanoparticles in conjunctival epithelium is dependent on the particle size: 100 nm particles exhibited the highest uptake as compared to larger particles (800 nm and 10 μm). The saturable particle uptake occurs via adsorptive-mediated endocytosis which is independent from clathrin- and caveolin-1-mediated pathways (8,34).

Some examples of PLA/PLGA particles for ocular purpose reported in literature are summarized in Table 3. Giannavola et al. changed the surface properties of PLA nanoparticles loaded with acyclovir by incorporating PEGylated 1,2-distearoyl-3-phosphatidylethanolamine (DSPE-PEG) into the polymer instead of coating the external surface as in the case of PACA nanoparticles (22,35). After

TABLE 3 Evaluation of Poly(D,L-Lactic Acid) and Poly(D,L-Lactide-Co-Glycolide) Particles for Ophthalmic Use in Animal Studies

Drug	Application	Observations	References
Acyclovir	Instillation	A 12.6-fold increase of aqueous humor AUC for PEG-coated nanoparticles compared with drug suspension	(35)
5-Fluorouracil	Conjunctival implantation	Therapeutic scleral levels during 7 days Low ocular toxicity and no irritation	(36)
Vancomycin	Instillation	A twofold increase of aqueous humor AUC with respect to drug solution and sustained release	(37)
rhVEGF	Subretinal and intravitreal in rats	Dose-dependent angiogenic response	(38)
Budesonide	Subconjunctival injection in rats	Sustained drug level in retina and other ocular tissues during 14 days	(39)

Note: Unless otherwise indicated, all in vivo tests were performed on rabbits.
Abbreviation: AUC, area under the curve.

administration of the nanoparticle suspension in the rabbit's eye, the AUC_{0-6} values in the aqueous humor were found to be significantly greater for the PEG-coated PLA nanospheres than for the uncoated particles. A drop of 48% in AUC value was observed when PEG-coated particles were administrated to the eye after removal of the mucus layer. This decrease was attributed to the absence of PEG–mucin interactions. Thus, differences in bioavailability of the drugs could be correlated with the different interactions between the nanoparticle's surface and the corneal epithelium.

Higher and prolonged vancomycin concentration was shown in the aqueous humor by incorporating the drug in PLGA microspheres. However, increasing the viscosity of the microsphere suspension by adding a viscosifying agent (hydroxypropyl cellulose) did not seem to improve any further drug absorption, probably because of the rapid ocular clearance of the highly hydrophilic drug. No irritation or ocular discomfort was observed in rabbits (37).

Microspheres have been investigated for use in delivering many ophthalmic drugs for intravitreal or subconjunctival injections. This includes retinoic acid, adriamycin, 5-fluorouracil, dexamethasone, cyclosporin A, and ganciclovir (9,33). It has been shown that intracellular drug delivery to retinal epithelial cells may be possible by coating the PLA microspheres with gelatin, probably via phagocytosis (9). Recent studies demonstrated that PLA/PLGA microspheres may be useful in sustained or even extended slow drug delivery targeted to the posterior segment of the eye for the treatment of chronic diseases or gene therapy (38,39).

As the integrity and activity of proteins and oligonucleotides is preserved when encapsulated within PLA, the nanoparticles were evaluated for delivering these molecules to the retina (9). After intravitreal injection in rats, transretinal movement of the nanoparticles with a preferential localization in the retinal epithelial cells was observed. A mild transient inflammatory reaction after injection was reported. The presence of nanoparticles within the retinal epithelium cells could be detected even after four months of a single injection. This suggests that a steady and continuous delivery of drugs could be achieved (40). However, interference with visual acuity due to floating of nanoparticles in the vitreous cavity could be a drawback. Before clinical implementation of the nanoparticles, the possible effects of the nanoparticles on the retinal function and the vision have to be investigated (9,40).

LIPIDS

Instead of using macromolecules, several lipids were proposed for use to prepare nanoparticles. Solid–lipid nanoparticles (SLNs) consist of a biocompatible lipid core and an amphiphilic surfactant as an outer shell. The advantages of SLNs are: scalable manufacturing process using hot or cold high-pressure homogenization, easy modulation of the drug-release profile, no organic solvents, the wide range of lipid/surfactant combinations, and the high drug payload (41). Cavalli et al. (42) evaluated the use of SLNs as carriers for tobramycin. Compared to commercial eye drops, the tobramycin-loaded SLNs produced a significantly higher bioavailability: a 1.5-fold increase in C_{max} and fourfold increase in AUC. The SLN dispersion was well tolerated, with no evidence of ocular irritation (42). The longer retention observed for SLNs on the corneal surface and in the cul-de-sac is probably related to their relatively small size. The nanoparticles are presumed to be entrapped and retained in the mucus layer.

CONCLUSIONS

The in vivo studies that were used to evaluate the use of nanoparticles for ocular drug delivery were primarily performed on animals. From the results to date, one could conclude that the nanoparticles should possess bio- or mucoadhesive properties in order to achieve a long precorneal retention time and to improve drug absorption. The intraocular use of biodegradable, slow-releasing nanoparticles looks very promising for drug delivery targeted to the tissues of the posterior segment in order to treat chronic diseases or for gene therapy.

REFERENCES

1. Lee VHL, Robinson JR. Review: topical ocular drug delivery: recent developments and future challenges. J Ocul Pharmacol 1986; 2:67.
2. Salminen L. Review: systemic absorption of topically applied ocular drugs in humans. J Ocul Pharmacol 1990; 6:243.
3. Baudouin C. Side effects of antiglaucomatous drugs on the ocular surface. Curr Opin Ophthalmol 1996; 7:80.
4. Le Bourlais C et al. Ophthalmic drug delivery systems—recent advances. Prog Retinal Eye Res 1998; 17:33.
5. Zimmer A, Kreuter J. Microspheres and nanoparticles used in ocular delivery systems. Adv Drug Deliv Rev 1995; 16:61.
6. Kreuter J. Nanoparticles. In: Colloidal Drug Delivery Systems. New York: Marcel Dekker, 1994 (Chapter 5).
7. Alonso MJ, Sanchez A. The potential of chitosan in ocular drug delivery. J Pharm Pharmacol 2003; 55:1451.
8. Rabinovich-Guilatt L et al. Cationic vectors in ocular drug delivery. J Drug Targeting 2004; 12:623.
9. Yasukawa T et al. Drug delivery systems for vitreoretinal diseases. Progr Retin Eye Res 2004; 23:253.
10. Arshady R. Albumin microspheres and microcapsules: methodology of manufacturing techniques. J Control Release 1990; 14:111.
11. Merodio M et al. Ganciclovir-loaded albumin nanoparticles: characterization and in vitro release properties. Eur J Pharm Sci 2001; 12:251.
12. Giunchedi P et al. Albumin microspheres for ocular delivery of piroxicam. Pharm Pharmacol Commun 2000; 6:149.
13. Merodio M et al. Ocular disposition of ganciclovir-loaded albumin nanoparticles after intravitreal injection in rats. Biomaterials 2002; 23:1587.
14. De Campos AM, Sanchez A, Alonso MJ. Chitosan nanoparticles: a new vehicle for the improvement of the delivery of drugs to the ocular surface. Application to cyclosporin A. Int J Pharm 2001; 224:159.
15. De Campos AM et al. Chitosan nanoparticles as new ocular drug delivery systems: in vitro stability, in vivo fate, and cellular toxicity. Pharm Res 2004; 21:803.
16. Di Colo G et al. Effect of chitosan on in vitro release and ocular delivery of ofloxacin from erodible inserts based on poly(ethylene oxide). Int J Pharm 2002; 248:115.
17. Giunchedi P et al. Pectin microspheres as ophthalmic carriers for piroxicam: evaluation in vitro and in vivo in albino rabbits. Eur J Pharm Sci 1999; 9:1.
18. Tuovinen L et al. Starch acetate microparticles for drug delivery into retinal pigment epithelium—in vitro study. J Control Release 2004; 98:407.
19. Bonferoni MC et al. Carrageenan-gelatin mucoadhesive systems for ion-exchanged based ophthalmic delivery: in vitro and preliminary in vivo studies. Eur J Pharm Biopharm 2004; 57:465.
20. Desai SD, Blanchard J. Pluronic F127-based ocular delivery systems containing biodegradable polyisobutylcyanoacrylate nanocapsules of pilocarpine. J Drug Deliv Target Ther Agents 2002; 7:201.

21. Fresta M et al. Ocular tolerability and in vivo bioavailability of poly(ethylene glycol) (PEG)-coated polyethyl-2-cyanoacrylate nanospheres-encapsulated acyclovir. J Pharm Sci 2001; 90:288.

22. Durrani AM, Farr SJ, Kellaway IW. Precorneal clearance of mucoadhesive microspheres from the rabbit eye. J Pharm Pharmacol 1995; 47:581.

23. Langer K et al. Methylmethacrylate sulfopropylmethacrylate copolymer nanoparticles for drug delivery. Part III. Evaluation as drug delivery system for ophthalmic applications. Int J Pharm 1997; 158:219.

24. Pignatello R, Bucolo C, Puglisi G. Ocular tolerability of Eudragit RS 100® and RL 100® nanosuspensions as carriers for ophthalmic controlled drug delivery. J Pharm Sci 2002; 91:2636.

25. Pignatello R et al. Eudragit RS 100® nanosuspensions for ophthalmic controlled delivery of ibuprofen. Eur J Pharm 2002; 16:53.

26. Pignatello R et al. Flurbiprofen-loaded acrylate polymer nanosuspensions for ophthalmic application. Biomaterials 2002; 23:3247.

27. Hsiue G-H et al. Preparation of controlled release ophthalmic drops, for glaucoma therapy using thermosensitive poly-N-isopropylacrylamide. Biomaterials 2002; 23:457.

28. De TK et al. Polycarboxylic acid nanoparticles for ophthalmic drug delivery: an ex vivo evaluation with human cornea. J Microencapsul 2004; 21:841.

29. Deshpande AA, Heller J, Gurny R. Bioerodible polymers for ocular delivery. Crit Rev Ther Drug Carrier Syst 1998; 15:381.

30. Calvo P, Vila-Jato JL, Alonso MJ. Evaluation of cationic polymer-coated nanocapsules as ocular drug carriers. Int J Pharm 1997; 153:41.

31. De Campos AM et al. The effect of a PEG versus a chitosan coating on the interaction of drug colloidal carriers with the ocular mucosa. Eur J Pharm Sci 2003; 20:73.

32. Bala I, Hariharan S, Kumar MNVR. PLGA nanoparticles in drug delivery: the state of the art. Crit Rev Therap Drug Carrier Syst 2004; 21:387.

33. Sintzel MB et al. Biomaterials in ophthalmic drug delivery. Eur J Pharm Biopharm 1996; 42:358.

34. Quaddoumi MG et al. The characteristics and mechanisms of PLGA nanoparticles in rabbit conjunctival epithelial cell layers. Pharm Res 2004; 21:641.

35. Giannavola C et al. Influence of preparations on acyclovir-loaded poly-D,L-lactic acid nanospheres and effect of PEG coating on ocular drug bioavailability. Pharm Res 2003; 20:584.

36. Chiang C-H et al. In vitro and in vivo evaluation of an ocular delivery system of 5-fluorouracil microspheres. J Ocular Pharmacol Therap 2001; 17:545.

37. Gavini E et al. PLGA microspheres for ocular delivery of a peptide drug, vancomycin using emulsification/spray-drying as preparation method: in vitro/in vivo studies. Eur J Pharm Biopharm 2004; 57:207.

38. Cleland JL et al. Development of poly-(D,L-lactide-coglycolide) microsphere formulations containing recombinant human vascular growth factor to promote local angiogenesis. J Control Release 2001; 72:13.

39. Kompella UB, Bandi N, Ayalasomayajula SP. Subconjunctival nano- and microparticles sustain retinal delivery of budesonide, a corticosteroid capable of inhibiting VEGF expression. Invest Ophthalmol Vis Sci 2003; 44:1192.

40. Bourges J-L et al. Ocular drug delivery targeting the retina and retinal epithelium using polylactide nanoparticles. Invest Ophthalmol Vis Sci 2003; 44:3562.

41. Mehnert W, Mäder K. Solid–lipid nanoparticles production, characterization and applications. Adv Drug Deliv Rev 2001; 47:165.

42. Cavalli R et al. Solid–lipid nanoparticles (SLN) as ocular delivery systems for tobramycin. Int J Pharm 2002; 238:241.

17 Nanoparticulate Systems for Central Nervous System Drug Delivery

Jean-Christophe Olivier and Manuela Pereira de Oliveira
Pharmacologie des Médicaments Anti-Infectieux, Faculty of Medicine and Pharmacy, and INSERM, ERI 023, Poitiers, France

INTRODUCTION

The central nervous system (CNS) is isolated from the whole body by the blood–brain barrier (BBB) which creates a strictly controlled extracellular fluid environment protecting the brain parenchyma from the blood composition variation and from blood-borne potentially CNS-toxic compounds. This tight physiological barrier limits drastically drug diffusion towards the brain parenchyma and is considered as the bottleneck in brain drug development and as an important limiting factor for the future applications of biotechnology-derived neurotherapeutics (1). The BBB can be circumvented by intraventricular or intracerebral administration. These invasive and risky techniques are limited to the treatments of restrained brain areas due to the poor tissue diffusion of injected materials from the administration sites. Postsurgical administrations are the usual administration routes for relatively large drug-delivery systems (DDSs), such as microspheres and wafers, and are presently limited in clinical practice to the adjuvant treatment of brain tumors after surgical resection (2,3). The noninvasive access from the blood compartment via the BBB is the most convenient and safest way to treat the entire brain space. There are indeed around 400 miles of blood capillaries in the average 1300-g human brain, which constitute a large interface of approximately 20 m² surface area (150 cm²/g) for blood-to-brain exchanges. Nanoparticulate DDSs (nano-DDSs), mostly liposomes and nanoparticles, have been investigated for the brain delivery of therapeutic agents which poorly diffuse through the BBB. Owing to their nanometric size, these nanocontainers freely circulate in blood capillaries and can be conveniently administered by the intravenous route. Table 1 summarizes the ideal properties that nano-DDS should possess for brain drug delivery. The transit within the blood compartment requires the nano-DDS to escape from the mononuclear phagocyte system (MPS). Once within the brain vasculature, nano-DDSs have to trigger their translocation through the BBB to deliver their content in the brain. This chapter reviews the various parameters that should be considered when designing nano-DDSs for brain delivery and the present achievements in the field.

THE BLOOD–BRAIN BARRIER AND THE NEED FOR BRAIN-SPECIFIC NANO-DRUG DELIVERY SYSTEMS

Normal Blood–Brain Barrier

A scientific consensus locates the BBB at the endothelia of brain capillaries which are in close relationship with the surrounding pericytes, actrocytes, neurons, and glial cells (Fig. 1). To summarize, the BBB results from the unique properties of

TABLE 1 Ideal Properties of Nano-Drug Delivery Systems for Drug Delivery Across the Blood–Brain Barrier

General for drug delivery
Nontoxic, biodegradable, and biocompatible
Amenable to small molecules, peptides, proteins, or nucleic acids (genes, antisense drugs)
Minimal nano-DDS excipient-induced drug alteration (chemical degradation/alteration, protein denaturation)
Modulation of drug-release profiles
Scalable and cost-effective manufacturing process
General for free circulation in blood
No capillary filtration: particle diameter <1 μm
Physical stability in blood (no aggregation, no dissolution, no interaction with blood cells)
Avoidance of the MPS, prolonged blood circulation time
Particular for brain delivery
Noninvasive delivery from the blood circulation into the brain parenchyma via the BBB without inducing BBB alteration, therefore by a transcytotic pathway
Particle diameter <100 nm to fit the loading capacity of transcytotic vesicles
Extra- or intracellular drug delivery to subset of brain cells or brain tumor cells

Abbreviations: BBB, blood–brain barrier; DDS, drug delivery system; MPS, mononuclear phagocyte system.

endothelial cells (1,4): (*i*) the tight junctions that connect adjacent endothelial cells and physically restrict solute flux between the blood and the brain with the consequence that passive diffusion towards brain is limited to small lipophilic compounds (optimal log $P_{o/w}$ is 1–3) of molecular weights below 400 to 500 Da, (*ii*) an elaborate system of transport proteins that allows the selective influx transport of hydrophilic solutes (generally by carrier-mediated transport or CMT) and macromolecules (by receptor-mediated transcytosis or RMT) necessary for CNS maintenance and extracellular fluid homeostasis, and that reject potentially CNS-toxic compounds or metabolites [by active efflux transport (AET) proteins], both influx and efflux transport proteins being the cause of the observed deviations from the precept of lipophilicity-based solute penetrability into the brain, (*iii*) a metabolic barrier which serves as a biotransformation and detoxification system, and (*iv*) a negligible pinocytotic activity. The high transendothelial electrical resistance value (~2000 Ω cm^2) measured across the brain capillary endothelium is indicative of the very low ionic permeability. As a consequence, BBB accounts for the restricted CNS access of more than 98% of all small-molecule drugs and of 100% of large-molecule drugs (4).

Blood–Brain Barrier Alteration in Pathology

In various brain pathologies, including brain trauma, stroke, septic encephalopathy, or neurodegenerative diseases, or in metabolic disorders such as diabetes mellitus, the alterations of the BBB permeability result in leakage of normally restrained plasma components and contribute to neuroinflammation and neuronal damage (5). It is still controversial whether the BBB permeability increase results from the opening of passageways through brain endothelial cells, defined as vesiculo-tubular systems or vesiculo-vacuolar organelles (6), or from tight junction degradation (5). Little is known on the degree of BBB permeabilization in inflammatory brain pathologies, but its actual impact on nano-DDS passive diffusion is likely to be low. In a rat model of cerebral ischemia and reperfusion, polystyrene nanoparticles (20 nm in diameter) were shown to extravasate into the brain interstitial fluid (7). In the case of larger nano-DDSs such as liposomes, the uptake by infiltrating

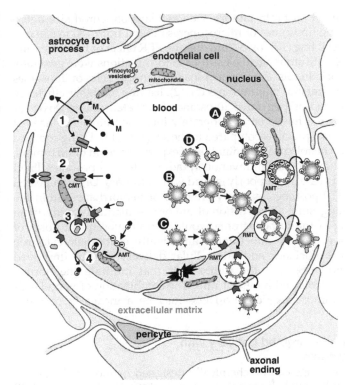

FIGURE 1 Schematic diagram of the neurovascular association forming the BBB together with the molecular transport pathways across the BBB (1–4) and proposed transcytotic brain-delivery mechanisms for nano-DDSs (A–D). Brain endothelial cells are characterized with tight junctions (tj) that lock the aqueous paracellular pathways, negligible pinocytotic activity, high transport, and metabolic activity. They are in close relationship with pericytes, astrocyte foot processes, axonal endings, and microglial cells (not represented). Passive diffusion across the endothelial cells is the passageway of small lipophilic molecules (M_w below 400–500 Da) (1). Restrained by tight junctions and the plasma membranes, hydrophilic compounds require specialized transport to reach brain: CMT systems for small molecules (2), RMT for macromolecules (3), or absorptive-mediated transcytosis (AMT) for cationic molecules (4). Compounds traversing endothelial cells may be rejected back into the blood compartment by AET systems as intact molecules or as metabolites (M). Proposed transcytotic pathways for nano-DDSs are AMT triggered by positively charged surfaces (A) or RMT triggered by natural substrate ligands such as transferrin (B) or peptidomimetic antibodies directed against exofacial epitopes of transferrin or insulin receptors (C). The hypothetic "differential protein adsorption mechanism" according to which the nano-DDS surface would adsorb, from blood, natural substrates of BBB receptors (e.g., apolipoproteins B or E, substrates low-density lipoprotein receptors) and then undergo endocytosis/transcytosis is also represented (D). *Abbreviations*: AET, Active efflux transport; AMT, absorptive-mediate transcytosis; BBB, blood–brain barrier; CMT, carrier-mediated transport; DDSs, drug delivery systems; RMT, receptor-mediated transcytosis.

macrophages is probably the mechanism for their increased distribution into inflammatory brain tissues (8).

In the case of brain tumors, the BBB integrity is locally compromised by the absence of tight junctions, allowing for tumor core penetration and retention of drugs, macromolecules, or nano-DDS otherwise excluded from normal brain (9). This phenomenon is known as the enhanced permeability and retention (EPR) effect of tumors. Generally, growing tumor margins and adjacent normal tissue remain unreachable. In experimental rat brain tumors, the vascular pore cutoff size determined with long-circulating liposomes or microspheres ranged from 100 to 550 nm, depending on the tumor cell line (10). By optimizing the EPR effect or by decreasing peripheral distribution of antitumor agents, nano-DDS formulations were generally more efficient than solutions. In rats, doxorubicin-loaded nanoparticles or liposomes increased delivery to experimental brain tumors (11,12), leading to higher efficiency (12). Doxorubicin formulated as pegylated liposomes (marketed under Doxil® or Caelyx® trademarks) showed, however, a moderately increased efficiency against high-grade gliomas in clinical practice, compared to the solution (13). Using confocal imaging, MR imaging, and histological examination of experimental rat brain tumors, Straubinger et al. (14) showed that intravenously administered liposomes lined tumor capillaries or blood vessels and poorly spread within tumors. Under repeated administrations of Doxil® liposomes, extensive regions of hemorrhage within the tumor tissue occurred, suggesting a destruction of tumor vasculature or underlying tumor cells. The opening of the tumor stroma would permit subsequent doses of liposomes to diffuse more deeply into tumors and finally exert their cytotoxic effect on margins. Uptake efficiency and intracellular delivery may be improved with tumor-specific nano-DDSs, but the tumor cells that infiltrate the normal brain parenchyma remain protected by intact BBB. The combination of nano-DDSs able to cross BBB with tumor-specific nano-DDSs may be a means to optimize antitumor therapy.

Candidate Drugs for Brain-Targeted Delivery with Nano-Drug Delivery Systems

Generally, small-molecule drugs can be chemically designed or modified (e.g., by prodrug synthesis) to be adequately lipophilic for passive diffusion through the BBB and do not need DDSs for brain delivery. However, drug lipidization is not always applicable or effective, especially when drugs are particular chemical entities that cannot be modified without losing their pharmacological activities and/or are substrates of efflux transport proteins present at the BBB, such as the P-glycoprotein. Furthermore, drug lipidization generally results in increased metabolism and peripheral distribution, which necessitates higher doses, potentially at the cost of more frequent adverse reactions. In such cases, or when small drug molecules undergo metabolization in brain endothelial cells, nano-DDS formulations should be considered as a means for improving brain delivery. Another group of molecules that necessitates nano-DDS formulations are the new large-molecule therapeutics potentially efficient to treat CNS: peptides, proteins, such as neurotrophic factors, antisense drugs, or genes (plasmids). Owing to their poor stability in biological fluids, rapid enzymatic degradation, unfavorable pharmacokinetic properties, and lack of diffusion towards the CNS, they could be advantageously formulated in brain-targeted protective nanocontainers. Compared to conventional drugs, they possess a high intrinsic pharmacological activity. The small dose needed for therapeutic efficiency would easily fit the loading capacity of nano-DDSs and avoid the administration of large amount of potentially toxic nano-DDS excipients. The choice between liposomes or nanoparticles will depend on formulation aspects, release kinetics, and stability upon storage. Proteins are generally unstable in the presence of organic solvent or solid interfaces. It may, therefore, be challenging to maintain their biological activities upon entrapment within nanoparticles that need solvents (polymeric NP) or heating steps (lipid NP) for preparation. Formulation additives may improve their stability (15), or liposome formulations may be more appropriate. Some drugs will require release into the brain interstitial fluid to be effective. Others, such as plasmid genes or antisense oligonucleotides, need to be delivered intracellularly for effectiveness, which means that after crossing the BBB nano-DDS should be also able to cross plasma membranes of targeted brain cells.

NANO-DRUG DELIVERY SYSTEMS FOR NONINVASIVE
DRUG BRAIN DELIVERY
Basic Principles

According to the pharmacokinetic rule, the percent of injected dose of a drug that is delivered per gram brain (%ID/g) is directly proportional to the BBB permeability–surface area (PS) product and the area under the plasma concentration curve (AUC, %ID min μL^{-1}): %ID/g = PS×AUC (1). This rule also stands for nano-DDS brain delivery. For optimal efficiency, nano-DDSs administered IV should remain in the blood compartment, avoiding useless peripheral distribution, in order to reach the brain vasculature and should possess an appropriate BBB PS in order to deliver their content beyond the BBB into the brain parenchyma. Owing to their size, nano-DDSs cannot cross the endothelium of brain capillaries by passive diffusion through normal BBB. Although effective for promoting liposome delivery into the brain parenchyma (16,17) and explored for improving antitumor drug diffusion into brain tumors (18), increasing BBB permeability using hyperosmolar solutions or the selective B_2 bradykinin Cereport (labradimil or RMP-7) should be limited to short-term therapy, as this promotes the non-selective entry of blood-borne compounds and may result in seizures and permanent neuropathological changes. With preserving the BBB integrity, the delivery of nano-DDSs into the brain parenchyma implies that nano-DDSs should not only recognize specific sites at the BBB, but also trigger their own transfer across the endothelial cells. Indeed intravenously administered pegylated immunoliposomes directed against brain astrocytes displayed long-circulating properties (elimination half-lives of 8–15 hours), but were unable to cross the BBB and missed their targets (19). On the basis of an already long research, both steps are being rationally apprehended and key parameters are well defined for liposomes. However, despite real achievements, optimization is still needed in the case of nanoparticles (20).

Circulating in the Blood Compartment

If not especially designed to escape from the MPS uptake, intravenously administered nano-DDSs are rapidly cleared from the blood stream (blood half-lives are generally around two to three minutes) and mostly accumulate in liver and spleen. It is generally admitted that opsonization, the first step for MPS recognition, is favored by hydrophobic surfaces, which promote protein adsorption, and negative surfaces, which are activators of the complement system (21). In contrast, hydrophilic coating sterically stabilizes nano-DDSs and reduces opsonization and MPS uptake. These rather simplistic views should, however, be tempered, as recent evidence showed that sterically stabilized particles were efficiently opsonized and activated the complement system, while keeping their stealth properties (22). Whatever the mechanism may be, the incorporation of polyethylene glycol (PEG) derivatized lipids into the phospholipids bilayer of liposomes resulted in long-circulating liposomes, generally referred to as sterically stabilized liposomes, with apparent terminal half-lives up to 90 hours in humans (23). Long-circulating nanoparticles are however still elusive. Pharmacokinetic studies are often contradictory, if not lacking. In the case of pegylated poly(lactide) or poly(lactide-co-glycolide) nanoparticles, the up-to-date most studied polymeric nano-DDSs, surface coating with PEG molecular weights of 5000 or over, were shown to be efficient at reducing opsonization, but blood half-lives were found to be very variable ranging from less than one to six hours (20). The variability in density-related PEG conformation may explain the rapid clearance of a significant fraction of intravenously injected "long-circulating" nanoparticles by the MPS (22). Contrary to liposomes, the variety in nanoparticle core nature (polymers or lipids) that characterizes the research on nanoparticles resulted in the dispersion of research effort which was probably at the origin of the limited achievements in the long-circulating nanoparticle design.

Nano-Drug Delivery System Transport Through Brain Endothelial Cells

The reasoned approaches presently under investigation for triggering nano-DDS translocation across BBB are based on AMT or RMT (Fig. 1). Unexpectedly, several research teams found that surfactant-coated nanoparticles delivered their contents to the brain. As they were not based on theoretical concept, these methods were referred to as "empirical" approaches.

Absorptive-Mediated Transcytosis

Cationized proteins (albumin, immunoglobulins) have been demonstrated to undergo absorptive-mediated endocytosis (AME) through the BBB in vivo (24). AME is triggered by an electrostatic interaction between the positively charged protein and the negatively charged plasma membranes. It is therefore not brain-specific, and cationized proteins also accumulate in liver, kidney, and/or lung tissues. However, the relatively high capacity of AME should be favorable to brain delivery (25). Preservation of appropriate pharmacokinetic profiles depends on the degree of cationization (24). As an application of such a concept, cationic bovine serum albumin-conjugated pegylated nano-DDSs [liposomes (26) and pegylated polylactide nanoparticles (27)] were shown to undergo endocytosis in in vitro BBB model. It is still to be demonstrated whether these cationic nano-DDSs will possess appropriate pharmacokinetic profiles by the intravenous administration route.

Receptor-Mediated Transcytosis

Owing to a high stereospecificity for their substrate, CMT requires drugs with molecular structures mimicking the endogenous nutrient and is not a realistic option for nano-DDS brain delivery (1,25). Only RMT may be used for transcytotic delivery of nano-DDSs through the BBB. Owing to the ubiquity of RMT, relative brain specificity may be achieved by targeting receptors that are overexpressed at the luminal side of brain endothelial cells compared to other organs, for example, the receptors of transferrin, insulin, insulin-like growth factor (IGF), or low-density lipoproteins (LDL) (4). Nano-DDSs should be less than 100 nm in diameter to fit the loading capacity of these transport systems and should have on their surface receptor-recognizing ligand (natural substrate or antibody) capable of triggering transcytosis. Transferrin ligand was investigated for liposome brain targeting with promising results (28), but an apolipoprotein E-derived peptide failed to trigger liposome endocytosis via LDL receptor (29). Antibodies directed against exofacial receptor epitopes that do not interfere with the natural ligand-binding sites should be preferred in order to avoid potential competition between targeted nano-DDSs and endogenous natural ligand (transferrin, apolipoproteins), pharmacological activity (insulin), or linkage to plasma-binding proteins (IGF) (4). The most advanced work based on this "Trojan horse" concept has been carried out by Pardridge and coworkers with pegylated immunoliposomes (4). The receptor-specific targeting ligands located at the tip of 1% to 2% of the PEG_{2000} strands are peptidomimetic monoclonal antibodies able to trigger the activation of transferrin or insulin receptors. After intravenous administration, these immunoliposomes delivered their content (small-drug molecules, plasmids) into the brain parenchyma without damaging the BBB (30–33). Owing to the presence of transferrin or insulin receptors on the neuronal plasma membrane, plasmid-loaded immunoliposomes permitted neuronal nuclear delivery, resulting in gene expression in the entire brain space (31–33). As RMT receptors are also abundant in some peripheral tissues, ectopic expression in nonbrain organs was eliminated using a brain-specific gene promoter (33). In a 6-hydroxydopamine rat model of Parkinson's disease, the selective gene expression in nigrostriatal neurons resulted in the restoration of tyrosine hydroxylase activity and in reversal of motor impairment (33). As immunoliposomes deliver their content quickly, as shown by the relatively short-lasting plasmid expression in brain (33), they would require monthly administrations to sustain a pharmacological effect (31). This potential inconvenience for the treatment of chronic brain disorders may be corrected using pegylated poly(lactide) immunonanoparticles with sustained-release properties (20,34).

Empirical Approaches
Various works reported on the beneficial effect of surfactant-coated lipid or polymeric nanoparticles for the brain delivery of drugs. No brain-targeting ligand is present on nanoparticle surface and the various mechanisms underlying increased brain uptake of entrapped compounds remain hypothetic.

Solid–Lipid Nanoparticles
Solid–lipid nanoparticles are basically constituted of a liquid or solid–lipid core (liquid glyceride or wax) surrounded by a solid shell made of an association of several anionic surfactants (polysorbates, PEG fatty acid ester, PEG fatty alcohol ether, poloxamers) and/or ionic surfactants (lecithin, etc.) and do not (generally) necessitate organic solvents for their preparation (35). Experimental demonstration of SLN "stealthness" is scarce and more often based on the presupposed antiopsonic effect of PEGylated surfactant rather than on experimental evidence (36). Several experimental works showed that surfactant-coated solid–lipid nanoparticles could increase the brain uptake of loaded drugs that poorly diffuse into the brain when administered as solutions. A prodrug of dioctanoylfluorodeoxyuridine had a significantly higher brain distribution when administered as pluronic F68-coated solid–lipid nanoparticle formulations compared to the solution (37). The authors proposed as brain uptake mechanisms either an increase in gradient concentration between blood and brain resulting from a higher plasma AUC (compared to the drug solution), or an endocytosis by endothelial cells. In other studies, intravenously administered to rats or rabbits, doxorubicin "stealth" SLN coated with PEG2000 stearate also increased brain uptake compared to the commercial solution (36,38). In an in situ rat brain perfusion model, paclitaxel brain uptake was increased when formulated in wax nanoparticles including polysorbate 60 and Brij 78 as surfactants, compared to the control solution (39). Control nanoparticles were shown to undergo a significant brain uptake (40) without altering BBB permeability (41,42). Unexpectedly, nanoparticle translocation through the BBB was not

retained as the mechanism for increased paclitaxel brain uptake, and the authors favored a modulation of paclitaxel efflux by P-glycoprotein transporter (39).

Polybutylcyanoacrylate Nanoparticles

Adsorbed onto polysorbate-coated polybutylcyanoacrylate (PBCA) nanoparticles administered intravenously, compounds with poor brain diffusion (doxorubicin, loperamide, tubocurarine, the hexapeptide dalargin) were successfully delivered to the brain where they induced pharmacological effects (for review, see Ref. 43). As these nanoparticles do not possess targeting ligands on their surface, the concept of "differential protein adsorption" was proposed by Müller (44). According to this concept, some blood proteins preferentially adsorb onto nanoparticle surfaces depending on their physicochemical properties. Apolipoproteins B and E would be the brain-targeting proteins that adsorb onto polysorbate-coated nanoparticles and permit nanoparticle endocytotic delivery into the brain vessel endothelia via LDL receptors (45). This mechanism may also account for polysorbate 80-coated poly(lactide) nanoparticle interaction with brain microvessels (46). However, it was shown that in rats treated with polysorbate 80-coated PBCA nanoparticles (polysorbate 80: 25 mg/kg, nanoparticles: 50 mg/kg) inulin spaces increased by 10% (nonsignificant) after 10 minutes and by 99% (significant) after 45 minutes compared to controls (47). A nanoparticle-induced nonspecific BBB permeabilization, resulting from the synergistic effect of nanoparticle toxicity and high polysorbate 80 concentrations, was proposed as an alternative mechanism to the brain translocation of nanoparticles across the BBB (48).

CONCLUSION

Technology now exists for designing safe brain-targeted long-circulating nano-DDSs. The PEGylated immunoliposomes based on the concept of molecular "Trojan horse" that targets the transcytotic BBB receptors and ferries the liposomes though the BBB permitted the efficient noninvasive, nonviral delivery of plasmid genes into the brain parenchyma cells. They constitute the present most convincing demonstration of successful brain delivery of complex macromolecules by nano-DDSs from the blood circulation through the BBB. The empirical use of simpler polymeric or lipid nanoparticles also resulted in promising results. The mechanisms underlying their still hypothetic translocation through the BBB need further investigations for validation. Thus, despite the complexity of the issue, there have been real achievements in nano-DDS brain delivery, but the way is still long from bench results to clinical applications.

REFERENCES

1. Pardridge WM. The blood–brain barrier: bottleneck in brain drug development. NeuroRx 2005; 2:3.
2. Benoit JP, Faisant N, Venier-Julienne MC, Menei P. Development of microspheres for neurological disorders: from basics to clinical applications. J Control Release 2000; 65:285.
3. Guerin C, Olivi A, Weingart JD, Lawson HC, Brem H. Recent advances in brain tumor therapy: local intracerebral drug delivery by polymers. Invest New Drugs 2004; 22:27.
4. Pardridge WM. Brain Drug Targeting: The Future of Brain Drug Development. Cambridge University Press, 2001.
5. Petty MA, Lo EH. Junctional complexes of the blood–brain barrier: permeability changes in neuroinflammation. Prog Neurobiol 2002; 68:311.

6. Lossinsky AS, Shivers RR. Structural pathways for macromolecular and cellular transport across the blood–brain barrier during inflammatory conditions. Histol Histopathol 2004; 19:535.
7. Yang CS, Chang CH, Tsai PJ, Chen WY, Tseng FG, Lo LW. Nanoparticle-based in vivo investigation on blood–brain barrier permeability following ischemia and reperfusion. Anal Chem 2004; 76:4465.
8. Rousseau V, Denizot B, Le Jeune JJ, Jallet P. Early detection of liposome brain localization in rat experimental allergic encephalomyelitis. Exp Brain Res 1999; 125(3):255–264.
9. Papadopoulos MC, Saadoun S, Binder DK, Manley GT, Krishna S, Verkman AS. Molecular mechanisms of brain tumor edema. Neuroscience 2004; 129(4):1011–1020.
10. Hobbs SK, Monsky WL, Yuan F, et al. Regulation of transport pathways in tumor vessels: role of tumor type and microenvironment. Proc Natl Acad Sci USA 1998; 95(8):4607–4612.
11. Brigger I, Morizet J, Aubert G, et al. Poly(ethylene glycol)-coated hexadecylcyanoacrylate nanospheres display a combined effect for brain tumor targeting. J Pharmacol Exp Ther 2002; 303(3):928–936.
12. Steiniger SC, Kreuter J, Khalansky AS, et al. Chemotherapy of glioblastoma in rats using doxorubicin-loaded nanoparticles. Int J Cancer 2004; 109:759.
13. Hau P, Fabel K, Baumgart U, et al. Pegylated liposomal doxorubicin-efficacy in patients with recurrent high-grade glioma. Cancer 2004; 100(6):1199–1207.
14. Straubinger RM, Arnold RD, Zhou R, Mazurchuk R, Slack JE. Antivascular and antitumor activities of liposome-associated drugs. Anticancer Res 2004; 24(2A):397–404.
15. Schwendeman SP. Recent advances in the stabilization of proteins encapsulated in injectable PLGA delivery systems. Crit Rev Ther Drug Carrier Syst 2002; 19:73.
16. Sakamoto A, Ido T. Liposome targeting to rat brain: effect of osmotic opening of the blood–brain barrier. Brain Res 1993; 26; 629(1):171–175.
17. Xie Y, Ye L, Zhang X, et al. Transport of nerve growth factor encapsulated into liposomes across the blood–brain barrier: in vitro and in vivo studies. J Control Release 2005; 105(1–2):106–119.
18. Kemper EM, Boogerd W, Thuis I, Beijnen JH, van Tellingen O. Modulation of the blood–brain barrier in oncology: therapeutic opportunities for the treatment of brain tumours? Cancer Treat Rev 2004; 30(5):415–423.
19. Chekhonin VP, Zhirkov YA, Gurina OI, et al. PEGylated immunoliposomes directed against brain astrocytes. Drug Deliv 2005; 12(1):1–6.
20. Olivier JC. Drug transport to brain with targeted nanoparticles. NeuroRx 2005; 2:108.
21. Moghimi SM, Hunter AC, Murray JC. Long-circulating and target-specific nanoparticles: theory to practice. Pharmacol Rev 2001; 53:283.
22. Moghimi SM, Szebeni J. Stealth liposomes and long circulating nanoparticles: critical issues in pharmacokinetics, opsonization and protein-binding properties. Prog Lipid Res 2003; 42:463.
23. Gabizon A, Shmeeda H, Barenholz Y. Pharmacokinetics of pegylated liposomal doxorubicin: review of animal and human studies. Clin Pharmacokinet 2003; 42:419.
24. Bickel U, Yoshikawa T, Pardridge WM. Delivery of peptides and proteins through the blood–brain barrier. Adv Drug Deliv Rev 2001; 46:247.
25. Tsuji A, Tamai II. Carrier-mediated or specialized transport of drugs across the blood–brain barrier. Adv Drug Deliv Rev 1999; 36(2–3):277–290.
26. Thole M, Nobmanna S, Huwyler J, Bartmann A, Fricker G. Uptake of cationizied albumin coupled liposomes by cultured porcine brain microvessel endothelial cells and intact brain capillaries. J Drug Target 2002; 10(4):337–344.
27. Lu W, Tan YZ, Hu KL, Jiang XG. Cationic albumin conjugated pegylated nanoparticle with its transcytosis ability and little toxicity against blood–brain barrier. Int J Pharm 2005; 295(1–2):247–260.
28. Omori N et al. Targeting of post-ischemic cerebral endothelium in rat by liposomes bearing polyethylene glycol-coupled transferring. Neurol Res 2003; 25:275.
29. Sauer I et al. An apolipoprotein E-derived peptide mediates uptake of sterically stabilized liposomes into brain capillary endothelial cells. Biochemistry 2005; 44:2021.
30. Huwyler J, Wu D, Pardridge WM. Brain drug delivery of small molecules using immunoliposomes. Proc Natl Acad Sci USA 1996; 93:14164–14169.
31. Schlachetzki F et al. Gene therapy of the brain: the trans-vascular approach. Neurology 2004; 62:1275.

32. Zhang Y, Schlachetzki F, Pardridge WM. Global non-viral gene transfer to the primate brain following intravenous administration. Mol Ther 2003; 7:11.
33. Zhang Y, Schlachetzki F, Zhang YF, Boado RJ, Pardridge WM. Normalization of striatal tyrosine hydroxylase and reversal of motor impairment in experimental parkinsonism with intravenous nonviral gene therapy and a brain-specific promoter. Hum Gene Ther 2004; 15(4):339–350.
34. Olivier JC, Huertas R, Lee HJ, Calon F, Pardridge WM. Synthesis of pegylated immunon-anoparticles. Pharm Res 2002; 19:1137–1143.
35. Mehnert W, Mader K. Solid–lipid nanoparticles: production, characterization and applications. Adv Drug Deliv Rev 2001; 47:165.
36. Fundaro A, Cavalli R, Bargoni A, Vighetto D, Zara GP, Gasco MR. Non-stealth and stealth lipid nanoparticles (SLN) carrying doxorubicin: pharmacokinetics and tissue distribution after i.v. administration to rats. Pharmacol Res 2000; 42(4):337–343.
37. Wang JX, Sun X, Zhang ZR. Enhanced brain targeting by synthesis of 3′,5′-dioctanoyl-5-fluoro-2′-deoxyuridine and incorporation into solid–lipid nanoparticles. Eur J Pharm Biopharm 2002; 54:285.
38. Zara GP, Cavalli R, Bargoni A, Fundaro A, Vighetto D, Gasco MR. Intravenous administration to rabbits of non-stealth and stealth doxorubicin-loaded solid–lipid nanoparticles at increasing concentrations of stealth agent: pharmacokinetics and distribution of doxorubicin in brain and other tissues. J Drug Target 2002; 10(4):327–335.
39. Koziara JM, Lockman PR, Allen DD, Mumper RJ. Paclitaxel nanoparticles for the potential treatment of brain tumors. J Control Release 2004; 99(2):259–269.
40. Koziara JM, Lockman PR, Allen DD, Mumper RJ. In situ blood–brain barrier transport of nanoparticles. Pharm Res 2003; 20(11):1772–1778.
41. Lockman PR, Koziara JM, Mumper RJ, Allen DD. Nanoparticle surface charges alter blood–brain barrier integrity and permeability. J Drug Target 2004; 12(9–10):635–641.
42. Lockman PR, Koziara J, Roder KE, et al. In vivo and in vitro assessment of baseline blood–brain barrier parameters in the presence of novel nanoparticles. Pharm Res 2003; 20(5):705–713.
43. Kreuter J. Nanoparticulate systems for brain delivery of drugs. Adv Drug Deliv Rev 2001; 47:65–81.
44. Müller RH, Keck CM. Drug delivery to the brain—realization by novel drug carriers. J Nanosci Nanotechnol 2004; 4:471.
45. Kreuter J et al. Apolipoprotein-mediated transport of nanoparticle-bound drugs across the blood–brain barrier. J Drug Target 2002; 10:317.
46. Sun W, Xie C, Wang H, Hu Y. Specific role of polysorbate 80 coating on the targeting of nanoparticles to the brain. Biomaterials 2004; 25(15):3065–3071.
47. Alyaudtin RN, Reichel A, Lobenberg R, Ramge P, Kreuter J, Begley DJ. Interaction of poly(butylcyanoacrylate) nanoparticles with the blood–brain barrier in vivo and in vitro. J Drug Target 2001; 9:209–221.
48. Olivier JC, Fenart L, Chauvet R, Pariat C, Cecchelli R, Couet W. Indirect evidence that drug brain targeting using polysorbate 80-coated polybutylcyanoacrylate nanoparticles is related to toxicity. Pharm Res 1999; 16(12):1836–1842.

18 Nanoparticles for Gene Delivery: Formulation Characteristics

Jaspreet K. Vasir and Vinod Labhasetwar
Department of Pharmaceutical Sciences, University of Nebraska Medical Center, Omaha, Nebraska, U.S.A.

INTRODUCTION

The recent advances in the field of molecular biology have highlighted gene therapy as a promising approach for the treatment of numerous diseases including genetic disorders, such as cystic fibrosis, hemophilia; many somatic diseases such as tumors, neurodegenerative diseases; and severe viral infections such as AIDS. Despite the considerable interest generated in gene therapy and the phenomenal pace at which research has advanced, "delivery" of genes to the target cells still remains the most formidable challenge. Polynucleotide molecules (e.g., DNA or RNA) are large, hydrophilic, macromolecules with a net negative charge. Unlike other drugs, these are very labile in the biological environment and do not cross biological membranes effectively. Thus, the need for an effective and safe gene-delivery system is quite obvious. In general, gene delivery/expression vectors can be broadly categorized into the viral and nonviral vectors. Viral vectors include the use of genetically engineered retroviruses, adenoviruses, adeno-associated viruses, and other viruses that have been used for gene-transfer procedures. Although the viruses are highly efficient for gene transfer to cells, their pote ntial to induce drastic immune responses such as with adenovirus or the risk of insertional mutagenesis in the host genome with retroviral vectors (1) has sparked a major debate over their safety for human gene therapy.

Thus, the current consensus is to develop suitable vector systems which are minimally invasive (safe) and highly efficient for gene therapy in humans. This has steered research towards the development of nonviral vectors for gene delivery. Nonviral vectors include nanoparticles (NPs), liposomes, and complexes prepared either using cationic lipids (lipoplexes) or polymers (polyplexes), and also mechanical methods such as electroporation or microneedle injections of plasmid, especially for transfection through the skin surface.

Among polymeric gene expression systems, biodegradable NPs offer certain advantages for gene delivery. These can be formed by encapsulating DNA into polymers or by complexing DNA to the surface of preformed NPs (Fig. 1). Plasmid DNA can be encapsulated in polymeric NPs (*i*) alone as naked plasmid DNA (2,3), (*ii*) condensed with some cationic polymers (4), or (*iii*) in noncondensed form with some protective excipients (5). Polynucleotide molecules can also be complexed with positively charged entities (cationic surfactants or polysaccharides) grafted on the surface of preformed polymeric NPs (6). Thus, there is a great degree of flexibility in developing biodegradable NPs as gene expression vectors.

POLY(LACTIC ACID)/POLY(D,L-LACTIDE-CO-GLYCOLIDE)-BASED NPS

Poly(lactic acid) (PLA) and poly(D,L-lactide-co-glycolide) (PLGA) are the biodegradable and biocompatible polymers used for formulating NPs and are approved

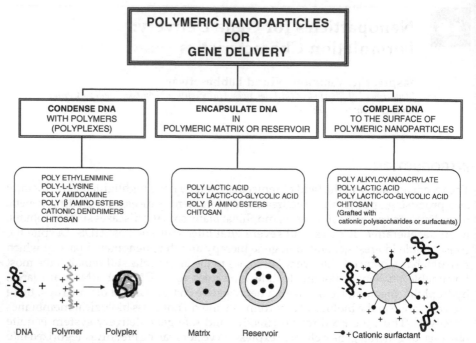

FIGURE 1 Schematic representation showing different types of polymeric nanoparticles for gene delivery.

for human use by the U.S. Food and Drug Administration. PLA/PLGA NPs with entrapped plasmid DNA are of special interest for gene delivery due to their non-viral and nonimmunogenic nature. Plasmid DNA is entrapped into the polymeric matrix, which not only protects DNA from nucleases, but also allows a control over the DNA-release kinetics from NPs. The main advantage of these NPs is the slow release of DNA from the NPs which facilitates sustained levels of gene expression. Moreover, the duration and levels of gene expression can be easily modulated by altering formulation parameters such as DNA:polymer ratio, or polymer molecular weight, and composition.

PLGA NPs are generally formulated using "water-in-oil-in-water" double-emulsion solvent evaporation technique, using polyvinyl alcohol (PVA) as an emulsifier (2). In brief, an aqueous solution of plasmid DNA is emulsified into the polymer solution in organic solvents (usually chloroform or methylene chloride) either by high-speed homogenization or sonication. This water-in-oil emulsion is then mixed into a second aqueous phase (usually an aqueous solution of surfactant/emulsifier, typically PVA is used). The double water-in-oil-in-water emulsion is then formed using sonication or homogenization. The organic solvent is then allowed to evaporate by stirring the emulsion at room temperature for approximately 18 to 20 hours. This results in the formation of polymeric NPs with entrapped plasmid DNA which are recovered by ultracentrifugation, washed with distilled water to remove PVA and unentrapped DNA. The NPs are suspended in water and lyophilized to form a dry powder. NPs prepared using this procedure are usually around 100 nm in diameter and have a negative zeta potential (7). DNA loading in these NPs has been reported around 0.5% to 2.5% (w/w) (3). The efficiency of DNA encapsulation using this process depends on the polymer composition, molecular weight of the polymer, and the nature and concentration of emulsifier used in the process (2). There are some concerns regarding the stability of DNA during the encapsulation process, due to the use of high-shear forces (generated using high-speed homogenization or sonication) and exposure of DNA to the organic solvents (8,9). These conditions may result in the transformation of DNA from its supercoiled form to the open-circular or linear forms. Preservation of the structural integrity of DNA is important, whereas the supercoiled form has the highest bioactivity and the linear form is least active (10). Studies have demonstrated that there is only a minimal loss of activity of DNA following nanoencapsulation as the DNA is mostly present in the supercoiled or open-circular forms in the NPs (11).

A cryopreparation method for the microencapsulation of plasmid DNA has been described, to reduce the loss of the supercoiled form of DNA during formulation and to improve the encapsulation of DNA (12). This method involves freezing the aqueous phase of the primary emulsion containing the plasmid DNA before subjecting it to homogenization. This has been shown to preserve the content of the supercoiled form of DNA, as DNA frozen in the aqueous phase is exposed to minimum shear stress. Addition of saccharides as cryoprotectants in the primary emulsion can also prevent the structural loss of DNA. Saccharides prevent crystal formation from the buffer salts (present in the primary emulsion) during lyophilization and thus consequently prevent nicking of DNA by such salt crystals.

Oster et al. (13) have described a gentle solvent displacement method, without the use of high-speed homogenization for the encapsulation of DNA. A new class of biodegradable polymers consisting of amine-modified PVA backbone grafted with PLGA side chains has been used in this procedure. The tertiary amino groups in the polymer backbone interact with DNA by electrostatic interactions and facilitate NP formation due to their amphiphilic character. These NPs exhibited positive zeta potential and high transfection efficiencies in cell culture comparable to polyethylenimine–DNA complexes. The high transfection efficiency may be due to the rapid polymer degradation rates and the preservation of DNA integrity and bioactivity during the NP formulation procedure.

Owing to their small size, PLGA NPs are taken up by cells (mainly by endocytosis) and facilitate intracellular delivery of plasmid DNA. As NPs come in direct contact with the cell membranes, the surface properties of NPs are critical in determining their intracellular fate and can potentially influence the gene transfection efficiencies (Fig. 2) (2). These include the surface-associated PVA in NPs, hydrophilicity, and the surface charge (zeta potential) of NPs. It has been shown that for NPs formulated using the double-emulsion solvent evaporation, a fraction of PVA used in the formulation remains associated with the NP surface, and cannot be removed even by multiple washings (14). This residual PVA on NP surface can alter its physical properties and affect the cellular uptake of NPs. NPs with lower amounts of surface-associated PVA show about threefold higher cellular uptake in vascular smooth muscle cells than the NPs with higher residual PVA (15). This could be due to shielding of the surface charge reversal of NPs by the presence of higher amount of surface-associated PVA, which could affect the endosomal escape of NPs. Further, the amount of PVA associated with the NP surface depends on its concentration used as an emulsifier during formulation, its molecular weight, and degree of hydroxylation (2). Cellular internalization of NPs also depends on their particle size and thus has been shown to affect the gene transfection. The smaller size

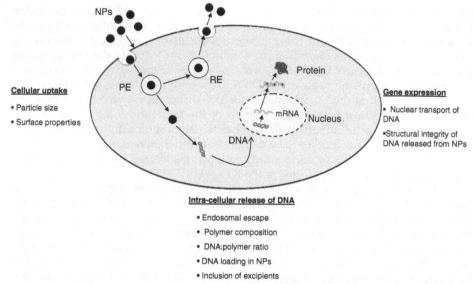

FIGURE 2 (*See color insert.*) Formulation factors influencing nanoparticle-mediated gene expression. *Abbreviations*: NPs, nanoparticles; PE, primary endosomes; RE, recycling endosomes.

(less than 100 nm) of NPs showed 27-fold higher gene transfection than the larger size (more than 100 nm) NPs (7). Thus, the smaller size with a uniform particle size distribution is expected to increase the gene transfection efficiency of NPs.

Other important formulation parameters which influence the gene transfection ability of NPs include the molecular weight of polymer and its composition (lactide to glycolide ratio) (2). NPs formulated with higher-molecular-weight polymer showed enhanced gene transfection. This may be attributed to the relatively higher DNA loading and its release from NPs prepared with high-molecular-weight polymer (Fig. 3). Higher viscosity and better emulsifying properties of the polymer solution facilitate higher loading of DNA in NPs and also lead to lower particle size of NPs. Polymer composition can affect the hydrophobicity of the polymer and thus can affect the DNA loading and release of DNA from the NPs. NPs prepared using more hydrophobic polymers (polylactides) demonstrated lower transfection than those formulated using copolymers of polylactide and glycolide (Fig. 4). The slow rate of release of DNA from the hydrophobic polymeric matrix may be responsible for the lower levels of gene transfection.

Although the levels of gene expression with NPs are lower than that achieved with lipid-based gene delivery, they are sustained for a prolonged period of time. Further NP-mediated gene transfection is not affected by the presence of serum in the cell culture media and thus PLGA NPs constitute a potential gene delivery vector for in vivo gene delivery. Prabha and Labhasetwar (16) have shown slow intracellular release of plasmid DNA from the PLGA NPs, which results in sustained retention of DNA inside the cells (Fig. 5). NPs loaded with *wt-p53* gene demonstrated higher mRNA levels for p53 as compared to that with a liposomal formulation at five days after transfection of MDA-MB-435S breast cancer cells. The sustained p53 expression levels resulted in greater and sustained inhibition of cell proliferation in vitro as compared to that with liposomal formulation or plasmid

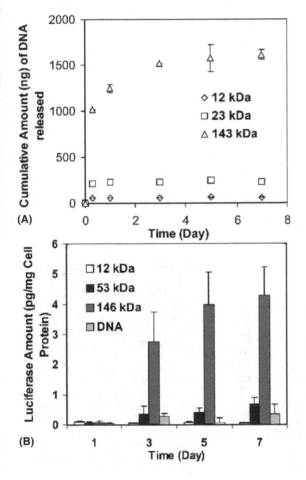

FIGURE 3 Effect of molecular weight of PLGA on (**A**) in vitro release of DNA from NPs and transfection of NPs in (**B**) MCF-7 cells. Cells (35,000 per well in 24-well plate) were incubated with NPs (444 μg/mL/well) for one day after which the medium in the wells was replaced with fresh medium (without NPs). Medium was changed on alternate days thereafter. NPs showed sustained gene transfection in MCF-7 cell line. Data as mean ± S.E.M., $n = 6$. *Abbreviation*: NPs, nanoparticles. *Source*: From Ref. 2.

DNA alone. Cohen et al. (3) have shown that despite the lower transfection levels observed in vitro with NPs as compared to liposomal formulations, the in vivo gene transfection with NPs was one to two orders of magnitude greater than that with liposomes at seven days after an intramuscular injection in mice. Their studies demonstrated gene expression sustaining over 28 days in vivo with a single dose of intramuscular injection of NPs. Such sustained gene expression is advantageous especially if the half-life of the expressed protein is very short and/or a chronic gene delivery is required for better therapeutic efficacy.

Although these NPs have been shown to release plasmid DNA at slower rates inside the cell, it is important that the DNA released as a result of polymer degradation retains its bioactivity. There are reports showing that the degradation of PLGA/PLA polymers into lactic and glycolic acids can produce highly acidic microenvironments in the NPs, which can compromise the stability and activity of DNA released from NPs (17). Additional excipients such as polyethylene oxide (PEO) can be coencapsulated with plasmid DNA in polymeric NPs in order to prevent the generation of extremely acidic microenvironments inside NPs on polymer degradation (18). Polymer blends of PLGA and polyoxyethylene derivatives have

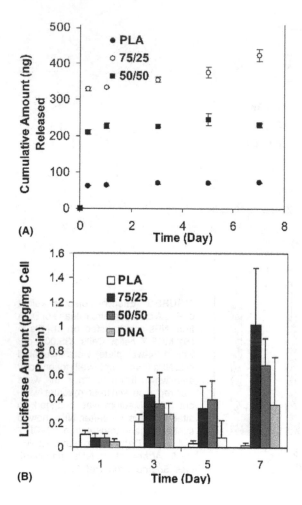

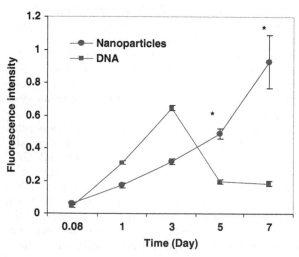

FIGURE 4 Effect of polymer composition on (**A**) in vitro DNA release from NPs and (**B**) transfection of NPs in MCF-7 cells. Cells (35,000/well in 24-well plate) were incubated with NPs (444 µg/mL/well) for one day, and then the medium was replaced with fresh medium (without NPs). Medium was changed on every alternate day thereafter, and transfection levels were determined at one, three, five, and seven days post-transfection in MCF-7 cell line. This figure represents lactide:glycolide ratio. Data shown as mean ± S.E.M., $n = 6$. *Abbreviation*: PLA, Poly(lactic acid). *Source*: From Ref. 2.

FIGURE 5 Quantitative determination of intracellular DNA levels cells transfected with YOYO-labeled DNA-loaded nanoparticles demonstrated sustained and increased intracellular DNA levels as opposed to transient DNA levels in the cells transfected with naked DNA. Data are represented as the mean ± the standard error of the mean (n = 6; $P < 0.001$ for points marked with asterisks). *Source*: From Ref. 16.

been used to prepare NPs entrapping plasmid DNA, using a modified emulsification-solvent diffusion technique (5). PLGA and poloxamer or poloxamine were mixed in different ratios and dissolved in methylene chloride. An aqueous solution of plasmid DNA can then be emulsified into this organic phase containing polymers using vortexing. The emulsion is then poured into a polar phase under moderate magnetic stirring, to allow immediate precipitation of the polymer. Thus, this modified technique avoids the use of high shear forces during nanoencapsulation of DNA, which can cause structural damages to the DNA. Moreover, the use of poloxamers and poloxamine facilitated DNA encapsulation and resulted in an increase in the encapsulation of DNA within the NPs. The nature and HLB value (hydrophilic/lipophilic balance) of the surfactant (poloxamer/poloxamine) can possibly affect the interaction of DNA with the hydrophobic polymers. Higher encapsulation of DNA with polymer blends made with surfactants of intermediate HLB values can be attributed to the improved compatibility of hydrophilic plasmid DNA with the hydrophobic PLGA polymer. The rate of release of plasmid DNA from the NPs also depends on the HLB value of the polyoxyethylene derivative used in the polymer blend. NPs prepared using hydrophilic poloxamers (Tetronic 908, HLB = 30.0) showed a continuous and fast release of DNA within one week, whereas the ones prepared with a more hydrophobic surfactant (Tetronic 904, HLB = 14.5) showed slow release of DNA over a period of two weeks (Fig. 6).

Attempts have been made to improve the encapsulation of DNA in biodegradable NPs. Condensing plasmid DNA prior to encapsulation can increase the encapsulation as compared to encapsulation of uncondensed DNA. Plasmid DNA condensed with polycations such as poly-L-lysine (PLL) or with cationic dendrons has also been encapsulated in the PLGA NPs. This allows for the protection of DNA inside the polymeric matrix and controlled delivery of plasmid DNA. Ribeiro et al. (4) have reported the encapsulation of plasmid DNA condensed with cationic PLL-based lipidic dendrons (dendriplexes) into PLGA NPs by double-emulsion method. The size of PLGA-dendriplex particles was a function of the molar charge ratios at which DNA was condensed with the dendriplexes. Plasmid DNA could be

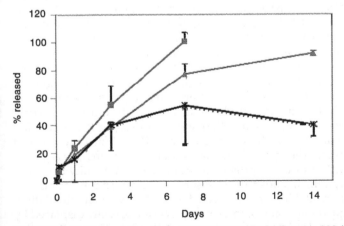

FIGURE 6 Release profiles of plasmid DNA from PLGA:Tetronic 908 (squares) and PLGA: Tetronic 904 (triangles) blend NPs and from the control PLGA (stars) NPs (mean ± S.D., n = 3). Abbreviations: PLGA, poly(D,L-lactide-co-glycolide); NPs, nanoparticles. Source: From Ref. 5.

fully condensed with cationic dendrons at high (10:1) molar charge ratios, resulting in dendriplexes with a positive zeta potential and a DNA loading of 15.0% (w/w).

PLGA NPs can be modified to generate cationic surfaces, to which negatively charged DNA molecules can be condensed. An emulsion–diffusion–evaporation technique using PVA–chitosan blend as a stabilizer has been described to produce cationically modified PLGA NPs (19). PVA helps in the stabilization of the particles, whereas chitosan owing to its positive charge provides a cationic surface to the NPs. Plasmid DNA can be complexed to the surface of these preformed cationic NPs by means of electrostatic interactions, thus avoiding the involvement of DNA during the NP formulation and hence preserving DNA integrity. Blends of the polymers PLA/PLGA with polyethylenimine (PEI) have also been used to prepare positively charged NPs by a diafiltration method (20). The use of diafiltration technique avoids the use of any surfactant in the NP formulation as the hydrophilic nature of PEI effectively reduces the interfacial energy between the hydrophobic NP surfaces and the aqueous media. Particle size and the zeta potential of these NPs can be controlled by the amount of PEI used in the polymer blends. Imine groups of PEI can be used to complex DNA to the surface of cationic NPs. The NPs produced using this method showed high adsorption capacity for plasmid DNA and a high dispersive stability.

Further, the surface of polymeric NPs based on PLGA/PLA can be functionalized to improve their biodistribution and also to conjugate targeting ligands which can direct NPs to specific cells/tissues where gene delivery is desired. Surface modification of NPs is achieved either by adsorbing amphiphilic excipients onto preformed NPs or by covalently linking excipients to the core-forming polymer prior to NP formulation. Biodegradable NPs have been prepared using PLL-graft-polysaccharide copolymers and poly(D,L-lactic acid) by using a solvent evaporation method or the diafiltration method (6). NPs prepared using these copolymers had bifunctional surfaces with positively charged amino groups of PLL and the polysaccharide moieties. This increased the adsorption capacity of NPs for polynucleotides and allowed introduction of ligand (carbohydrate) moieties on the NP surface for ligand-mediated recognition of specific receptors. The formulation resulted in NPs as small as 60 nm in diameter, and showed excellent dispersive stability in phosphate-buffered saline. A preferential distribution of dextran moieties over PLL was observed in the outer surface of NPs using a PLL-graft-dextran copolymer. Presence of dextran chains on NP surface can be potentially useful to prevent nonspecific interactions with serum proteins and also for receptor-mediated targeting to specific cells.

Subsequent to intravenous injection of the NPs, the major problem is to avoid their opsonization by plasma proteins and subsequent uptake by the phagocytic cells. PEO/PEG has been used to coat the polymeric NPs to provide a protective hydrophilic sheath, which prevents the rapid opsonization of the otherwise hydrophobic NPs by reticuloendothelial system (RES) and thus prolong the circulation time of NPs in blood stream (21). The hydrophobic part of PEO/PEG polymers can adsorb to NP surface, whereas the hydrophilic chains protrude towards the aqueous medium. PEG coats on NP surface also provide an attractive opportunity to chemically conjugate active-targeting ligands to the NP surface (22,23). These coatings can modify the biodistribution of NPs when injected into the systemic circulation. However, it has been argued that some of these polymers can be easily displaced by serum proteins, which can lead to aggregation of NPs (24). Thus, alternative approaches of synthesizing copolymers of PLA/PLGA with PEG (25,26) and coencapsulation of PEG with plasmid DNA inside PLGA NPs have been tried (27).

CHITOSAN NANOPARTICLES

Chitosan is a linear cationic polysaccharide, obtained by partial alkaline deacetylation of chitin, a polymer found in the exoskeleton of crustaceans. Chitosans are biodegradable and biocompatible polymers and thus can be potentially safe and nontoxic carriers for gene delivery. Moreover, derivatives of chitosan can be synthesized, with relative ease, to hydrophobically modify chitosan or to conjugate different chemical entities for targeting chitosan NPs to specific tissues or organs.

NPs for gene delivery can be prepared by (*i*) complexing plasmid DNA with chitosan (28) or (*ii*) by encapsulating DNA inside chitosan NPs (29). The high density of amino groups present in the glucosamine backbone of chitosan can be protonated and thus offers the opportunity to complex chitosans with negatively charged DNA molecules, owing to the electrostatic interactions.

Self-assembling chitosan/DNA complexes, in the size range of 150 to 500 nm, were first prepared by mixing a solution of chitosan with plasmid DNA (30). The particle sizes of the complexes depend on the molecular weight of chitosan used, but not on the buffer compositions. Chitosan, hydrophobically modified using deoxycholic acid, can form spherical self-aggregates with a mean diameter of 160 nm in aqueous media (28). Charge complexes formed between these self-aggregates of modified chitosan and plasmid DNA have been shown to transfect COS-1 cells in culture. The transfection efficiency of chitosan self-aggregate/DNA complexes was reported to be more than that achieved with plasmid DNA alone, but lower than liposomal formulations.

DNA can be encapsulated in chitosan NPs, prepared by a complex coacervation method, yielding particle sizes in the range of 200 to 500 nm. Mao et al. (29) have studied the influence of various parameters of NP preparation on the size of chitosan–DNA NPs. The size of the particles was optimized to 100 to 250 nm using an N/P ratio of three to eight. The zeta potential of these particles was +12 to +18 mV at a pH lower than 6.0 and nearly zero at pH 7.2. Chitosan NPs could partially protect DNA from nucleases. The transfection efficiency was found to be cell-dependent and lower than that achieved with Lipofectamine–DNA complexes in HEK 293 cells. However, the presence of serum in the cell culture medium did not interfere with the transfection using chitosan NPs. Chitosan–DNA NPs are also considered a very appealing carrier choice for oral gene-delivery strategies, owing to the mucoadhesive properties of chitosan. Orally administered chitosan–DNA NPs can adhere to the gastrointestinal epithelium and transfect epithelial or immune cells present in the gut-associated lymphoid tissue (31).

POLY(β-AMINO ESTER)-BASED NANOPARTICLES

Poly(β-amino esters) constitute a relatively new class of synthetic biodegradable cationic polymers with tertiary amines in their backbone. Unlike other cationic polymers, these are hydrolytically degradable polymers and are generally less cytotoxic than the polycations such as PEI (32). Using MTT assay, these polymers and their degradation products have been shown to be nontoxic relative to PEI in NIH 3T3 cell line.

These polymers have been shown to possess pH-dependent solubility, and thus are suitable for the preparation of DNA NPs which can trigger the polymer degradation and release of encapsulated DNA in the acidic pH in endosomal vesicles inside cells (33). Owing to their polycationic nature, these polymers can condense

DNA into complexes of the order of 50 to 200 nm and thus can be used for gene transfection.

POLY(ALKYLCYANOACRYLATE) NANOPARTICLES

Poly(alkylcyanoacrylate) (PACA) NPs were first prepared by Couvreur et al. in 1979 (34). PACA NPs have been used for intracellular delivery of various oligonucleotide sequences. PACA NPs can be coated with cationic surfactants (cetyltrimethylammonium bromide) or polymers (DEAE-dextran) which can be used for complexing oligonucleotides via electrostatic interactions (35). Alternatively, oligonucleotides can be associated with the PACA NPs by covalently linking to a hydrophobic molecule (cholesterol) which can then be anchored at the NP surface (36). In earlier studies, it has been shown that the PACA NPs are taken up by the RES system of the body and thus can be used for targeting DNA delivery to the RES organs such as liver, spleen, lungs, and bone marrow (37).

MAGNETIC NANOPARTICLES

Magnetic NPs usually incorporate magnetic-responsive materials such as magnetite, iron, nickel, cobalt, and so on. In contrast to the conventional polymeric NPs, magnetic NPs can be directed and preferentially localized in the diseased tissue upon application of an external localized magnetic field.

The magnetic NPs can be modified with different chemical compounds to facilitate a change in the surface charge or particle size of the NPs. Magnetic NPs for gene delivery involve associating naked plasmid DNA or DNA vectors (such as DNA complexed with polycations or packaged in viral vectors) to the surface of the NPs. This technique of gene transfection is commonly referred to as "magneto-fection." The magnetic field can improve the vector concentration near the cells to be transfected and thus has been shown to reduce the vector dose and incubation time with vector required to achieve high transfection efficiency in vitro (38). The surface of superparamagnetic iron-oxide NPs coated with PEI has been used to associate PEI–DNA complexes (38). The basic principle used for the formulation of these magnetic NPs is that of salt-induced aggregation of colloidal particles. PEI-coated magnetic NPs, PEI, and plasmid DNA are mixed in salt-containing solutions to form the magnetic vectors for gene transfection. PEI–DNA complexes (polyplexes) associated with superparamagnetic NPs can be guided to accumulate selectively in the target tissue, by the use of an external magnetic field focused at the tissue. Magnetic-field-guided local transfection in the gastrointestinal tract and in blood vessels has also been reported (38).

Another report of using magnetic NPs for gene delivery involves association of magnetic (maghemite) NPs with the DNA vector hemagglutinating virus of Japan-envelope (HVJ-E) (39). This can potentially enhance the gene transfection efficiency of the vector by promoting its cell association, using magnetic force. The magnetic NPs were coated either with protamine sulfate or heparin to produce a cationically charged surface of the NPs. The DNA-carrying vector—HVJ-E—was associated with the modified NPs and used for gene transfection. These magnetic NPs promote gene transfection, mediated by cell fusion of the HVJ-E vectors. Cationically charged magnetic NPs can be speculated to promote greater association of the vector with the cells, which then carry DNA into the cells under the influence of magnetic force, thus enhancing the transfection efficiency of the vectors.

Thus, the use of magnetic NPs in conjunction with DNA alone or DNA polyplexes is an emerging gene transfection technique, which can effectively increase the gene transfection efficiency of these vectors. However, it is important that such magnetic NPs for gene transfection be water-based, biocompatible, nontoxic, and nonimmunogenic.

SUMMARY

Biodegradable NPs constitute safer and versatile gene-delivery systems that allow ligand conjugation for targeted gene therapy as well as modulation of the DNA release to control the level and duration of gene expression. Although we have achieved some success in overcoming the cellular barrier of DNA delivery, the nuclear membrane still stands as a rate-limiting factor for efficient gene expression using nonviral vectors (40). Incorporation of cationic peptides such as nuclear localizing signaling peptides, protein transduction domain from the transactivator of transcription, and protamine have been shown to enable nuclear transport of DNA, and hence conjugating these to a carrier system may prove to be an effective strategy to enhance gene expression of nonviral systems (41). For in vivo applications, it is important to restrict the gene transfection to the treated (target) tissue, and thus, targeting of NPs can potentially increase the efficacy and reduce the toxicity of gene therapy. Approaches such as decorating the surface of NPs with cell-specific ligands and use of magnetic force to target the NPs to specific tissues or organs for targeted gene delivery, though in early stages of development, constitute promising efforts at improving gene delivery. To successfully develop such formulation approaches for targeted gene delivery, it is essential to add to our basic understanding of the cellular barriers and mechanisms of intracellular sorting of NPs, and ultimately define rational formulation strategies to overcome these barriers (42).

ACKNOWLEDGMENTS

Grant support from the National Institutes of Health (R01 EB003975) and a predoctoral fellowship to J.K.V. from the American Heart Association, Heartland Affiliate (Award #0515489Z). Author (V.L.) acknowledges his former laboratory members, Dr. Swayam Prabha and Dr. Sanjeeb K. Sahoo, whose data are cited in this chapter.

REFERENCES

1. Li Z, Dullmann J, Schiedlmeier B, et al. Murine leukemia induced by retroviral gene marking. Science 2002; 296(5567):497.
2. Prabha S, Labhasetwar V. Critical determinants in PLGA/PLA nanoparticle-mediated gene expression. Pharm Res 2004; 21(2):354–364.
3. Cohen H, Levy RJ, Gao J, et al. Sustained delivery and expression of DNA encapsulated in polymeric nanoparticles. Gene Ther 2000; 7(22):1896–1905.
4. Ribeiro S, Hussain N, Florence AT. Release of DNA from dendriplexes encapsulated in PLGA nanoparticles. Int J Pharm 2005; 298(2):354–360.
5. Csaba N, Caamano P, Sanchez A, Dominguez F, Alonso MJ. PLGA:poloxamer and PLGA: poloxamine blend nanoparticles: new carriers for gene delivery. Biomacromolecules 2005; 6(1):271–278.
6. Maruyama A, Ishihara T, Kim JS, Kim SW, Akaike T. Nanoparticle DNA carrier with poly(L-lysine) grafted polysaccharide copolymer and poly(D,L-lactic acid). Bioconjug Chem 1997; 8(5):735–742.

7. Prabha S, Zhou WZ, Panyam J, Labhasetwar V. Size-dependency of nanoparticle-mediated gene transfection: studies with fractionated nanoparticles. Int J Pharm (2002); 244(1–2):105–115.
8. Kuo JH, Jan MS, Sung KC. Evaluation of the stability of polymer-based plasmid DNA delivery systems after ultrasound exposure. Int J Pharm 2003; 257(1–2):75–84.
9. Lengsfeld CS, Anchordoquy TJ. Shear-induced degradation of plasmid DNA. J Pharm Sci 2002; 91(7):1581–1589.
10. Middaugh CR, Evans RK, Montgomery DL, Casimiro DR. Analysis of plasmid DNA from a pharmaceutical perspective. J Pharm Sci 1998; 87(2):130–146.
11. Labhasetwar V, Bonadio J, Goldstein S, Levy RJ. Gene transfection using biodegradable nanospheres: results in tissue culture and a rat osteotomy model. Colloid Surf B 1999; 16:281–290.
12. Ando S, Putnam D, Pack DW, Langer R. PLGA microspheres containing plasmid DNA: preservation of supercoiled DNA via cryopreparation and carbohydrate stabilization. J Pharm Sci 1999; 88(1):126–130.
13. Oster CG, Wittmar M, Unger F, et al. Design of amine-modified graft polyesters for effective gene delivery using DNA-loaded nanoparticles. Pharm Res 2004; 21(6):927–931.
14. Murakami H, Kobayashi M, Takeuchi H, Kawashima Y. Preparation of poly(D,L-lactide-co-glycolide) nanoparticles by modified spontaneous emulsification solvent diffusion method. Int J Pharm 1999; 187(2):143–152.
15. Sahoo SK, Panyam J, Prabha S, Labhasetwar V. Residual polyvinyl alcohol associated with poly (D,L-lactide-co-glycolide) nanoparticles affects their physical properties and cellular uptake. J Control Release 2002; 82(1):105–114.
16. Prabha S, Labhasetwar V. Nanoparticle-mediated wild-type p53 gene delivery results in sustained antiproliferative activity in breast cancer cells. Mol Pharm 2004; 1(3):211–219.
17. Fu K, Pack DW, Klibanov AM, Langer R. Visual evidence of acidic environment within degrading poly(lactic-co-glycolic acid) (PLGA) microspheres. Pharm Res 2000; 17(1):100–106.
18. Tobio M, Nolley J, Guo Y, Mciver J, Alonso MJ. A novel system based on a poloxamer/PLGA blend as a tetanus toxoid delivery vehicle. Pharm Res 1999; 16(5):682–688.
19. Ravi Kumar MN, Bakowsky U, Lehr CM. Preparation and characterization of cationic PLGA nanospheres as DNA carriers. Biomaterials 2004; 25(10):1771–1777.
20. Kim IS, Lee SK, Park YM, et al. Physicochemical characterization of poly(L-lactic acid) and poly(D,L-lactide-co-glycolide) nanoparticles with polyethylenimine as gene delivery carrier. Int J Pharm 2005; 298(1):255–262.
21. Redhead HM, Davis SS, Illum L. Drug delivery in poly(lactide-co-glycolide) nanoparticles surface modified with poloxamer 407 and poloxamine 908: in vitro characterisation and in vivo evaluation. J Control Release 2001; 70(3):353–363.
22. Otsuka H, Nagasaki Y, Kataoka K. PEGylated nanoparticles for biological and pharmaceutical applications. Adv Drug Deliv Rev 2003; 55(3):403–419.
23. Benns JM, Kim SW. Tailoring new gene delivery designs for specific targets. J Drug Target 2000; 8(1):1–12.
24. Neal JC, Stolnik S, Schacht E, et al. In vitro displacement by rat serum of adsorbed radiolabeled poloxamer and poloxamine copolymers from model and biodegradable nanospheres. J Pharm Sci 1998; 87(10):1242–1248.
25. Stolnik S, Dunn SE, Garnett MC, et al. Surface modification of poly(lactide-co-glycolide) nanospheres by biodegradable poly(lactide)–poly(ethylene glycol) copolymers. Pharm Res 1994; 11(12):1800–1808.
26. Hawley AE, Illum L, Davis SS. Preparation of biodegradable, surface engineered PLGA nanospheres with enhanced lymphatic drainage and lymph node uptake. Pharm Res 1997; 14(5):657–661.
27. Perez C, Sanchez A, Putnam D, et al. Poly(lactic acid)–poly(ethylene glycol) nanoparticles as new carriers for the delivery of plasmid DNA. J Control Release 2001; 75(1–2):211–224.
28. Lee KY, Kwon IC, Kim YH, Jo WH, Jeong SY. Preparation of chitosan self-aggregates as a gene delivery system. J Control Release 1998; 51(2–3):213–220.

29. Mao HQ, Roy K, Troung-Le VL, et al. Chitosan–DNA nanoparticles as gene carriers: synthesis, characterization and transfection efficiency. J Control Release 2001; 70(3): 399–421.
30. Mumper RJ, Wang J, Claspell JM, Rolland AP. Novel polymeric condensing carriers for gene delivery. Proc Int Symp Control Rel Bioact Mater 1995; 22:178–179.
31. Bernkop-Schnurch A, Krajicek ME. Mucoadhesive polymers as platforms for peroral peptide delivery and absorption: synthesis and evaluation of different chitosan–EDTA conjugates. J Control Release 1998; 50(1–3):215–223.
32. Lynn DM, Langer R. Degradable poly(beta-amino esters): synthesis, characterization, and self-assembly with plasmid DNA. J Am Chem Soc 2000; 122:10761–10768.
33. Lynn DM, Amiji MM, Langer R. pH-responsive polymer microspheres: rapid release of encapsulated material within the range of intracellular pH. Angew Chem Int Ed Engl 2001; 40(9):1707–1710.
34. Couvreur P, Kante B, Roland M, et al. Polycyanoacrylate nanocapsules as potential lysosomotropic carriers: preparation, morphological and sorptive properties. J Pharm Pharmacol 1979; 31(5):331–332.
35. Chavany C, Le Doan T, Couvreur P, Puisieux F, Helene C. Polyalkylcyanoacrylate nanoparticles as polymeric carriers for antisense oligonucleotides. Pharm Res 1992; 9(4): 441–449.
36. Godard G, Boutorine AS, Saison-Behmoaras E, Helene C. Antisense effects of cholesterol-oligodeoxynucleotide conjugates associated with poly(alkylcyanoacrylate) nanoparticles. Eur J Biochem 1995; 232(2):404–410.
37. Lenaerts V, Nagelkerke JF, Van Berkel TJ, et al. In vivo uptake of polyisobutyl cyanoacrylate nanoparticles by rat liver Kupffer, endothelial, and parenchymal cells. J Pharm Sci 1984; 73(7):980–982.
38. Scherer F, Anton M, Schillinger U, et al. Magnetofection: enhancing and targeting gene delivery by magnetic force in vitro and in vivo. Gene Ther 2002; 9(2):102–109.
39. Morishita N, Nakagami H, Morishita R, et al. Magnetic nanoparticles with surface modification enhanced gene delivery of HVJ-E vector. Biochem Biophys Res Commun 2005; 334(4):1121–1126.
40. Munkonge FM, Dean DA, Hillery E, Griesenbach U, Alton EW. Emerging significance of plasmid DNA nuclear import in gene therapy. Adv Drug Deliv Rev 2003; 55(6):749–760.
41. Park YJ, Liang JF, Ko KS, Kim SW, Yang VC. Low molecular weight protamine as an efficient and nontoxic gene carrier: in vitro study. J Gene Med 2003; 5(8):700–711.
42. Labhasetwar V. Nanotechnology for drug and gene therapy: the importance of understanding molecular mechanisms of delivery. Curr Opin Biotechnol 2005; 16(6):674–680.

19 Gastrointestinal Applications of Nanoparticulate Drug-Delivery Systems

Maria Rosa Gasco
Nanovector srl, Torino, Italy

EXCITING REASONS FOR STUDYING THE APPLICATION OF NANOPARTICULATE SYSTEMS TO THE GASTROINTESTINAL TRACT

The uptake of nanoparticulate systems (NPSs) through the gastrointestinal tract (GIT) is today a well-known and accepted phenomenon, and excellent reviews of the intestinal uptake of particles have been published (1–5). NPS uptake from the gut can provide an additional drug administration route; each system has its own pharmacokinetic parameters and specific drug-carrying ability. The bioactive molecule is transported into the GIT by carriers whose chemicophysical characteristics must be taken into account, although the chemicophysical and pharmacological characteristics of the drug remain intact. This chapter will concentrate particularly on the translocation of NPSs via the lymphatic system, and briefly consider the hitherto less widely studied colonic targeting of NPSs.

Lymphatic Targeting

Peyer's patches are the most important structural units of the gut associated with lymphoid tissue (GALT); they are characterized by M-cells that overlie the lymphoid tissue and are specialized for endocytosis and transport into intraepithelial spaces and adjacent lymphoid tissue. Nanoparticulates bind to the apical membrane of M-cells, after which they are rapidly internalized and "shuttled" to the lymphocytes (3,5). The lymphatic absorption of a drug via the GALT has an advantage over the portal blood route, because it avoids presystemic metabolism by the liver (hepatic first-pass effect). Florence (6) has suggested a simplified diagram of pre- and postabsorption processes (Fig. 1).

The requisites enabling NPS to be absorbed via the GALT not only concern the loaded drug, but also and more specifically the carrier's physical characteristics, such as size, shape, specific surface, surface charge, chemical stability of both NPS and loaded drug, potential interactions with gut contents, transit time through the GIT, transport through the mucosa, adhesion to epithelial surfaces, and aggregation of the particulates in contact with the fluid content of the gut. The transit and translocation of NPSs depend to a considerable extent on their mean diameter, surface charge, and release characteristics (2,3). Some phenomena, such as aggregation, adsorption, and adhesion, can alter the zeta potential, hydrophilicity, and size of the NPS.

From the pharmaceutical standpoint, the measure of any feasible application of a drug-delivery system is its efficacy, that is, its ability to exert a pharmacological effect. Indeed, besides the different properties of NPS listed above, a critical aspect is the loading capacity of the nanoparticulates. The higher the loading, the higher is the bioavailability per particle absorbed (2). Another important issue is biocompatibility and biodegradability of the NPS components.

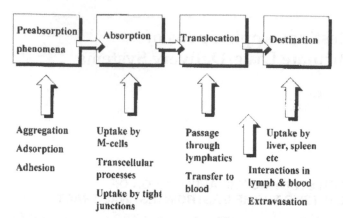

FIGURE 1 A simplified schematic of pre-absorption and post-absorption processes in nanoparticle-dependent drug delivery to gastrointestinal sited following oral administration, highlighting the variety of processes involved in the journey of a nanoparticle from delivery to target. *Source*: From Ref. 6.

Lymph targeting of NPSs can permit (2,3,5): (*i*) oral delivery of labile molecules protected by the carrier; (*ii*) oral delivery of poorly soluble molecules following their nanosolubilization in NPSs; (*iii*) improved bioavailability of drugs with poor absorption characteristics, due both to the large specific surface of NPSs and to their increased residence time; (*iv*) oral delivery of vaccine antigens to gut-associated lymphoid tissue; (*v*) translocation of antineoplastic drugs for treatment of lymphomas; (*vi*) delivery of diagnostics for the lymphatic system; (*vii*) sustained/controlled drug release, particularly important for toxic drugs (e.g., antineoplastic drugs); (*viii*) reduction of drug-related GI mucosa irritation; and (*ix*) avoidance of the hepatic first-pass effect.

Colonic Targeting

Lymphatic tissue in the colon, rectum, and appendix vermiform is usually not found in discrete patches, but is diffusely present in aggregate masses at irregular intervals. Despite the fact that the colon and rectum contain the most abundant lymphoid intestinal tissue, there is a lack of research examining lymphatic absorption from these sites (2). The presence of M-cells (7) suggests that NPSs may also be absorbed in this region of the GIT. Colon-specific drug delivery systems can be used to improve drug bioavailability at the colon, particularly in the case of proteins and peptides, targeting them to the less proteolytically active colon (8). Nanoparticulates targeted to the colon have been studied with the aim of treating some types of colon disease, but also to investigate transport and release of some labile molecules such as peptides and proteins as some early studies showed.

Colonic targeting of nanoparticulates can permit therapeutic intervention in pathological processes of the gut, such as ulcerative colitis or Crohn's disease (2), and possible targeting of labile molecules (such as peptides and small proteins) to the colon (8).

DEVELOPMENT OF NANOPARTICULATE SYSTEMS FOR LYMPHATIC TARGETING

The following NPSs are considered.

Dendrimers

Although the first reports on dendrimers were published more than two decades ago, their potential biological applications have only been explored in the past few years (2,9,10).

Dendrimer chemistry has been used to prepare monodisperse nanoparticles (diameter below 50 nm) in order to investigate the relation between nanoparticle diameter and uptake from the GIT (3). The study examined both dendrimers with lipidic external character and a series of cationic dendrimers, and investigation of dendrimer absorption in rats through Peyer's patches and enterocytes showed their preferential uptake through Peyer's patches.

5-Fluorouracil (11) can be entrapped in polyamidoamine dendrimers that have been coated with phospholipids; in vivo studies in albino rats have shown phospholipid-coated dendrimers to be more effective orally than free drug. Lymphatic uptake also increased, indicating absorption of the formulation via the lymphatic route.

Polymeric Nanoparticulates (Nanoparticles and/or Nanocapsules)

Polymeric nanoparticulates are particles of diameter below 1 µm, prepared from natural or synthetic polymers. Natural polymers (i.e., proteins or polysaccharides) have not been widely used for this purpose, as they may vary in purity and often require cross-linking, which could denature the embedded drug (5). Synthetic biodegradable polymers have received much more attention; the most widely used polymers have been poly(lactic acid), poly(glycolic acid), their copolymers poly(lactide-co-glycolide acid) (PLGA) (12), and polyalkylcyanoacrylates (PACA) (13). The bioactives are well protected in these polymers, which offer the advantage of delivering drugs in a sustained fashion, avoiding repeated administration. Nanoparticles were first developed for the parenteral route; more recently, they have also been studied as oral delivery vehicles. The major interest is in the lymphatic uptake of nanoparticles by Peyer's patches in the GALT (12). Microparticles remain in Peyer's patches, while nanoparticles are disseminated systemically (5). Clearly, a wide variety of drugs can be delivered via the oral route using polymeric nanoparticulate carriers. Much of the research has focused on the absorption enhancement of peptides (14), proteins, and vaccine antigens.

Mucoadhesive ability can be conferred to NPSs by coating their surface with microadhesive polymers such as chitosan or Carbopol®; action is more effective and prolonged, confirming the usefulness of mucoadhesive properties (15). Insulin entrapped in PACA nanospheres dispersed in an oily phase containing a surfactant produces prolonged hypoglycemia (16). The fate of poly(isobutylcyanoacrylate) nanocapsules carrying insulin administered to rats was monitored by fluorescence and transmission electron microscopy (TEM) and evidenced intestinal absorption through the epithelial mucosa (17). A luminescent polymer was used as a visible tracer to monitor the oral fate of PLGA microspheres containing insulin (18). The therapeutic effects of another peptide, octreotide, can be improved and prolonged on incorporation into PACA nanocapsules (19).

Biodegradable PLGA nanoparticles containing salmon calcitonin (sCT), complexed with amphiphilic molecules, afford high loading efficiency; absorption was good on oral administration to rats (20). Positively charged nanoparticles incorporating cyclosporin A (21) have been prepared by the emulsification solvent diffusion method; the bioavailability in beagle dogs increased 1.2-fold over that of Neoral®.

The same peptide was encapsulated by nanoprecipitation within nonbiodegradable polymers, and different formulations were prepared; oral absorption of the peptide nanoparticulates in rabbits was compared to that of Neoral® capsule. The relative bioavailability of cyclosporin A from various formulations ranged from 20% to 35% that of Neoral® (22).

Heparin has no oral bioavailability, and is thus generally administered by the parenteral route. Heparin-loaded polymeric nanoparticles, prepared with biodegradable poly-ε-caprolactone and PLGA and nonbiodegradable positively charged polymers, used alone or in combination, were administered orally to rabbits (23); with each formulation anti-Xa activity and activated partial thromboplastin time (aPTT) were detected. In particular, anti-Xa activity was detected for a longer period than when a heparin solution was administered intravenously.

A delivery system allowing oral administration of vaccines would be ideal. An antigen is taken up into the Peyer's patches mostly through the M-cells, which appear to be the main site for uptake of antigens after oral administration, and it is generally accepted that limited doses of antigen are sufficient for mucous immunization. Oral delivery of antigens may be considered the most convenient means of producing an IgA antibody response (24). The use of micro- and nanoparticles for the oral delivery of antigens can be efficient if these systems are able to protect the antigen molecule. Oral administration of antigens incorporated in particulates induces a stronger antigen-specific immune response than do antigens in the water-soluble form, because incorporation in NPSs protects them from the low pH of the stomach and from proteolytic enzymes (25,26).

The immune response has been studied after subcutaneous, oral, and intranasal administration to mice of PLGA nanospheres loaded with bovine serum albumin (BSA), evaluating some factors affecting the immune response, such as size, surface hydrophobicity, zeta potential, adjuvants, or excipients used in the formulations (27).

Liposomes

Oral delivery of liposomes would be the simplest and most convenient route for drug administration (28,29), but it is important to examine their stability in the acid pH of the stomach environment and in the gastrointestinal medium. Stability in the physiological conditions affecting oral drug delivery has been studied to determine which components have the best chance of surviving through the GIT (30).

Liposomes coated with polyethylene glycol containing recombinant human epidermal growth factor were administered orally to rats and the area under the concentration–time curve (AUC) was evaluated and compared to that of the solution. It increased 1.7- and 2.5-fold for phosphatidylcholine and dipalmitoylphosphatidylcholine liposomes, respectively (31).

Liposomes containing an extract of natural marine lipids containing large amounts of N-3-polyunsaturated fatty acids (PUFA) were prepared with the aim of increasing PUFA bioavailability. Thoracic lymph duct-cannulated rats were fed intragastrically with these liposomes, and absorption of fatty acids was higher than with fish oil (32).

The effect of liposomes coated with chitosan or Carbopol® on rats' intestinal absorption of calcitonin has been studied, testing negatively and positively charged liposomes. The overall pharmacological efficacy of coated liposomes was more than double that of noncoated liposomes (33). Absorption of sCT from the intestine is poor because of its high molecular weight and rapid degradation by enzymes in the

GIT. Double liposomes (i.e., liposomes containing smaller liposomes) with different charges were investigated as carriers of sCT, administered to rats, and compared to the solution. The highest hypocalcemic effect was obtained with cationic charged liposomes (34).

Self-(Micro)Emulsifying Drug-Delivery Systems

Self-(micro)emulsifying Drug-Delivery Systems (S(M)EDDSs) are isotropic mixtures of oils, surfactants, solvents, and cosolvents/surfactants; they are used solely for the purpose of improving oral absorption of highly lipophilic drugs. The principal characteristic of these systems is their ability to form fine oil-in-water emulsion or microemulsion upon mild stirring, following dilution by the aqueous phase (35,36).

A supersaturable (S-SEDDS) formulation of paclitaxel, developed using hydroxypropylcellulose as precipitation inhibitor (37), in a pharmacokinetic study on rats achieved fivefold oral bioavailability versus an orally dosed Taxol® formulation.

An S(M)EDDS of paclitaxel was administered to rats with and without the use of P-glycoprotein inhibitors (38). Compared to commercial Taxol®, the oral bioavailability of paclitaxel S(M)EDDS increased at the various doses. The bioavailability was significantly improved for paclitaxel S(M)EDDS when cyclosporin A, as inhibitor of P-glycoprotein, was coadministered. An S(M)EDDS system loaded with simvastatin, orally administered to beagle dogs, increased bioavailability 1.5-fold versus the conventional oral tablet (39).

Solid–Lipid Nanoparticles

Solid–lipid nanoparticles (SLNs) are in the submicron size range and usually consist of biocompatible and biodegradable materials, such as triglycerides and fatty acids; the production and properties of SLNs have been reviewed (40–42). Various preparation methods are possible: one depends on the application of mechanical high-pressure homogenization to a melted lipid dispersed in an aqueous solution of surfactants (40). When camptothecin-loaded SLNs, produced by high-pressure homogenization, were administered perorally to rats, the concentration–time curves in plasma and in organ tissues showed enhanced availability of the drug compared to solution: AUC and mean residence time (MRT) increased significantly (43). Piribedil SLNs, administered orally to rabbits, increased drug bioavailability more than twofold compared to pure piribedil (44). SLNs loaded with all-*trans* retinoic acid, as a poorly soluble model drug, can be prepared by high-pressure homogenization; administered orally to rats, they significantly enhanced *trans* retinoic acid absorption (45). The bioavailability of clozapine formulated in SLNs prepared by the hot homogenization method was determined after intravenous (IV) and intraduodenal administration and compared to those of a clozapine suspension. The area under the curve (AUC) increased by about three times in the case of the IV route, and up to 4.5 times for the intraduodenal route (46). Clear solutions of cyclosporin A, a solid triglyceride, a water-miscible organic solvent, and a mixture of surfactants and emulsifiers were dispersed by mixing in water to produce a suspension of nanoparticles of sizes between 25 and 400 nm depending on the formulations. The oral bioavailability was determined on humans; the best results were similar to the Neoral® reference formulation and were obtained for the formulations forming nanoparticles below 60 nm (47). Other preparation methods for SLNs are the solvent emulsification technique (48) and the solvent diffusion method (49).

SLNs can also be produced by dispersing warm microemulsions in cold water (50,51). SLNs are the solidified droplets of microemulsions with a mean diameter of 80 to 200 nm; they can incorporate both hydrophilic and lipophilic drugs. Many drugs have been incorporated in SLNs, and different administration routes have been studied in laboratory animals. Stealth SLNs have been prepared for the purpose of avoiding reticuloendothelial system recognition; after IV administration, SLNs and stealth SLNs are able to cross the blood–brain barrier, increasing the MRT (to a greater extent with stealth than with nonstealth SLNs) of the loaded drug compared to solution (52). SLNs are taken up within a few minutes by neoplastic (53,54) and nonneoplastic cell lines (55).

The gastrointestinal uptake and transport in the lymphatic circulation of drug-unloaded SLNs was initially studied; labeled and unlabeled SLNs were administered duodenally to rats, at two different amounts in equal volumes. After a few minutes, TEM evidenced SLNs in the lymph; the size of the particles in the lymph (130–140 nm) was practically unchanged after administration. Labeled SLNs were used to evaluate lymphatic uptake and the radioactivity data confirmed transport of SLNs in lymph and blood. SLN concentration versus time increased out of proportion to the increased amount administered, being very much higher with the higher concentration of SLNs (56).

Successively, tobramycin was incorporated in SLNs as a model drug; it was chosen because it is not absorbed at the gastrointestinal level and is therefore still administered by the parenteral route. Tobramycin-loaded SLNs (Tobra-SLN) were administered to rats into the duodenum and compared to Tobra-SLN and tobramycin solution, both administered IV (57). The AUC of IV Tobra-SLN was 1710 min µg mL^{-1}, whereas that of Tobra-solution administered IV was 352 min µg mL^{-1}. The AUC of Tobra-SLNs administered duodenally was over 100 times that of the solution and over 20 times that of Tobra-SLN, both administered IV. Pharmacokinetic parameters showed a marked difference between Tobra-SLNs administered duodenally and IV, in the former case providing a sufficiently high level of the drug even after 24 hours. Most of the difference between the two administration routes is due to the transmucosal transport of SLNs to the lymph rather than to the blood. Tobra-SLN administered duodenally act as a sustained-release system.

SLNs containing three different percentages (1.25%, 2.5%, and 5%) of tobramycin were prepared, and the same dose of Tobra of each of the three types was administered intraduodenally to rats (58). Figure 2 shows the tobramycin plasma concentrations versus time for the three types of SLNs. The pharmacokinetic

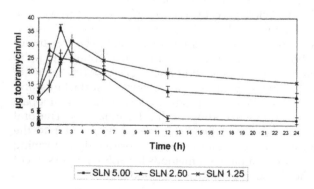

FIGURE 2 Tobramycin plasma concentrations versus time ± standard deviation after duodenal administration of the three types of Tobra-SLN. *Abbreviation*: SLN, solid–lipid nanoparticle. *Source*: From Ref. 58.

TABLE 1 Apparent Pharmacokinetic Parameters[a]

Formulation	C_{max} (mg/L)	MRT (min)	$T_{1/2\beta}$ (min)	AUC (min·mg/L)	V_d (L)	Cl (L/h)
Tobra-SLN 1.25	31.5[b,e] ± 1.9	2964[c,f] ± 858	1901[c,f] ± 310	74880[d,f] ± 2047	0.094 ± 0.010	0.002[d,f] ± 0.0001
Tobra-SLN 2.50	28.5 ± 0.4	1544 ± 304	998 ± 21	37469 ± 1516	0.096 ± 0.009	0.004 ± 0.0002
Tobra-SLN 5.00	36.3[h] ± 1.2	439[g] ± 138	291[g] ± 16	13817[h] ± 707	0.073 ± 0.020	0.010[i] ± 0.0003

[a]"Apparent" pharmacokinetic parameters are so named because they refer to the drug incorporated into SLN and not to the free drug; data expressed as mean ± SD; MRT, mean residence time; $T_{1/2\beta}$, elimination half-life; AUC, area under the curve of plasma concentration versus time; Cl, total body clearance; V_d, volume of distribution; statistical significances are;
SLN 1.25 versus SLN 2.50
[b]$p < 0.05$.
[c]$p < 0.01$.
[d]$p < 0.001$;
SLN 1.25 versus SLN 5.00
[e]$p < 0.01$.
[f]$p < 0.001$;
SLN 2.5 versus SLN 5.00
[g]$p < 0.05$.
[h]$p < 0.01$.
[i]$p < 0.001$.
Abbreviations: AUC, area under the curve; SLN, solid–lipid nanoparticle.
Source: From Ref. 57.

parameters varied considerably with the percentage of Tobra (Table 1). This finding is probably due to the differences among the three types of SLNs, in particular, the number of SLNs administered, average diameter, total surface area, and drug content in each nanoparticle. The highest percentage of Tobra in SLNs corresponded to the highest release rate, whereas the lowest percentage produced the most prolonged release. Sustained drug release by the oral route could thus be obtained by appropriately mixing SLNs loaded with different percentages of the drug. Tobramycin was still determined in lymph mesenteric nodes 21 hours after duodenal administration of 2.5% Tobra SLNs, as confirmed also by TEM. The amounts of Tobra in the kidneys after Tobra-SLN administration, duodenally or IV, were lower than after IV administration of the solution (59).

Idarubicin is an anthracycline administered by the IV or the oral route. Its efficacy has been demonstrated in the treatment of different tumors. SLNs incorporating idarubicin (Ida-SLNs) (60) were administered IV and duodenally to rats in a comparative study versus solution, the aim being to determine whether drug bioavailability can be improved. After duodenal administration of Ida-SLN and of Ida solution, idarubicin and its main metabolite idarubicinol were determined over time, as shown in Figure 3A and B; the AUC and elimination half-life of idarubicin were, respectively, about 21 and 30 times higher than those with solution. Again the AUC of Ida-SLNs administered intravenously was lower than when administered duodenally. Pharmacokinetics and biodistribution of Ida-SLNs differ from those of the solution. These changes could be exploited to reduce toxicity and increase clinical efficacy of the drug.

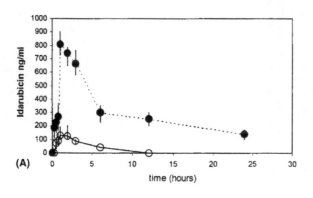

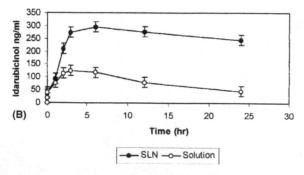

FIGURE 3 (A) Idarubicin plasma concentrations versus time after duodenal administration of the two formulations. (B) Idarubicinol plasma concentrations versus time after duodenal administration of the two formulations.

COLONIC DRUG TARGETING USING NANOPARTICULATES

One way to target the colon is to incorporate drugs in appositely studied nanoparticulates. In one such study, coated calcium-alginate-gel beads were used to entrap liposomes (61). Bee venom peptide was taken as a model drug, and investigated in vitro and then in vivo: gamma-scintigraphy was used in a human study to determine colonic arrival time, which was found to be four to five hours.

Bioadhesion of NPSs to inflamed colonic mucosa was shown to be size-dependent, using fluorescent particles, in a rat study taking nonulcerated tissue as comparison (62). PLGA nanoparticles (63) carrying an antiinflammatory drug, Rolipram, were thus studied for the treatment of inflammatory bowel disease. Experimental colitis was induced in rats with trinitrobenzenesulfonic acid, which produced significant damage of the intestinal tissue. Nanoparticles containing Rolipram with a diameter between 200 and 500 nm were prepared; for better targeting, they combined efficient drug loading with an appropriate size range (64). The particles were administered for five days and compared with the drug solution. After five days, when drug treatment was discontinued, the drug solution group underwent a severe relapse, whereas the nanoparticle group continued to show reduced inflammation levels; the solution group had a higher adverse effect index than the nanoparticle group.

SPECIFIC ADVANTAGES

Many adverse conditions in the GIT must be overcome to obtain the desired results after administration of nanoparticulates. Both academia and industry have made great efforts in this direction over the last 10 to 15 years, but more studies are required to achieve the results that so many groups are working for. From the pharmaceutical standpoint, most nanoparticulates targeted to the lymph have increased bioavailability versus the referee drug; this is particularly appreciable for labile drugs and molecules with poor solubility. One factor requiring improvement for some NPSs is incorporation efficiency, which must be increased in order to reach the required dose. Studies are also necessary with regard to storage stability.

With regard to the different NPSs, the history of some of them, such as dendrimers, is short and thus there are relatively few in vivo on the oral route. Some polymeric biodegradable nanoparticles are already on the market, although to date only for the parenteral route. Studies on the oral route have chiefly addressed the administration of vaccine antigens, peptides, and small proteins. Provided that the polymer is selected appropriately (type, molecular weight, kind of preparation), the results obtained in vivo have been promising. Lipid-based systems have achieved some of the desired results; some antiprotease drugs, ritonavir, and saquinavir, carried by S(M)EDDS, are now on the market and provide better bioavailability than the referee drug (34). Some production methods of SLNs do not use any solvent, their feasibility is relatively good, and their components are physiologically compatible.

SLNs loaded with a drug (Tobramycin or Idarubicin) and administered duodenally show better pharmacokinetic parameters than the same drug administered IV as a solution. Tobra-SLN administered duodenally permitted absorption of tobramycin by the GIT, interestingly, as this is a drug still only administered by the parenteral route.

Interest in the oral administration of chemotherapeutics has been stimulated by the discovery that oral fluoropyrimidines have at least equivalent efficacy, as well as the potential to reduce toxicity, compared to administration by the IV route; using rational nanoparticulate design, several antineoplastic drugs could be developed for oral use (65). Although studies on nanoparticulates targeting the colon are relatively few, some interesting results have been achieved using liposomes (61) and PLGA nanoparticles (63).

EVALUATION AND FUTURE PERSPECTIVES

The main goal of administration of NPSs by the oral route is to lower the dose of the drug (and consequently to diminish its toxicity) as well as to improve patient compliance and supply an easy administration route. Other aims may be to decrease the fed/fasted variability and patient-to-patient variability. Efficient incorporation of bioactive molecules in NPSs requires in-depth study. Factors that must be examined in order to obtain the best formulation for the type of NPSs selected are: (*i*) sufficient drug loading to achieve therapeutic levels; (*ii*) good translocation of NPSs to lymph (i.e., small size, biocompatible, biodegradable components, chemicophysical stability of carrier and drug, zeta potential, etc.); (*iii*) sustained/controlled drug release from NPSs; and (*iv*) increased oral bioavailability to enhance efficacy.

Many steps have already been taken in these directions, but research must continue, varying the surface properties of NPSs, improving their drug-loading capacity, and testing new materials with little or no toxicity for use as carriers; this last requisite is particularly important for drugs to be taken chronically. An innovative oral-delivery reformulation of a drug could extend its patent life; development of new delivery systems for old, well-known molecules, whether natural or out of patent, could lead to reduced side effects and to more efficient therapy, with evident social benefits.

REFERENCES

1. Kreuter J. Peroral administration of nanoparticles. Adv Drug Deliv Rev 1991; 7:71.
2. Hussain N, Jaitely B, Florence AT. Recent advances in understanding the uptake of microparticulates across the gastrointestinal lymphatics. Adv Drug Deliv Rev 2001; 50:107.
3. Florence AT, Hussain N. Trancytosis of nanoparticle and dendrimer systems: evolving vistas. Adv Drug Deliv Rev 2001; 50:S69.
4. Nishioka Y, Yoshino H. Lymphatic targeting with nanoparticulate systems. Adv Drug Deliv Rev 2001; 47:55.
5. Hans ML, Lowman AM. Biodegradable nanoparticles for drug delivery and targeting. Curr Opin Sol St Mater Sci 2002; 6:319.
6. Florence AT. Issues in oral nanoparticles: drug carrier uptake and targeting. J Drug Target 2004; 12:65.
7. Uchida J. Electron microscopic study of microfold cells (M cells) in normal and inflamed human appendix. Gastroenterol Jpn 1988; 23:251.
8. Watts PJ, Illum L. Colonic drug targeting. Drug Dev Ind Pharm 1997; 23:893.
9. Patri AK, Majoros IJ, Baker JR. Dendritic polymer carriers for drug delivery. Curr Opin Chem Biol 2002; 6:466.
10. Gillies ER, Frachet JM. Dendrimers and dendritic polymers in drug delivery. Drug Discov Today 2005; 10:35.
11. Tripathi PK, Khopade AS, Nagaich S, et al. Dendrimer grafts for delivery of 5-fluorouracil. Pharmazie 2002; 57:261.
12. Bala I, Hariharan S, Kumar R. PLGA nanoparticles in drug delivery: the state of the art. Crit Rev Ther Drug Carrier Syst 2004; 21:387.
13. Vauthier C, Dubernct C, Fattal E, et al. Poly(alkylcyanoacrylates) as biodegradable materials for biomedical applications. Adv Drug Deliv Rev 2003; 55:519.

14. Delie F, Blanco-Prieto MJ. Polymeric particulates to improve oral bioavailability of peptide drugs. Molecules 2005; 10:65.
15. Takeuki H, Yamamoto H, Kawashima Y. Mucoadhesive nanoparticulate systems for peptide drug delivery. Adv Drug Deliv Rev 2001; 47:39.
16. Damge C, Vranks H, Balschmit P, et al. Poly(alkylcyanoacrylate) nanospheres for oral administration of insulin. J Pharm Sci 1997; 86:1403.
17. Pinto-Alphandary H, Aboubakar M, Jallar D, et al. Visualization of insulin loaded nanocapsules: in vitro and in vivo studies after oral administration to rats. Pharm Res 2003; 20:1071.
18. Li Y, Jang HL, Jin JE, et al. Bioadhesive fluorescent microspheres as visible carriers for local delivery of drugs—uptake of insulin loaded PCEFB/PLGA microspheres by the gastrointestinal tract. Drug Deliv 2004; 11:335.
19. Damge C, Aphrahamian, Marchais H, et al. Poly(alkylcyanoacrylate) nanocapsules as a delivery system for octreotide, a long acting somatostatin analogue. J Pharm Pharmacol 1997; 49:949.
20. Sang Yoo H, Gwan Park T. Biodegradable nanoparticles containing protein–fatty acid complexes for oral delivery of salmon calcitonin. J Pharm Sci 2004; 93:488.
21. El-Shabouri MH. Positively charged nanoparticles for improving the oral bioavailability of cyclosporin-A. Int J Pharm 2002; 249:101.
22. Ubrich N, Schmidt C, Bodmeier R, et al. Oral evaluation in rabbits of cyclosporin-loaded Eudragit RS or RL nanoparticles. Int J Pharm 2005; 288:169.
23. Jiao Y, Ubrich N, Marchand-Arvier M, et al. In vitro and in vivo evaluation of oral heparin-loaded polymeric nanoparticles in rabbits. Circulation 2002; 105:230.
24. Foster N, Hirst BH. Exploiting receptor biology for oral vaccination with biodegradable particulates. Adv Drug Deliv Rev 2005; 57:431.
25. Fooks AR. Development of oral vaccine for human use. Curr Opin Mol Ther 2000; 2:80.
26. Tabata Y, Inoue Y, Ikada Y. Size effect on systemic and mucosal immune responses induced by oral administration of biodegradable microspheres. Vaccine 1996; 14:1667.
27. Gutierro I, Hernandez RH, Igartua H, et al. Size dependent immune response after subcutaneous, oral and intranasal administration of BSA loaded nanospheres. Vaccine 2002; 21:67.
28. Allen TM. Liposomes opportunity in drug-delivery. Drugs 1997; 54(suppl 4):8.
29. Barratt GM. Therapeutic applications of colloidal drug carriers: physical structure to therapeutic applications. Pharm Sci Technol Today 2000; 3:163.
30. Taira MC, Chiaramonti NS, Fecuch KM, et al. Stability of liposomal formulations in physiological conditions for oral drug delivery. Drug Deliv 2004; 11:123.
31. Cansell M, Nacka F, Combe N. Marine lipid-based liposomes increase in vivo FA bioavailability. Lipids 2003; 38:551.
32. Takeuchi H, Matsui Y, Yamamoto H, et al. Mucoadhesive properties of carbopol or chitosan-coated liposomes and their effectiveness in oral administration of calcitonin to rats. J Control Release 2003; 86:235.
33. Li H, Son JH, Park JS, et al. Polyethylene glycol-coated liposomes for oral delivery of recombinant human epidermal growth factor. Int J Pharm 2003; 258:11.
34. Yamabe K, Kato Y, Onishi H, et al. Potentiality of double liposomes containing salmon calcitonin as an oral dosage form. J Control Release 2003; 89:429.
35. Gershanik T, Benita S. Self-dispersing lipid formulations for improving oral absorption of lipophilic drugs. Eur J Pharm Biopharm 2000; 50:179.
36. Lawrence MJ, Rees GD. Microemulsion-based media as novel delivery systems. Adv Drug Deliv Rev 2000; 45:89.
37. Gao P, Rush PD, Pfund W, et al. Development of a supersaturable SEDDS formulation of paclitaxel with improved bioavailability. J Pharm Sci 2003; 92:2386.
38. Gursoy RN, Benita S. Self-emulsifying drug delivery systems (SEDDS) for improved oral delivery of lipophilic drugs. Biomed Pharmacother 2004; 58:173.
39. Kang BK, Lee JS, Chron SK, et al. Development of self-microemulsifying drug delivery systems (SMEDDS) for oral bioavailability enhancement of simvastatin in beagle dogs. Int J Pharm 2004; 274:65.
40. Muller RH, Karsten M, Sven G. Solid–lipid nanoparticles (SLN) for controlled drug delivery—a review of the state of the art. Eur J Pharm Biopharm 2000; 50:161.

41. Bummer PM. Chemical consideration of lipid-based oral drug delivery—solid–lipid nanoparticles. Crit Rev Ther Drug Carrier Syst 2004; 21:1.
42. Manjunath K, Reddy JS, Venkateswarlu V. Solid–lipid nanoparticles as drug delivery systems. Methods Find Exp Clin Pharmacol 2005; 27:127.
43. Yang S, Zhu J, Lu Y, et al. Body distribution of camptothecin solid–lipid nanoparticles after oral administration. Pharm Res 1999; 16:751.
44. Demirel M, Yazan Y, Muller RH, et al. Formulation and in vitro–in vivo evaluation of piribedil solid–lipid micro and nanoparticles. J Microencapsul 2001; 18:359.
45. Hu L, Tang X, Cui F. Solid–lipid nanoparticles to improve bioavailability of poorly soluble drugs. J Pharm Pharmacol 2004; 56:1527.
46. Manjunath K, Venkateswarlu V. Pharmacokinetics, tissue distribution and bioavailability of clozapine solid–lipid nanoparticles after intravenous and intraduodenal administration. J Control Release 2006;14:632
47. Bekerman T, Golenser J, Domb A. Cyclosporin nanoparticulate lipospheres for oral administration. J Pharm Sci 2004; 93:1264.
48. Siekman B, Westesen K. Investigation on solid–lipid nanoparticles prepared by precipitation in o/w emulsion. Eur J Pharm Biopharm 1996; 43:104.
49. Hu FQ, Yuan H, Zhang RH, et al. Preparation of solid–lipid nanoparticles with clobetasol propionate by a novel solvent diffusion method in aqueous system and physicochemical characterization. Int J Pharm 2002; 239:121.
50. Gasco MR. Method for producing solid–lipid microspheres having narrow size distribution. US Patents 1993;5,250,236.
51. Gasco MR. Solid–lipid nanospheres from warm microemulsions. Pharm Tech Eur 1997; 9:52.
52. Gasco MR. Solid–lipid nanoparticles for drug delivery. Pharm Tech Eur 2000; 13:32.
53. Serpe L, Laurora S, Pizzimenti S, et al. Cholesteryl butyrate solid–lipid nanoparticles as a butyric acid pro-drug: effects on cell proliferation, cell-cycle distribution and c-myc expression in human leukemic cells. Anticancer Drugs 2004; 15:525.
54. Serpe L, Catalano MG, Cavalli R, et al. Cytotoxicity of anticancer drugs incorporated in solid–lipid nanoparticles on HT-29 colorectal cancer cell line. Eur J Pharm Biopharm 2004; 58:673.
55. Dianzani C, Cavalli R, Zara GP, et al. Cholesteryl butyrate nanoparticles enhances butyrate inhibition of neutrophils adhesion to endothelium. Br J Pharmacol. 2006;148:648
56. Bargoni A, Cavalli R, Caputo O, et al. Solid–lipid nanoparticles in lymph and plasma after duodenal administration to rats. Pharm Res 1998; 15:745.
57. Cavalli R, Zara GP, Caputo O, et al. Transmucosal transport of tobramycin incorporated in SLN after duodenal administration to rats. Part I. A pharmacokinetic study. Pharmacol Res 2000; 42:541.
58. Cavalli R, Bargoni A, Podio V, et al. Duodenal administration of solid–lipid nanoparticles loaded with different percentages of tobramycin. J Pharm Sci 2003; 92:1085.
59. Bargoni A, Cavalli R, Zara GP, et al. Transmucosal transport of tobramycin incorporated in solid–lipid nanoparticles (SLN) after duodenal administration to rats. Part II. Tissue distribution. Pharmacol Res 2001; 43:497.
60. Zara GP, Bargoni A, Cavalli R, et al. Pharmacokinetics and tissue distribution of idarubicin loaded solid–lipid nanoparticles after duodenal administration to rats. J Pharm Sci 2002; 91:1024.
61. Xing L, Dawei C, Liping X, et al. Oral colon-specific drug delivery for bee venom peptide: development of a coated calcium alginate gel beads-entrapped liposome. J Control Release 2003; 93:293.
62. Lamprecht A, Ubrich N, Yamamoto H, et al. Size dependent targeting of micro and nanoparticulate carriers to the inflamed colonic mucosa. Pharm Res 2001; 18:788.
63. Lamprecht A, Ubrich N, Yamamoto H, et al. Design of rolipram loaded nanoparticles: comparison of two preparation methods. J Control Release 2001; 71:297.
64. Lamprecht A, Ubrich N, Yamamoto H, et al. Biodegradable nanoparticles for targeted drug delivery in treatment of inflammatory bowel disease. J Pharmacol Exp Ther 2001; 299:775.
65. Royce ME, Hoff PM, Pazdur R. Novel oral chemotherapy agents. Curr Oncol Rep 2000; 2:31.

20 Nanoparticles as Adjuvant-Vectors for Vaccination

Socorro Espuelas
Department of Pharmacy and Pharmaceutical Technology, University of Navarra, Pamplona, Spain

Carlos Gamazo
Department of Microbiology, University of Navarra, Pamplona, Spain

María José Blanco-Prieto and Juan M. Irache
Department of Pharmacy and Pharmaceutical Technology, University of Navarra, Pamplona, Spain

INTRODUCTION

Looking for successful vaccines has become one of the driving forces in global health. The history of vaccination is rich in many trials to treat numerous infectious diseases. Vaccinations are responsible for approximately 25% of global mortality, especially in children younger than five years (1). Live attenuated vaccines are still by far the most utilized for their efficiency with respect to inactivated (i.e., bacterins) and acellular or subunit ones, but is it necessary to run the risk of using live vaccinal strains? Are there not other safer alternatives? Consequently, the need for better vaccines clearly exists, but in spite of the progress made during the last few years, "the ideal vaccine" against many severe infectious diseases still is not available.

The ideal live vaccine has to comply, at least, with the following requisites: (*i*) innocuous for the vaccinated host, (*ii*) provide long-term protection with a single vaccination, (*iii*) minimize the long-term production of antibodies, which may interfere with the current serodiagnosis tests of natural field infections, (*iv*) avoid the contamination of food or any effect in the environment, (*v*) nonpathogenic for humans or any other plant or animal host, and (*vi*) be biologically stable. In consequence, the actual tendencies are oriented towards the development of new vaccines containing perfectly characterized antigens, rigorously controlled during all the steps concerning their preparation, and safe. However, the new vaccines of the new biotechnology era suffer, in general, from immunogenicity, requiring the use of adjuvants (2,3).

The adjuvants have various functions, such as facilitate the passage through cellular barriers and the stimulation of the cells of the immune system. The nanoparticles may be considered as adjuvants that can accomplish these requisites, being able even to induce a response at the mucosa level given their capacity to interact with it. We will review these carrier adjuvants in this chapter.

IMMUNOADJUVANTS

Adjuvants are compounds that enhance or modulate the immunogenicity of coadministered antigens. Specific antigen/adjuvant combinations preferentially induce type 1 or type 2 cytokine responses. The Th1 subset secretes cytokines, including interleukin-2 (IL-2) and interferon-γ (IFN-γ), to assist in cell-mediated immune response. The Th2 subset assists preferentially in antibody immune responses after secreting cytokines including interleukin-4 (IL-4). The mechanism of the adjuvant action is in some cases, still unknown (4). In spite of large lists of compounds and strategies described as adjuvants, the only FDA-approved adjuvant is alum, a general name for the aluminum-based mineral salt (5). It yields a reasonable antibody response (Th2), but it does not induce a Th1 profile. Th1 immunity is essential for protection against many infective organisms (e.g., intracellular parasites, including virus and some prokaryotic and eukaryotic microorganisms) and even to limit allergenic processes (6). Moreover, aluminum adjuvants have shown limitations in their applicability in vaccines based on small-sized peptides or antigen-expressing DNA (7,8). Another limitation lies in the fact that aluminum-adsorbed vaccines are frost-sensitive and thus not lyophilizable. Therefore, a large number of new adjuvants are under investigation, such as the particulate-delivery systems.

It is well established that adjuvants can enhance the specific immune response of the coadministered antigens by two major mechanisms (3,9):

1. They increase the antigen uptake by antigen-presenting cells (APCs) ("delivery"). The adjuvants are directly engulfed by APCs or they form a depot of the antigens that prolong their exposure and so the chance to be taken up by APCs.
2. Another group of adjuvants ("immunopotentiators") directly activates innate immune cells. To this category belong inflammatory stimuli (frequently associated with vaccine administration), cytokines, CD40L, and pattern-associated molecular pathogens (PAMPs: molecular patterns shared by multiple microorganisms, not presented in mammalian cells, that activate immune cells through interaction with pattern-recognition receptors). Lipopolysaccharide, murine, flagellin, and other main structural components of bacterial cells are examples of PAMPs used empirically for a long time (4).

Particulate-delivery systems belong to the first category of adjuvants (10,11), although their activity as immunopotentiators cannot be completely discarded.

NANOPARTICLES AND ANTIGEN-PRESENTING CELLS

Numerous reports indicate that particulate antigens are naturally captured by APCs, but also that size is a decisive factor for an adequate uptake. Dendritic cells (DCs), a paradigm of APCs, are able to capture particles in vitro and in vivo but to a lesser extent than macrophages and the optimal size is smaller than that described for macrophages (in the range of 500 nm or below) (12,13). In addition, the surface charge and hydrophobicity of nanoparticles also modify their uptake (14). Once inoculated, the particle surface changes by the adsorption of endogenous proteins presented in serum and in the interstitial fluid at the administration site. The more hydrophobic the surface is, the easier the coating process by the dominant proteins (opsonins as IgG or C3 complement factors) can be (15). Macrophages and DCs have receptors for Fc fraction of IgG, C3 complement component, or the C-lectins family, such as mannose receptors (16). Coating nanocarriers with these ligands has been proven a good strategy for improving antigen delivery and targeting. Furthermore, these ligands have influence in the profile of the elicited immune response (17).

THE FATE OF NANOPARTICLES AFTER ADMINISTRATION
Parenteral Immunization

Nanoparticles administered intramuscularly (IM) or subcutaneously (SC) are expected to remain essentially at the site of administration and control the release of the loaded antigen. Slowly degradable polymers [i.e., poly(lactide acid) (PLA), poly(lactide-co-glycolide) (PLGA), poly(methylmethacrylate) (PMMA), poly(alkylc yanoacrylates), or caprolactone polymers (PEC)] are suitable for this application as they provide adequately prolonged antigen release. Nanoparticles of PMMA were claimed to be biodegradable after SC or IM injection and shown to exhibit very powerful adjuvant properties for a number of antigens. Thus, they were able to improve the antibody response and the protection against influenza challenge in comparison to the classical adjuvant aluminum hydroxide (18).

Desai and coworkers (19) have demonstrated adjuvant properties of PLGA nanoparticles containing encapsulated staphylococcal enterotoxoid B. However, the systemic antibody immune response elicited in the animals injected SC with these nanoparticles was comparable to that obtained following injection of alum. The same group (20) showed in a further study with tetanus toxoid (TT), that coinjecting subcutaneously to rats TT-alum along with TT-loaded PLGA nanoparticles induces a synergistic immune response. The combination induced a fourfold greater mean serum anti-TT IgG response than a single injection of TT nanoparticles alone.

In another study, a single immunization of PLA nanoparticles entrapping immunoreactive TT administered IM to rats elicited anti-TT antibodies that persisted for more than five months (21).

Recently, Schöll et al. (22,23) demonstrated the effectiveness of PLGA nanoparticles in immunotherapy of allergy to birch pollen (Bet-v1) in BALB/c mice. PLGA nanoparticles loaded with Bet-v1, the major allergen, enhanced the right immunogenicity of the allergen and did not lead to novel sensitization of naïve animals. The authors assumed that vaccination with PLGA nanoparticles can counterbalance an ongoing Th2 response to Bet-v1, readdressing it to a Th1-protective response.

Mucosal Immunization

Although most vaccines traditionally have been administered by IM or SC injection, mucosal administration of vaccines offers a number of important advantages, including easier administration, reduced adverse effects, and the higher mucosal immune response achieved. Another important advantage is that the vast majority of infections are from a mucosal surface and protection at this port of entry level is essential (gastrointestinal, respiratory, and urogenital tracts).

Oral Route

The most attractive, easiest, and most acceptable route for mucosal immunization is the oral one. However, as a result of the acidity in the stomach, an extensive range of digestive enzymes in the intestine, and a protective coating of mucus that limits access to the mucosal epithelium, the oral delivery of vaccines remains a challenge where it is difficult to achieve high and reproducible effects. In order to solve these difficulties, nanoparticles may be useful to protect antigens and facilitate the interaction with components of the gut mucosa by a mechanism of bioadhesion.

In mice, oral immunization with PLGA nanoparticles has been shown to induce potent mucosal and systemic immunity to entrapped antigens (24,25). For instance, the encapsulation of *Helycobacter pylori* antigens in PLGA nanoparticles induced significantly specific mucosal IgA response as well as serum IgG1 and IgG2b responses (24). Another interesting study was based on the use of TT associated with sulfobutylatedpoly(vinyl alcohol)-graft-poly(lactide-co-glycolide) nanoparticles, that a given by peroral (PO) or intranasal (IN) route induced specific IgG and IgA in mice in a reproducible manner (26).

Oral vaccination using chitosan nanoparticles as vector for *Toxoplasma gondii* GRA 1 pDNA primed an antibody-mediated immune response, although not the cellular protective one (25). Similarly, it was shown that mucosal immunity towards Tat protein could be triggered in mice by oral or rectal route when this protein is loaded in chitosan nanoparticles. Tat protein plays an essential role in HIV-1 replication and also participates in T-cell immunosuppression (27). In fact, sera from mice immunized with chitosan nanoparticles inhibited the activity of Tat protein, which is a prerequisite for the development of an anti-AIDS-protective vaccine (28). In addition, this vaccine also induced cell-mediated immunity (28).

More recently, chitosan nanoparticles have also been proved effective as adjuvant immunotherapy (29,30). Thus, DNA encoding allergens from house mites were complexed with chitosan and delivered orally, inducing a successfully specific Th1-immune response (30). Finally, of special interest in immunotherapy of allergy and treatment of diseases induced by a disbalance in the Th1/Th2 response such as autoimmune disorders, is the capacity of the adjuvant to induce IL-10 (31,32). Thus, pegylated nanoparticles containing ovalbumin were able to induce significant and sustained levels of IL-10 for at least six weeks in mice (33).

In any case, it appears that "conventional" nanoparticles offer a limited ability as adjuvants for oral vaccination. An interesting strategy to solve this problem may be the use of nanoparticles coated with bacterial adhesins in order to obtain a similar distribution within the gut to that observed for the pathogen. In this context, we have evaluated the properties of Gantrez nanoparticles coated with flagellin from *Salmonella enteritidis* (34). In vivo, these carriers displayed a similar distribution within the gut as the whole bacteria interacting strongly with the enterocytes and Peyer's patches (Fig. 1).

Nasal Route

In contrast to oral administration, nasally administered vaccines have to be transported over a very small distance and are not exposed to low pH values and degrading enzymes. In addition, the nasal mucosa shows a relatively good permeability for proteins, compared to the gastrointestinal tract. Furthermore, nasal delivery of antigens allows a direct access to the nasal-associated lymphoid tissue (NALT), the major site of antigen uptake and presentation, whereas oral delivery requires diffusion of the antigen carriers to extensively widespread lymphoid aggregates.

Various authors have studied the nasal mucosa as a potential route of vaccination against tetanus, as nanoparticles have been demonstrated to be a useful vector

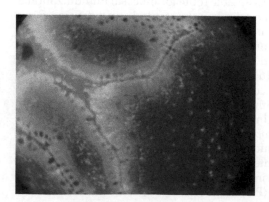

FIGURE 1 (*See color insert.*) Visualization of flagellin-coated nanoparticles (*red dots*) in the follicle-associated epithelium of Peyer's patches by fluorescence. Flagellin of *S. enteritidis* was used to coat Gantrez nanoparticles (labeled with rhodamine B isothiocyanate) and, thus, obtained adjuvant vectors able to spread within the gut in a way similar to the whole bacteria. *Source*: From Ref. 34.

system for TT. The intranasal application of that formulation resulted in significantly increased IgG and IgA levels compared to nontreated animals (26,35,36). For other clinically relevant antigens, it was found that, in general, intranasal vaccination requires fewer administrations at lower dosing levels to stimulate immune responses than orally. This fact can be explained by a lower efficient particle uptake from the gut and a more destructive gastrointestinal environment for proteins (26). Table 1 summarizes these experimental works.

TABLE 1 Some of Studies Using Nanoparticles as Vaccine Adjuvants for Nasal Administration

Formulation	Antigen	Species	Results	References
SB-PVAL-g-PLGA NP	Tetanus toxoid	Mice	Smallest particles induced the most significant antibody responses	(28)
Chitosan NP, CS-PLGA NP, PLA–PEG NP	Tetanus toxoid	Rat	Intranasal administration of chitosan NP formulation provided high and long-lasting immune response	(37)
PLA NP, PLA–PEG NP	Tetanus toxoid	Mice	Pegylation increases the stability of resulting nanoparticles and elicited higher antibody levels	(36)
Chitosan NP	Tetanus toxoid	Mice	6 months postadministration, the IgA response was significantly higher than for a control vaccine	(38)
PLA–PEG NP	Tetanus toxoid	Rat	A decrease in the size improves the transport across the nasal mucosa	(35)
PLGA NP	Influenza virus antigens	Rat	Smaller nanoparticles provided better immunization than larger ones	(39)
PLGA NP, PMMA NP	Bovine para-influenza type 3 proteins	Mice	Encapsulation of antigen in PLGA NP provided higher levels of specific antibodies than adsorption in PMMA NP	(40)
Polystyrene NP	Concanavalin A-inactivated HIV-1	Mice, macaque	Vaccines provided high immune responses and provided significant protection against intravaginal challenge	(41,42)
Calcium phosphate NP	Herpes simplex virus type-2 glycoprotein	Mice	Induction of protective immunity against intravaginal challenge	(43)
Chitosan NP	pDNA expressing either hemagglutinin HA or nuclear protein of the influenza A virus	Mice	Immunization induced protection against challenge with influenza A virus	(44)

Abbreviations: CS-PLGA NP, chitosan-coated poly(lactic acid–glycolic acid) nanoparticles; PLA NP, poly(lactic acid) nanoparticles; PLA–PEG, poly(ethylene glycol)-coated poly(lactic acid) nanoparticles; PLGA, poly(lactide-co-glycolide) nanoparticles; PMMA NP, polymethylmethacrylate nanoparticles; SB-PVAL-g-PLGA NP, sulfobutylated poly(vinyl alcohol)-graft-poly(lactide-co-glycolide) nanoparticles.

In contrast, pegylation appears to be a good strategy to enhance the ability of nanoparticles as adjuvants for nasal vaccination. In fact, IgG levels elicited by TT loaded in PLA–PEG nanoparticles were significantly higher and longer-lasting than those corresponding to both the fluid vaccine and conventional nanoparticles (45). Moreover, this potential of pegylated nanoparticles was also demonstrated for a model DNA nasal vaccine, where a single nasal dose of DNA PEG-nanoparticles led to a significant antibody response to the encoded protein (37,38). All of these results concerning pegylated nanoparticles can be directly related to the ability of PEG coating to facilitate the internalization of nanoparticles through a given epithelium (33,37,46). It appears that the PEG coating has a role in stabilizing nanoparticles in mucosal fluids, facilitating the transport of the nanoencapsulated antigen and, hence, eliciting a high and long-lasting immune response.

Comparing PEG-nanoparticles with chitosan-coated nanoparticles, it was observed that PEG-nanoparticles were more efficient than chitosan-coated nanoparticles in facilitating the transport of the associated antigen (TT) through the mucosa. The explanation was found in the different interaction mechanisms of both types of modified nanoparticles with the nasal epithelium (35). In particular, PEG-nanoparticles did not interact with the mucin, whereas those coated with chitosan were designed to stick to the mucus layer (47,48), impeding the transport across the nasal epithelium. Again, modification of the physicochemical characteristics of nanoparticles may facilitate the diffusion of nanoparticles through the protective mucus layer and their interaction with the NALT. In this context, it has been described that a decrease on the size of PLGA nanoparticles resulted in an increase in their ability to reach the NALT and to potentiate the immune response (39). In another interesting work, two different types of nanoparticles were evaluated as adjuvants for nasal immunization against bovine parainfluenza type 3 virus. In this work, viral proteins were either encapsulated in PLGA nanoparticles or adsorbed in PMMA nanoparticles (44). Mice immunized with a single dose of PLGA nanoparticles developed higher levels of virus-specific antibody than mice immunized with the PMMA vaccine or with the viral proteins alone. In any case, these results can be due to the method of association between antigen and nanoparticle (encapsulation vs. adsorption) or to the intrinsic ability of the polymer to act as adjuvant (PLGA vs. PMMA) (44).

Miyake and coworkers described the ability of polystyrene nanoparticles coated with Concanavalin A to efficiently capture HIV-1 particles (40). After intranasal immunization, this formulation induced a high vaginal IgA antibody response in mice. In macaques, after a series of six intranasal immunizations with this formulation and intravaginal challenge, only 33% of animals became infected. Similar results were obtained with a derived vaccine obtained by mixing ConA-NP with inactivated HIV-1 particles (41).

In mice, nasal immunization with herpes simplex virus type-2 glycoprotein in calcium phosphate nanoparticles induced protective immunity against an intravaginal challenge (42). Also in mice, mucosal immunization with chitosan–DNA nanoparticles induced protection against challenge with influenza A virus (43). Recently, a chitosan-influenza vaccine was found effective in humans when administered by the nasal route (49).

Overall, it is reasonable to consider that the nasal route seems to be more promising for vaccination in mice than the oral one for nanoparticle vaccine administration (26).

Other Mucosal Routes

Few recent studies have focused on pulmonary immunization and the involvement of the pulmonary immune system in eliciting protective immune responses against inhaled pathogens. In this context, the pulmonary administration of pDNA (encoding protective epitopes from *Mycobacterium tuberculosis*) loaded in chitosan nanoparticles induced increasing levels of interferon-gamma compared to either a control formulation or the more frequently used intramuscular immunization route (50).

In contrast, calcium phosphate (CP) nanoparticles, containing HSV-2 viral proteins, have been proved effective in enhancing the mucosal immune response against the virus. In mice, immunized intravaginal immunization with HSV-2 loaded in CP nanoparticles induced high levels of HSV-specific mucosal IgA and IgG in vaginal lavage fluids. Furthermore, mice vaccinated with this formulation were protected against challenge, with higher survival rates and less clinical infection than unvaccinated controls (42).

In summary, nanoparticles containing entrapped or adsorbed antigens are being investigated as vaccine adjuvant alternatives to the currently used alum with the objective of developing better vaccine adjuvants and minimizing the frequency of immunization. However, little success has been proved by the oral administration of antigens or allergens in nanoparticles. Accumulated experimental evidence suggests that simple encapsulation of vaccines into nanoparticles is unlikely to result in the successful development of oral vaccines, and improvements in the current technology are clearly needed. In contrast, the nasal route seemed to be more promising for vaccination than the oral one for nanoparticle vaccine-based administration.

REFERENCES

1. Kieny MP, Excler JL, Girard M. Research and development of new vaccines against infectious diseases. Am J Public Health 2004; 94:1931.
2. Lima KM, dos Santos SA, Rodrigues JM, et al. Vaccine adjuvant: it makes the difference. Vaccine 2004; 22:2374.
3. O'Hagan DT, Valiante NM. Recent advances in the discovery and delivery of vaccine adjuvants. Nat Rev Drug Discov 2003; 2:727.
4. Sheikh NA, al-Shamisi M, Morrow WJ. Delivery systems for molecular vaccination. Curr Opin Mol Ther 2000; 2:37.
5. Clements CJ, Griffiths E. The global impact of vaccines containing aluminium adjuvants. Vaccine 2002; 20:24.
6. Lindblad EB, Elhay MJ, Silva R, et al. Adjuvant modulation of immune responses to tuberculosis subunit vaccines. Infect Immun 1997; 65:623.
7. Francis MJ, Fry CM, Rowlands DJ, et al. Immune response to uncoupled peptides of foot-and-mouth disease virus. Immunology 1987; 61:1.
8. Kwissa M, Lindblad EB, Schirmbeck R, et al. Co-delivery of a DNA vaccine and a protein vaccine with aluminium phosphate stimulates a potent and multivalent immune response. J Mol Med 2003; 81:502.
9. Schijns VE. Immunological concepts of vaccine adjuvant activity. Curr Opin Immunol 2000; 12:456.
10. Kersten G, Hirschberg H. Antigen delivery systems. Expert Rev Vaccines 2004; 3:453.
11. Ulmer JB. Enhancement of vaccine potency through improved delivery. Expert Opin Biol Ther 2004; 4:1045.
12. Thiele L, Merkle HP, Walter E. Phagocytosis of synthetic particulate vaccine delivery systems to program dendritic cells. Expert Rev Vaccines 2002; 1:215.
13. Thiele L, Merkle HP, Walter E. Phagocytosis and phagosomal fate of surface-modified microparticles in dendritic cells and macrophages. Pharm Res 2003; 20:221–228.

14. Reece JC, Vardaxis NJ, Marshall JA, et al. Uptake of HIV and latex particles by fresh and cultured dendritic cells and monocytes. Immunol Cell Biol 2001; 79:255.

15. Allemann E, Gravel P, Leroux JC, et al. Kinetics of blood component adsorption on poly(D,L-lactic acid) nanoparticles: evidence of complement C3 component involvement. J Biomed Mater Res 1997; 37:229.

16. Geijtenbeek TB, van Vliet SJ, Engering A, et al. Self- and non self-recognition by C-type lectins on dendritic cells. Annu Rev Immunol 2004; 22:33.

17. Foged C, Sundblad A, Hovgaard L. Targeting vaccines to dendritic cells. Pharm Res 2002; 19:229.

18. Desai M, Hilfinger J, Amidon G, et al. Immune response with biodegradable nanospheres and alum: studies in rabbits using staphylococcal enterotoxin B-toxoid. J Microencapsul 1999; 17:215.

19. Katare YK, Panda K, Lalwani K, et al. Potentiation of immune response from polymer-entrapped antigen: toward development of single dose tetanus toxoid vaccine. Drug Deliv 2003; 10:231.

20. Kreuter J. Nanoparticle-based drug delivery systems. J Control Release 1991; 16:169.

21. Raghuvanshi RJ, Mistra A, Talwar GP, et al. Enhanced immune response with a combination of alum and biodegradable nanoparticles containing tetanus toxoid. J Microencapsul 2001; 18:723.

22. Schöll I, Weissenböck A, Förster-Waldl E, et al. Allergen-loaded biodegradable poly(D,L-lactic-co-glycolic) acid down-regulate an ongoing Th2 response in the BALB/c mouse model. Clin Exp Allergy 2004; 34:315.

23. Schöll I, Boltz-Nitulescu G, Jensen-Jarolim E. Review of novel particulate antigen delivery systems with special focus on treatment of type I allergy. J Control Release 2005; 104:1.

24. Ensoli B, Barillari G, Salahuddin SZ, et al. Tat protein of HIV-1 stimulates growth of cells derived from Kaposi's sarcoma lesions of AIDS patients. Nature 1999; 345:84.

25. Le Buanec H, Vetu C, Lachgar A, et al. Induction in mice of anti-Tat mucosal immunity by the intranasal and oral routes. Biomed Pharmacother 2001; 55:316.

26. Kim SY, Doh HJ, Jang MH, et al. Oral immunization with *Helicobacter pylori*-loaded poly(D,L-lactide-co-glycolide) nanoparticles. Helicobacter 1999; 4:33.

27. Bivas-Benita M, Laloup M, Versteyhe S, et al. Generation of *Toxoplasma gondii* GRA1 protein and DNA vaccine loaded chitosan particles: preparation, characterization, and preliminary in vivo studies. Int J Pharm 2003; 266:17.

28. Jung T, Kamm W, Breitenbach A, et al. Tetanus toxoid loaded nanoparticles from sulfo-butylated poly(vinyl alcohol)-graft-poly(lactide-co-glycolide): evaluation of antibody response after oral and nasal application in mice. Pharm Res 2001; 18:352.

29. Chew JL, Wolfowicz CB, Mao HQ, et al. Chitosan nanoparticles containing plasmid DNA encoding house dust mite allergen, Der p 1 for oral vaccination in mice. Vaccine 2003; 21:2720.

30. Roy K, Mao HQ, Huang SK, et al. Oral gene delivery with chitosan–DNA nanoparticles generates immunologic protection in a murine model of peanut allergy. Nat Med 1999; 5:387.

31. Adorini L. Cytokine-based immunointervention in the treatment of autoimmune diseases. Clin Exp Immunol 2003; 132:185.

32. Blaser K, Akdis A. Interleukin-10, T regulatory cells and specific allergy treatment. Clin Exp Allergy 2004; 34:328.

33. Yoncheva K, Gómez S, Campanero MA, et al. Bioadhesive properties of pegylated nanoparticles. Expert Opin Drug Deliv 2005; 2:205.

34. Salman H, Gamazo C, Campanero MA, et al. *Salmonella*-like bioadhesive nanoparticles. J Control Release 2005; 106:1.

35. Vila A, Sanchez A, Evora C, et al. PLA–PEG particles as nasal protein carriers: the influence of the particle size. Int J Pharm 2005; 292:43.

36. Vila A, Sanchez A, Evora C, et al. PEG–PLA nanoparticles as carriers for nasal vaccine delivery. J Aerosol Med 2004; 17:174.

37. Vila A, Sanchez A, Tobio M, et al. Design of biodegradable particles for protein delivery. J Control Release 2002; 78:15.

38. Vila A, Sanchez A, Janes K, et al. Low molecular weight chitosan nanoparticles as new carriers for nasal vaccine delivery in mice. Eur J Pharm Biopharm 2004; 57:123.
39. Lemoine D, Deschuyteneer M, Hogge F, et al. Intranasal immunization against influenza virus using polymeric particles. J Biomater Sci Polym Ed 1999; 10:805.
40. Shephard MJ, Todd D, Adair BM, et al. Immunogenicity of bovine parainfluenza type 3 virus proteins encapsulated in nanoparticle vaccines, following intranasal administration to mice. Res Vet Sci 2003; 74:187.
41. Akagi T, Kawamura M, Ueno M, et al. Mucosal immunization with inactivated HIV-1-capturing nanospheres induces a significant HIV-1-specific vaginal antibody response in mice. J Med Virol 2003; 69:163.
42. Miyake A, Akagi T, Enose Y, et al. Induction of HIV-specific antibody response and protection against vaginal SHIV transmission by intranasal immunization with inactivated SHIV-capturing nanospheres in macaques. J Med Virol 2004; 73:368.
43. He Q, Mitchell A, Morcol T, et al. Free in PMC calcium phosphate nanoparticles induce mucosal immunity and protection against herpes simplex virus type 2. Clin Diagn Lab Immunol 2002; 9:1021.
44. Illum L, Jabbal-Gill I, Hinchcliffe M, et al. Chitosan as a novel nasal delivery system for vaccines. Adv Drug Deliv Rev 2001; 51:81.
45. Vila A, Gill H, McCallion O, et al. Transport of PLA–PEG particles across the nasal mucosa: effect of particle size and PEG coating density. J Control Release 2004; 98:231.
46. Vila A, Sánchez A, Pérez C, et al. PLA–PEG nanospheres: new carriers for transmucosal delivery of proteins and plasmid DNA. Polym Adv Technol 2002; 13:51.
47. Tobio M, Gref R, Sanchez A, et al. Stealth PLA–PEG nanoparticles as protein carriers for nasal administration. Pharm Res 1998; 15:270.
48. Behrens I, Peña AI, Alonso JM, et al. Comparative uptake studies of bioadhesive and non-bioadhesive nanoparticles in human intestinal cell lines and rats: the effect of mucus on particle adsorption and transport. Pharm Res 2002; 19:1185.
49. Bivas-Benita M, van Meijgaarden KE, Franken KL, et al. Pulmonary delivery of chitosan–DNA nanoparticles enhances the immunogenicity of a DNA vaccine encoding HLA-A*0201-restricted T-cell epitopes of *Mycobacterium tuberculosis*. Vaccine 2004; 22:169.
50. Read RC, Naylor SC, Potter CW, et al. Effective nasal influenza vaccine delivery using chitosan. Vaccine 2005; 23:4367.

21 Transdermal Applications of Nanoparticulates

Jongwon Shim
*Nanotechnology Research Team, Skin Research Institute, R&D Center,
Amorpacific Corporation, Kyounggi, South Korea*

INTRODUCTION

As the principal purpose of using nanoparticulates lies on increasing bioavailability of drugs, the more accurate definition of transdermal applications should be the applications of transdermal drug delivery with nanoparticulates. The pharmaceutical industries have applied these nanoparticulates to deliver drugs requiring acute treatment or to formulate the nonsoluble drugs into the practical formula enabling the in vivo applications. Of course, there are some topical applications of nanoparticulates targeted to the skin organ, but most of the pharmaceutical applications with nanoparticulates have been developed to give systemic effects to the body by penetrating the full thickness of skin layers (1,2). For these purposes, the drugs encapsulated by nanoparticulates have to penetrate various regions of the body. Many mechanical and electrical delivery systems for nanoparticulates are available using injection, patch, and electrophoresis methods other than the simple topical administration of spreading the drug onto skin surface (3). However, the use of nanoparticulates in the cosmetic industry has led to expectation of the efficacy of drugs on the skin itself in most cases. It is used to make the skin tones elegant, to prevent the formation of melanin by UV light, to degrade callous layers, to remove wrinkles, and to moisturize skin. The typical difference of a nanoparticulate system applied in the cosmetic industry from that of the pharmaceutical industry is that the major delivery method is very limited to the topical application of spreading onto skin surfaces, and it also serves the emotional function of provided beauty and psychological satisfaction.

But it is certain that the current major trend of interdisciplinary research is conducted without any limitations, and the same trend is applied in all industries. From the above, the application of nanoparticulates has been discussed by using two industry categories for convenience, but it is true that such classification seems to get more obscure as time goes by. The newly emerging cosmeceutical products in the cosmetic industry propose more enhanced efficacy than previous products. These products are available not only for skin whitening, hair removal, hair growth, antiwrinkle, anticellulite, and acne treatments, but also for atopic dermatitis and cosmetic supplementary foods for skin health. The same trend is going on in pharmaceutical industry in the form of noninvasive treatment in the dermatological area for cosmetic purposes. Namely, the treatment methods such as some laser therapy for the pore-tightening, chemical peeling, and ion-treatment methods have been performed to enhance the skin condition or texture and to provide a semipermanent makeup by penetrating colorants in epidermal layers. In the past, only the efficacy of a product was appreciated in pharmaceutical product development but, now, the development of pharmaceutical products that were only differentiated by color,

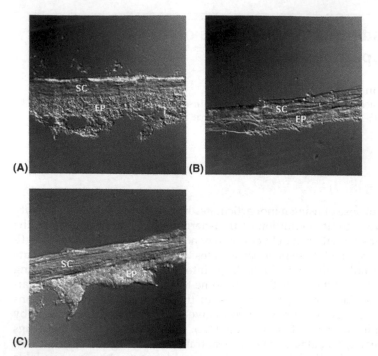

FIGURE 1 (*See color insert*.) Cryo-sectioned images of the fluorescent labeled nanoparticulate with porcine epidermal skin layer after in vitro skin permeation test. (**A**) Stratum corneum outer layer adsorption of 200 nm-sized polysturene nanoparticulate. (**B**) Percutaneous absorption of 40 nm-sized polystyrene nanoparticulate. (**C**) Epidermal layer penetration of the modified nanoparticulate. *Abbreviations*: EP, epidermis; SC, stratum corneum.

fragrance, taste, and texture are currently expected to meet the consumer's complex demands. Accordingly, it seems not desirable to classify the nanoparticulate system for transdermal delivery in cosmetics by terms used to describe its transdermal delivery of drugs. So, the current chapter is intended to describe the transdermal applications of nanoparticulate by the depth of skin to which nanoparticulates are delivered: stratum corneum adsorption, percutaneous absorption, and whole skin penetration (Fig. 1).

CLARIFICATIONS IN THIS CHAPTER
Permeation
The terminology in skin delivery indicates the phenomenon of molecular movement of active ingredients into skin. As in the case of delivering some ingredients by spreading onto a skin surface, these molecules are generally dissolved in some type of liquid-phase vehicles or they should have fluidity by themselves, and this mass transfer follows Fick's diffusion law. The required driving force for the diffusion is the thermodynamic energy of the concentration gradient (4).

Penetration
The term "penetration" indicates the skin delivery of particulates by colloidal movement, and this particulate is homogeneously dispersed in some medium. The

status of particulates dispersed in a medium could be dependent on the particulate properties including its size and mass. As if particulates belong to the region that is not affected by gravity like molecules, they seem to diffuse by thermodynamic energy and the diffusion is in a direction that can reduce the overall entropy value of the system.

Nanoparticulates

Nanoparticulates indicate various types of subsidiary concepts of particulates that can be represented as capsules, aggregates, powders, crystals, micelles, emulsions, complex, and vesicles. It is usually used to designate a particulate whose range size reaches a submicron level. However, the current chapter uses the terminology not only to indicate particulates with submicron size, but also to indicate the system showing a colloidal dispersion within appropriate vehicles.

STRATUM CORNEUM ADSORPTION

The stratum corneum is the location where the transdermal delivery is initiated, and as in the most molecules, it is also poweful barrier to nanoparticulates (5). Physically considered, skin has irregular surfaces showing elevation differences between surfaces, which makes it difficult for large materials greater than the elevation differences to have enough contact area on the skin surfaces, and an external force can easily detach them (6). Primarily, there are application areas that utilize the small sizes of nanoparticulates to achieve even dispersion and strong adhesion onto the skin surface (7). These nanoparticulate applications are widely developed in the cosmetic industry to be used as organic or inorganic pigments to manufacture cosmetics for color makeup, and there are inorganic nanoparticulates proposed for UV light protection. However, it is never desirable for such inorganic nano-sized materials to be penetrated under the stratum corneum, but rather it is recommended they be removed naturally by the turn-over period of stratum corneum or by washing (8–10).

In the aspect of drug delivery, it is most ideal for drugs dissolved in a liquid-phase vehicle at the molecular level to be evenly spread onto skin surfaces to achieve the high transdermal delivery efficiency. But if such ideal solvents or vehicles do not exist or these molecules are repulsive to the skin surface, it is advantageous to use a nanoparticulate system that has high affinity for skin. So, the use of solid–lipid nanoparticles or a polymeric nanoparticulate that was modified to have a surface to be easily adsorbed by skin surface is appropriate (11,12). By using such materials, the nanoparticulate encapsulating the drugs can be evenly spread onto skin surfaces, and after the medium is either evaporated or absorbed, the strong adhesion force between nanoparticulates produces membrane-like substrates, which function as a type of patch with high drug concentration (11). On the basis of this, the drug concentration in the skin surface is rapidly elevated and the strong driving force of the concentration gradient stimulates the drug delivery. For such a mechanism, it is essential to assume that the drug encapsulated by the nanoparticulates should be released into skin easily. The appropriate kind of drugs for such a nanoparticulate application is determined by the characteristics of molecular weight or hydrophilic property of the drugs, which have a moderate range of skin absorption availability, but no affinity with skin surface. The drugs for commonly used pharmaceutical patch products could be the appropriate level of drugs that can apply in this type of nanoparticulate applications.

PERCUTANEOUS ABSORPTION

In cases when the drug molecules can penetrate stratum corneum, and molecules showing rapid molecular dispersion in water phase could be dispersed into whole skin without many problems due to the high moisture level with low cell density under the epidermal layer (14). So, the penetration of drugs or particulates into stratum corneum becomes the most important task in the transdermal delivery, and currently two approaches are available:

1. The use of materials that can disturb or remove the barrier function of stratum corneum or the mixed use of particulates with mechanical devices or with electrical devices.
2. The noninvasive applications of special particulates that can enhance the penetration without damaging the barrier function of skin.

The first method could be reclassified into passive and active approaches. The passive method delivers the drug molecules through simple diffusion by disturbing the barrier function of the stratum corneum with permeation enhancers that can perturb, extract, and exchange the molecules which comprise the lipid bilayer of stratum corneum, with solvents that can solubilize lipids, or with surface-active agents appropriate to skin use (15,16). As the most representative formulations in cosmetic products, emulsions and micelles can be the particulate systems that apply to the first method. As they are comprised by oils and surface-active agents having affinity to skin, the effective perturbation of stratum corneum is available when being spread onto skin, which will facilitate easier drug delivery down into the epidermal layer. The drug property that fits this delivery system can be water-soluble or oil-soluble ingredients, or they can be micellized by using surfactants and appropriate solvents. Furthermore, if the droplet size of the emulsion particulate can be uniformly made to nanoscale, this emulsion of nanoparticulates can enhance drug permeation and systemic efficiency of drugs (17,18). However, because of the difficulty of isolating drugs from external environments for these emulsion or micelle particulates, the ability to prevent the drug degradation can be hardly expected. So, if the drug to be captured is unstable in oil or water phase, it is not the appropriate system to be used. For such drugs, various stabilizers and antioxidants should be blended to acquire enough stability to achieve effective drug delivery during the period of use. In addition, it is hard to achieve the enhancement of drug delivery under the epidermal layers by the active transport of particulates because these two types of particulates release drug as they contact skin surface by the absorption of surfactants or oils onto skin surface, or by losing their particulate shape due to the surface energy change (19). Meanwhile, the active approach enables the powder type of drug particulates to be directly transported by applying instantaneously strong pressure of fluid onto skin surface. Also, the use of surface-charged particulates and the use of iontophoresis or electrophoresis to enhance the penetration of drugs are also available. Although these types of methods could enhance the drug's skin delivery very effectively by minimizing the damage on skin stratum corneum, it is absolutely necessary to use specially manufactured instruments for the operations, and the additional cost and the usability depreciation have to be considered (20,21). Contrary to the emulsion or micelle system, the second method is a drug-delivery method without causing skin damage by using nanoparticulate which does not lose its original property of particulate while penetrating the stratum corneum of the skin surface. The special types of liposomes and polymeric nanoparticulates could be suggested as its most representative examples. As a special type of liposome, there is lipid vesicle system that could be represented as Transfersome™. It has been known as the vesicle membrane that has ultradeformability and can overcome the instability of typical liposomes in skin surface, which can penetrate skin appendages and even the intracellular space of skin smaller than the size of vesicle itself (22,23). As in the case of polymeric nanoparticulate dispersed in a water phase, recent studies have revealed that most of the particulates penetrate through the skin appendages and shunts that have been known to be the pathways for large hydrophilic molecules (24,25). Especially the hair follicles were regarded as the major pathway, and transport efficiency seems to be determined by the average particulate size. So, the smaller size of nanoparticulate could transport the drug more easily under the epidermal layer (26–28) (Fig. 2). As the polymeric nanoparticulates have different absorption characteristics due to the material property of polymers, the drug encapsulation and release behavior within the nanoparticulate should be expected to be different from that of microparticulate systems. Previously, the skin absorption tendency of the drug by nanoparticulate was enhanced or delayed depending upon the drug types, questioning the true efficacy of the nanoparticulate (29–31), but it is more appropriate to interpret the problem by the way that the chemical property or surface characteristics like the partition coefficient of captured molecules cannot be completely covered by the nanoparticulate encapsulation. But yet, there are no proven results regarding this matter, and further studies to resolve the problem should be made. If any of these methods has been selected to deliver the drug to the epidermal layer, the suitable drugs should be active materials with similar functions as keratinocytes and melanocytes in cosmetic products. Namely, these active materials can degrade melanin or inhibit the formation of it from melanocytes. As a pharmaceutical product, the steroidal drug of hydrocortisone could be suggested as its example, which alleviates the atopic symptom by the action on Langerhans cells existing in the epidermal layer. It also shows its effectiveness on erythema, psoriasis, and dermatorrhea. However, the long-term use of this drug can causes severe side effects. So, the delicate design has to be made to maximize its efficacy by using an effective delivery system and to minimize the side effects.

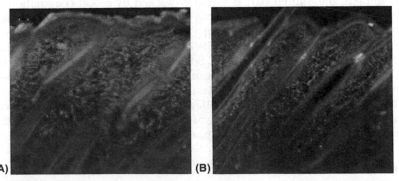

(A)   **(B)**

FIGURE 2 (*See color insert.*) CLSM images of the nanoparticulate penetration with a guinea pig skin (cryo-sectioned). Fluorescent-labelled nanoparticulate (*green region*), nuclei-labeled DAPI (*blue region*). **(A)** 40 nm size of nanoparticles, **(B)** 130 nm size of nanoparticles (10 pieces of z-direction sectioning image of cross sectioned tissue are merged). Nanoparticulate: Polycaprolactone-polyethyleneglycol block copolymer aggregates. Fluorescent: Rubrene. *Source*: From Ref. 27.

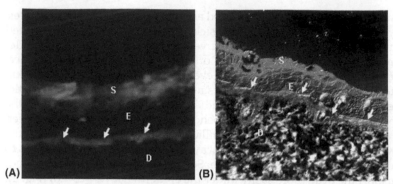

FIGURE 3   (*See color insert.*) Images of the liposome nanoparticulate with fluorescent by in vitro permeation test with a guinea pig skin. (**A**) RITC saturated solution (**B**) RITC with the modified liposome. (*Red region*), hydrophilic fluorescent dye (RITC); (*blue region*), DAPI for nuclei; basal layer (*white arrows*).

As mentioned previously, if all material delivery and diffusion can be easily achieved after penetrating the stratum corneum, it seems to be not required for nanoparticulates to penetrate the epidermal layer. However, some kind of drugs could not penetrate the epidermal permeability barrier (EPB) which has the basal layer (dermal–epidermal junction layer). EPB is thought to act as the barrier to water loss, intestinal fluid, and infection of microorganisms (32). It is supposed that the high cell density and abundant amounts of materials comprising the extra-cellular matrix and tight junction between cells in this layer might affect drug-permeation behavior. So, the particulate that can penetrate the whole epidermal layer should be used when delivering drug to the dermal layer (Fig. 3). As for the cosmetics to be used on the dermal layer level, the antiwrinkle application to enhance the collagen synthesis and the anticellulite application to be used to destroy and to remove the irregularly presenting subfats under the dermis could be suggested as appropriate products for use, and applications for deep wound healing could be suggested for effective use in pharmaceutical products. Although it is differentiated by the depth of wound and the degree of its seriousness, if a part of skin was injured, the injured part is initially blocked by blood coagulation to prevent blood and body fluids loss, and rapid epidermal cell divisions are carried out to recover the injured skin surface. But the recovery for the injured dermis takes more time to progress. At that time, the insufficiency or over-multiplication of dermal cells can cause the scar in the skin. So, if the nanoparticulates are directly delivered down to the dermal layer to release the drug in concentrative manner, the resulting rapid multiplication of fibroblast cells will increase cell density, and can stimulate the normal synthesis of collagen to have the wrinkle-free skin promised by cosmetic products; the application of it seems appropriate for the restoration of scar-free skin as promoted in pharmaceutical products.

WHOLE SKIN PENETRATION

The particulate system designed for whole skin penetration has the purpose of enhancing the overall bioavailability of drug molecules which are required to be delivered to the target organs in spite of low permeability due to large molecular weight and low partition coefficient on skin. For the nanoparticulate systems, needed to penetrate the skin, nearly identical particulate characteristics are required to deliver the drugs to dermal or epidermal layer as just discussed above. Considered from the aspect of drugs to be absorbed, material partitioning into skin can be inhibited by corneocytes and by various compositions of lipids and fatty acids that fill up the gap. That is why the particulate system is primarily formulated to penetrate the stratum corneum, but once penetration below stratum corneum is accomplished, free diffusion is allowed by the abundant amount of humoral fluid in skin tissue that can be delivered into the whole body through the circulation system. Although the nanoparticulate system may succeed in penetrating the stratum corneum, the efficiency of delivering the drug into the circulation system can be downgraded if the drug cannot permeate the epidermal and dermal layer or cannot avoid various types of existing defense systems in skin. Otherwise, if the drugs have lipophilic property and low molecular weight, the initial partitioning onto lipid compositions in the outermost layer of skin can be easily achieved, but delivery under the stratum corneum layer with the relatively high moisture content in epidermal and dermal layers will get more difficult for the mass transfer of the molecules. So, these molecules will be clusterized due to the decreased solubility in the environment, and eventually the mobility of these molecules could be nearly disabled by diffusion.

Even if nanoparticulates can penetrate whole skin layer and can avoid various immune systems presenting in the skin organ after dispersion, they have to face the highly developed and more complex defense system in the body such as the blood–brain barrier, Langerhans cells and T-cells in liver, Peyer's patches in the gut-associated lymphoid tissue, and so on (33,34). So, a high delivery efficiency could not be expected unless a proper counterplan for this is prepared. As in the case of percutaneous absorption, the particulate for skin penetration should not be destroyed by external environments between the early steps of skin penetration and the delivery into the circulation system, and must have material properties that can suppress drug release and avoid degradation of the encapsulated drugs. Although there is much unclarified information, if the particulate types of micelles, emulsions, and generally manufactured liposome vesicles were applied by spreading onto skin surfaces, it is difficult to maintain their original particulate shape due to the absorption behavior between skin surface and molecules comprising the particulates and by the difference of surface energy (35). In some cases of their practical uses, it was reported that the particulates were destroyed by the salts existing on exudates or sweat ducts in the skin surface. There are many cases that cannot maintain the stability of the system due to the rapid evaporation of water or other solvents in the skin surface, and if the product requires spreading action by users, the external physical stress of spreading may cause the structural destruction of the particulate to occur. So, these systems are not an appropriate system because the particulate cannot be maintained until it reaches the destination due to burst-releasing the drug premature (Fig. 4).

To avoid such problems, the most easily applied method is injection administration. The material is delivered down to the dermal layer in the skin barrier by using a mechanical device. This method is not strictly restricted by particulate size, and it also allows direct injection into blood vessels to have immediate efficiency of the drug. Additionally, it can avoid the particulate disruption caused by environmental change and by the primary protection mechanisms existing in skin. However, the injection administration method is stressful to the user and its use is difficult, which seems disadvantageous in long-term and repeated use. The method has

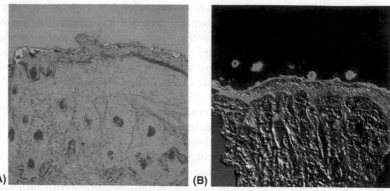

FIGURE 4 *(See color insert.)* Fluorescent images of in vivo permeation study with Albino Hartley guinea pig. **(A)** O/W emulsion formulation. **(B)** Modified polymeric nanoparticulate.

been improved to create the patch formulation method, but it also has some disadvantages due to the action of barrier function in skin by swelling and by the aspect of having relatively low delivery efficiency. As for the system to be used easily, to minimize skin damage and to deliver a higher concentration of drug to the circulation system, the use of particulate that can penetrate the whole skin layer such as the polymeric particulate, other solid type nanoparticulates, or special lipid vesicle particulate seems appropriate. Ethosome™ has been known as a liposome system that can maintain high ethanol content, which can effectively disturb the skin lipids without losing its particulate property to enhance the drug-delivery efficiency (36,37). In addition, the previously mentioned Transfersome™ has shown high efficiency of drug delivery for whole body application in addition to the function of delivering drugs to skin layers. However, it is still difficult to find a commercialized polymeric nanoparticulate for external skin use as well as for whole body functions of a drug. Its limited delivery pathway other than hair follicles make it difficult to increase the delivery efficiency, its inability to capture hydrophilic drugs, and the very limited amount of applicable materials are thought to be the appropriate reasons.

THE LIMITATIONS OF NANOPARTICULATE SYSTEM FOR TRANSDERMAL APPLICATIONS

First, there are limitation of acquiring stable materials. Most of the nanoparticulates and their debris that penetrate deep into skin layers might cause an immune response. So, materials that can be disintegrated by appropriate mechanisms to be absorbed into body have to be used. However, very limited numbers of materials exist for a nanoparticulate system, which can be degraded within skin to be absorbed naturally into the body. This could be suggested as the major topic that researchers speculate, the conventionally used U.S. Food and Drug Administration (FDA)-approved materials of poly(lactic acid) (PLA), poly(glycolic acid) (PGA), and polydioxanone (PDS) that are using lecithin or biocompatible polymeric biomaterials; these have nearly reached their maximum capacity to enlarge their field of application. Similar degradable polyester-type polymers of poly(anhydride), polyphosphonate, polyamide and polyiminocarbonate, polycaprolactone, polyphosphazene, and poly(phosphate ester) are available, but cannot be used because their official approvals have not been granted. For these reasons, many investigators currently make every effort to find and to apply materials that can be as safe as lecithin in the human body and materials having clear degradation mechanisms that can be synthesized and purified such as PLA (38,39). Although these nanoparticulates will be formulated from safe materials for human body, consideration for a different aspect of the material not shown in the bulk phase might be necessary when these materials are formulated in the form of nanoparticulates and when these nanoparticulates are actually used by encapsulating drugs. As an example, some kind of nanoparticulate system is proposed for skin penetration, and the enhanced skin absorption rate has the risk of causing strong irritation or immune response due to the overstimulation of the skin immune system by the drug. So, the nanoparticulate system for transdermal delivery should be investigated in the appropriate concentration ranges to represent its safety and efficacy from the following four aspects: drugs, raw materials comprising nanoparticulate, drug-encapsulated nanoparticulate, and the empty nanoparticulate.

Secondly, a limited delivery pathway could be suggested. In spite of the excellent skin absorption rate of general skin products of external use, there are still some problems remaining to be solved. Especially for the nanoparticulates to penetrate lower than the stratum corneum, use injured skin parts, hair follicles, and auxiliary skin systems as the pathway to move. But the area of the pathways provided by these auxiliary skin systems make up a very small portion compared to the total skin area. The skin absorption of the drug using the limited pathways essentially requires a larger range of administration and repeated use to reach the desired drug concentration in a body compared to the oral and injection administration methods.

Thirdly, there is an absence of proper stabilization functions for unstable active ingredients. Because of the relatively thin wall thickness of nanoparticulate compared to microparticulate, it is beyond the capability of nanoparticulate to prevent the material degradation by reactive oxygen species, UV light, and heat. Practically, the active ingredients of cosmetic products are easily degradable by oxygen and heat (40). If a nanoparticulate system is applied to enhance bioavailability of actives to the skin, it is often necessary to add various additives, like antioxidants and anti-fading agents, or highly air-tight containers should be used.

THE FUTURE OF NANOPARTICULATE APPLICATIONS FOR TRANSDERMAL DELIVERY

Simply considered, the research can overcome the limitation of nanoparticulate systems as described in this chapter. As mentioned above, the advantages of nanoparticulate applications should be maximized and the disadvantages should be overcome. The ultimate nanoparticulate applications for transdermal delivery that will be developed in the future can deliver nearly all types of drugs including macromolecules into target sites by simply spreading onto the skin surface to provide concentrative and long-term release of the drug. To enlarge the applicable scopes of nanoparticulate for transdermal delivery, it is absolutely necessary to develop new nanoparticulate systems to enhance the skin absorption and not be affected by the active ingredients to be encapsulated. Above all, the material diversification of nanoparticulate by the development of material science should be solved initially, and the analysis methods to analyze the chemical and physical properties of nanoparticulate should be developed along with the development of analytical instruments which will enable the above goals.

REFERENCES

1. Muller RH, Jacobs C, Kayser O. Nanosuspensions as particulate drug formulations in therapy rationale for development and what we can expect for the future. Adv Drug Deliv Rev 2001; 47:3–17.
2. Panyam J, Labhasetwar V. Biodegradable nanoparticles for drug and gene delivery to cells and tissue. Adv Drug Deliv Rev 2003; 55:329–347.
3. Barry BW. Is transdermal drug delivery research still important today? DDT 2001; 6(19):967–971.
4. Hadgraft J. Skin deep. Eur J Pharm Biopharm 2004; 58(2):291–299.
5. Shah VP, Flynn GL, Yacobi A, et al. Bioequivalence of topical dermatological dosage forms—methods of evaluation of bioequivalence. Skin Pharmacol Appl Skin Physiol 1998; 11:117–124.
6. Fiedler M, Meier W-D, Hoppe U. Texture analysis of the surface of the human skin. Skin Pharmacol 1995; 8:252–265.
7. Muller RH, Radtke M, Wissing SA. Solid–lipid nanoparticles (SLN) and nanostructured lipid carriers (NLC) in cosmetic and dermatological preparations. Adv Drug Deliv Rev 2002; 54(suppl 1):S131–S155.
8. Auton TR, Westhead DR, Woolen BH, Scott RC, Wilks MF. A physiologically based mathematical model of dermal absorption in man. Hum Exp Toxicol 1994; 13:51–60.
9. Reddy MB, Guy R, Bunge AL. Does epidermal turnover reduce percutaneous penetration? Pharm Res 2000; 17(11):1414–1419.
10. Kwon SS, Nam YS, Lee JS, et al. Preparation and characterization of coenzyme Q10-loaded PMMA nanoparticles by a new emulsification process based on microfluidization. Colloid Surf A 2002; 210:95–104.
11. Schreier H, Bouwstra J. Liposomes and niosomes as topical drug carriers: dermal and transdermal drug delivery. J Control Release 1994; 30:1–15.
12. Morganti P, Ruocco E, Wolf R, Ruocco V. Percutaneous absorption and delivery systems. Clin Dermatol 2001; 19: 489–501.
13. Lan Honeywell-Nguyen P, De Graaff AM, Wouter Groenink HW, Bouwstra JA. The in vivo and in vitro interactions of elastic and rigid vesicles with human skin. Biochim Biophys Acta 2002; 1573:130–140.
14. Ritschel WA, Hussain AS. The principles of permeation of substances across the skin. Methods Find Exp Clin Pharmacol 1988; 10(1):39–56.
15. Smith EW, Maibach HI, eds. Percutaneous Penetration Enhancers. New York: CRS Press, 1995.
16. Hadgraft J. Modulation of the barrier function of the skin. Skin Pharmacol Appl Skin Physiol 2001; 14:72–81.
17. Stiess M, ed. Mechanische Verfahrenstechnik 1. Berlin: Springer, 1995:59–62.
18. de Vringer T, de Ronde HAG. Preparation and structure of a water-in-oil cream containing lipid nanoparticles. J Pharm Sci 1995; 84:466–472.
19. Müller RH, Mäder K, Gohla S. Solid–lipid nanoparticles (SLN) for controlled drug delivery—a review of the state of the art. Eur J Pharm Biopharm 2000; 50:161–177.
20. Barry BW. Breaching the skin's barrier to drugs. Nat Biotechnol 2004; 22(2):165–167.
21. Mark R, Prausnitz, Mitragotri S, Langer R. Current status and future potential of transdermal drug delivery. Nat Rev Drug Discov 2004; 3:115–124.
22. Cevc G, Blume G, Schatzlein A. Transfersomes-mediated transepidermal delivery improves the region-specificity and biological activity of corticosteroids in vivo. J Control Release 1997; 45:211–226.
23. Cevc G, Schatzlein A, Blume G. Transdermal drug carriers: basic properties, optimization and transfer efficiency in the case of epicutaneously applied peptides. J Control Release 1995; 36:3–16.
24. Cevc G. Lipid vesicles and other colloids as drug carriers on the skin. Adv Drug Deliv Rev 2004; 56:675–711.

25. Barry BW. Drug delivery routes in skin: a novel approach. Adv Drug Deliv Rev 2002; 54(1):S31–S40.
26. Alvarez-Roman R, Naik A, Kalia YN, Guy RH, Fessi H. Skin penetration and distribution of polymeric nanoparticles. J Control Release 2004; 99:53–62.
27. Shim J, Kang HS, Park W-S, Han S-H, Kim J, Chang I-S. Transdermal delivery of minoxidil with block copolymer nanoparticles. J Control Release 2004; 97:477–484.
28. Prabha S, Zhou W-Z, Panyam J, Labgasetwar V. Size-dependency of nanoparticle-mediated gene transfection: studies with fractionated nanoparticles. Int J Pharm 2002; 244:105–115.
29. Muller B, Kreuter J. Enhanced transport of nanoparticle associated drugs through natural and artificial membranes—a general phenomenon? Int J Pharm 1999; 178:23–32.
30. Markus J. Cappel, Kreuter J. Effect of nanoparticles on transdermal drug delivery. J Microencapsul 1991; 8(3):369–374.
31. Hassan Lboutaunne Jean-François Chaulet, Christine Ploron, François Falson and Fabrice Pivot. Sustainel ex vivo skin antiseptic activity of chlorhexidine in poly(ε-caprolactone) nanocapsule encapsulated from as a digluconate. J Control Release 2002; 82:319–334.
32. Troya T-C, Rahbara R, Arabzadeh A, Cheunga RM-K, Turksena K. Delayed epidermal permeability barrier formation and hair follicle berrations in Inv-Cldn6 mice. Mech Dev 2005; 122:805–819.
33. Florence AT. The oral absorption of micro- and nanoparticulates: neither exceptional nor unusual. Pharm Res 1997; 14(3):259–266.
34. Florence AT, Hussain N. Transcytosys of nanoparticle and dendrimer delivery systems: evolving vistas. Adv Drug Deliv Rev 2001; 50:69–89.
35. Zellmer S, Pfeil W, Lasch J. Interaction of phosphatidylcholine liposomes with the human stratum corneum. Biochim Biophys Acta 1995; 1237:176–182.
36. Touitou E, Dayan N, Bergelson L, Godin B, Eliaz M. Ethosomes-novel vesicular carriers for enhanced delivery: characterization and skin penetration properties. J Control Release 2000; 65:403–418.
37. Touitou E, Godin B, Weiss C. Enhanced delivery of drugs into and across the skin by ethosomal carriers. Drug Dev Res 2000; 50:406–415.
38. Drotleffa S, Lungwitza U, Breuniga M et al. Biomimetic polymers in pharmaceutical and biomedical sciences. Eur J Pharm Biopharm 2004; 58:385–407.
39. Soppimatha KS, Aminabhavia TM, Kulkarnia AR, Rudzinski WE. Biodegradable polymeric nanoparticles as drug delivery devices. J Control Release 2001; 70:1–20.
40. Jenning V, Gysler A, Schafer-Korting M, Gohla SH. Vitamin A loaded solid–lipid nanoparticles for topical use: occlusive properties and drug targeting to the upper skin. Eur J Pharm Biopharm 2000; 49(3):211–218.

Index

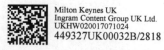

9 780367 453114